ISLAMIC PERSPECTIVES ON THE PRINCIPLES OF BIOMEDICAL ETHICS

Intercultural Dialogue in Bioethics

Series Editor: Alireza Bagheri
(Tehran University of Medical Sciences, Iran)

Published

Vol. 1 Islamic Perspectives on the Principles of Biomedical Ethics
edited by Mohammed Ghaly

Forthcoming

Islamic Bioethics: Current Issues and Challenges
by Alireza Bagheri and Khalid Abdulla Al-Ali

■ Intercultural Dialogue in Bioethics — Vol. 1
Series Editor: Alireza Bagheri

ISLAMIC PERSPECTIVES ON THE PRINCIPLES OF BIOMEDICAL ETHICS

Muslim Religious Scholars and Biomedical Scientists in Face-To-Face Dialogue with Western Bioethicists

Editor

Mohammed Ghaly
Hamad Bin Khalifa University, Qatar

World Scientific
ICP Imperial College Press

Published by

World Scientific Publishing (UK) Ltd.
57 Shelton Street, Covent Garden, London WC2H 9HE
Head office: 5 Toh Tuck Link, Singapore 596224
USA office: 27 Warren Street, Suite 401-402, Hackensack, NJ 07601

Library of Congress Cataloging-in-Publication Data
Names: Ghaly, Mohammed, editor.
Title: Islamic perspectives on the principles of biomedical ethics / Mohammed Ghaly.
Description: New Jersey : World Scientific, [2016] | Series: Intercultural dialogue in bioethics ; v. 1 | Includes bibliographical references and index.
Identifiers: LCCN 2016000558 | ISBN 9781786340474 (hc : alk. paper)
Subjects: LCSH: Medical ethics--Religious aspects--Islam--Congresses. | Bioethics--Religious aspects--Islam--Congresses. | Islamic ethics--Congresses.
Classification: LCC R725.59 .I854 2016 | DDC 174.2--dc23
LC record available at http://lccn.loc.gov/2016000558

British Library Cataloguing-in-Publication Data
A catalogue record for this book is available from the British Library.

In-house Editors: Chandrima/Mary Simpson

Typeset by Stallion Press
Email: enquires@stallionpress.com

Printed in Singapore by B & Jo Enterprise Pte Ltd

In memory of my father, Mustafa

His life full of meaningful experiences has played a role in guiding me to the field of bioethics

Contents

About the Authors/Participants in the Seminar Deliberations ix

Introduction xv

Part I: Methodological Issues **1**

Deliberations within the Islamic Tradition
on Principle-Based Bioethics: An Enduring Task 3
Mohammed Ghaly

The "Bio" in Biomedicine: Evolution, Assumptions,
and Ethical Implications 41
Muna Ali

A *Maqāṣid*-Based Approach for New Independent Legal
Reasoning (*Ijtihād*) 69
Jasser Auda

Part II: Principles of Biomedical Ethics **89**

The Principles of Biomedical Ethics as Universal Principles 91
Tom L. Beauchamp

Response by Ali Al-Qaradaghi to Tom Beauchamp's Paper 121
Ali Al-Qaradaghi

The Principles of Biomedical Ethics Revisited 133
Annelien L. Bredenoord

Script of Oral Discussions (Day 1, Session 3) 153

Script of Oral Discussions (Day 2, Session 3) 177

Part III: Islamic Perspectives on the Principles of Biomedical Ethics 209

Ethics in Medicine: A Principle-Based Approach in Light of the Higher Objectives (*Maqāṣid*) of Sharia 211
Ahmed Raissouni

Response by Hassan Chamsi-Pasha to Raissouni's Paper 233
Hassan Chamsi-Pasha

Script of Oral Discussions (Day 1, Session 2) 241

Governing Principles of Islamic Ethics in Medicine 263
Abdul Sattar Abu Ghuddah

Response by Hassan Chamsi-Pasha to Abu Ghuddah's Paper 293
Hassan Chamsi-Pasha

Script of Oral Discussions (Day 1, Session 1) 301

Formulating Ethical Principles in Light of the Higher Objectives of Sharia and Their Criteria 317
Ali Al-Qaradaghi

Script of Oral Discussions (Day 3, Session 3) 341

Script of Concluding Discussions: Part One (Day 2: Session 1 and Session 2) 359

Script of Concluding Discussions: Part Two (Day 3: Session 1 and Session 2) 385

Conclusion: Critical Remarks 413
Tariq Ramadan

Glossary 419

Index 425

About the Authors/Participants in the Seminar Deliberations

Abdul Sattar Abu Ghuddah: Abdul Sattar Abu Ghuddah is a prominent contemporary Muslim jurist and has written on Islamic medicine and biomedical ethics. He obtained his B.A. in Islamic Law (1964) from Damascus University and earned another B.A. in Law (1965) from the same university. He continued his postgraduate studies in Egypt and received his M.A. in Islamic Law (1966) and another M.A. in Hadith sciences (1967). He earned a Ph.D. (1975) in Comparative Fiqh (Jurisprudence) from Al-Azhar University, Egypt. He is a member of the International Islamic Fiqh Academy, Jeddah and also of the European Council for Fatwa and Research. He is currently chairman and member of the Sharia Supervisory Boards of several Islamic financial institutions. He has authored books about the Islamic jurisprudence and rulings of contemporary issues and is a regular speaker at Islamic conferences and forums.

Mohammed Ali Al-Bar: Mohammed Al-Bar received from Cairo University his MBBS degree with honors (1964) and his Diploma of Internal Diseases (1969). He received membership in the Royal College of Physicians (London, Edinburgh, and Glasgow) in February 1971 and became a fellow of the Royal College of Physicians, London in 1994. After his studies, he developed an interest in bioethics from an Islamic perspective and has since participated in meetings and discussions on Islamic jurisprudence and ethics, including those of International Islamic Fiqh Academy, Jeddah; Islamic Fiqh Academy, Mecca; and the Islamic Organization for Medical Sciences (IOMS), Kuwait. Dr. Al-Bar serves as Director of the Medical Ethics Center, International Medical Center in Jeddah and is an internal medical consultant and advisor of the Islamic Medicine Department, King Fahd Center for Medical Research, King Abdul-Aziz University, Jeddah. He has authored numerous publications on bioethical questions, including organ transplantation, stem cell research, sperm banks, AIDS, artificial insemination, abortion, contraception, embryology, brain death, and Prophetic medicine. He has written numerous books, one of which is the celebrated work known in English under the title *Human Development as Revealed in the Holy Qur'an and Hadith* (2002).

Ali Al-Qaradaghi: Ali Al-Qaradaghi has founded numerous charitable organizations and international Islamic jurisprudence bodies. He is Secretary General of the International Union of Muslim Scholars. He also serves as member of the Sharia Supervisory Boards of several banks in the Muslim world. He headed the Department of Islamic Jurisprudence in the College of Sharia and Islamic Studies at Qatar University. Al-Qaradaghi has authored eight books, with several more in various stages of publication, on topics including Islamic jurisprudence and Islamic thought. He completed his Ph.D. in Contracts and Financial Transactions from Al-Azhar University in Cairo, Egypt, in 1985.

Jasser Auda: Jasser Auda is the Executive Director of the Maqasid Institute, a global think tank based in London, and a Visiting Professor of Islamic Law at Carleton University in Canada. He is a founding and board member of the International Union of Muslim Scholars, Member of the European Council for Fatwa and Research, Fellow of the Islamic Fiqh Academy of India, and General Secretary of Yaqazat Feker, a popular youth organization in Egypt. He has a Ph.D. in the philosophy of Islamic law from University of Wales in the UK and a Ph.D. in systems analysis from University of Waterloo in Canada. Early in his life, he memorized the Qur'an and studied Fiqh, Usul, and Hadith in the *halaqas* of Al-Azhar Mosque in Cairo. He previously worked as: Founding Director of the Maqasid Center in the Philosophy of Islamic Law in London; Founding Deputy Director of the Center for Islamic Legislation and Ethics (CILE) in Doha; Professor at the University of

Waterloo in Canada, Alexandria University in Egypt, Islamic University of Novi Pazar in Sanjaq, Qatar Faculty of Islamic Studies, and the American University of Sharjah. He has lectured and trained on Islam, its law, spirituality, and ethics in dozens of other universities and organizations around the world. He has written numerous books in Arabic and English, some of which were translated to 20 languages.

Tom Beauchamp: Tom Beauchamp is a Professor of philosophy and is Senior Research Scholar at Kennedy Institute of Ethics. He holds graduate degrees from Yale University and Johns Hopkins University, where he received his Ph.D. in 1970. In 1975, he joined the staff of the National Commission for the Protection of Human Subjects of Biomedical and Behavioral Research, where he wrote the bulk of the *Belmont Report* (1978). Dr. Beauchamp's research interests include the ethics of human-subjects research, the place of universal principles and rights in biomedical ethics, and methods of bioethics. He has coauthored *Principles of Biomedical Ethics* (6th edn., 2009), *A History and Theory of Informed Consent* (Oxford, 1986), and *The Human Use of Animals* (Oxford, 2nd edn., 2008, with four coauthors). Many of his articles on biomedical ethics were collected and republished in 2010 by the Oxford University Press under the title *Standing on Principles*: *Collected Works*.

Abdullah Bin Bayyah: Abdullah Bin Bayyah was born in 1935 in the East of Mauritania. He studied in the Mauritanian centers of learning known as *Mahadhir*. He was later sent to study law at the Faculty of Law in Tunisia and was trained in the Tunisian courts in 1961. Sheikh Bin Bayyah is currently Professor of Islam at King Abdul-Aziz University in Jeddah and Director of the Global Center for Renewal and Guidance, UK. He is former Vice President of International Union of Muslim Scholars (IUMS). He previously served as Minister of Education, Minister of Justice, and one of the first Vice Presidents in Mauritania. He is a member of the International Islamic Fiqh Academy affiliated with the Organization of Islamic Cooperation, Jeddah. He has authored numerous publications and spoken at length about the endurance of the Islamic legal tradition.

Annelien Bredenoord: Annelien Bredenoord is an Associate Professor of Biomedical Ethics at UMC Utrecht, the Netherlands, where she teaches ethics at the Medical School. She received a VENI-grant to study the ethics of pluripotent stem cell research. She is member of several committees, including the Young Health Council of the Netherlands, the Ethics Committee of the Dutch Association for Clinical Genetics, UMC Utrecht's Research Ethics Committee (METC), and the International Stem Cell Forum Ethics Working Party. Her interests include biomedical ethics with an emphasis on ethical issues in regenerative medicine, stem cell research, genetics/genomics, biobanking, and novel reproductive technology. She studied theology and political science at Leiden University and obtained her Ph.D. at Maastricht University.

Hassan Chamsi-Pasha: Hassan Chamsi-Pasha is Consultant Cardiologist and Head of Non-Invasive Cardiology at King Fahd Armed Forces Hospital in Jeddah, Saudi Arabia and a Fellow of the Royal College of Physicians in Ireland, Glasgow, and London. He is the author of 52 books on diverse health issues and 60 papers in peer-reviewed medical journals. He was an advisory member to the Board of Directors of the Saudi Heart Association and served as a member of the Board of Directors of the Saudi Heart Association for 10 years. He serves as Expert in the International Islamic Fiqh Academy, Jeddah. He is also a member of the Editorial Board of *Saudi Medical Journal* and the Editorial Board of the *Journal of Heart Health.*

Mohammed Ghaly: Mohammed Ghaly is currently Professor of Islam and Biomedical Ethics at the research Center for Islamic Legislation & Ethics (CILE), Qatar. In 1999, he did Islamic Studies in English at Al-Azhar University in Cairo, Egypt and was awarded his Bachelor's degree with *cum laude*. In 2002, he completed his M.A. degree in Islamic Studies also with *cum laude* from Leiden University, the Netherlands, and in 2008 he received his Ph.D. from the same university. During the period 2007–2013, Dr. Ghaly was a faculty member of Leiden University and since 2011 he has been a faculty member of the Erasmus Mundus Program; the European Master of Bioethics jointly organized by a number of European universities. In 2012, Dr. Ghaly was awarded the prestigious VENI grant (2012–2016) from the Netherlands Organization for Scientific Research (NWO) for his research project "Islam and Biomedical Ethics: The Interplay of Islam and the West." In 2015, he received another prestigious grant from the Qatar National Research Fund (QNRF) for conducting the research project "Indigenizing Genomics in the Gulf Region (IGGR): The Missing Islamic Bioethical Discourse." Besides his strong record of peer-reviewed publications on a wide range of topics in the field of Islam and Biomedical Ethics, Dr. Ghaly serves on the editorial board of a number of academic journals and is the research consultant of a number of research projects as well. He has been invited to lecture on Islamic bioethics at many universities worldwide including Imperial College London, Oxford University, University of Oslo, University of Chicago, and Georgetown University. During the academic year 2014–2015, he was Visiting Researcher of the Kennedy Institute of Ethics at Georgetown University, USA.

Ahmed Raissouni: Besides serving as Chairman of the League of Sunni Scholars, Ahmed Raissouni is a member of the International Islamic Fiqh Academy, Jeddah and is Vice President of the International Union of Muslim Scholars. He is a Visiting Professor at Qatar Faculty of Islamic Studies and was formerly a Professor of Fundamentals of Islamic Jurisprudence (Usul Al-Fiqh) and Higher Objectives of Sharia (Maqasid Al-Sharia) at Mohammed Al-Khamis University in Rabat, Morocco. His works include those on the higher objectives of Sharia, Islamic political theories, and issues of religious revival. He earned a degree in Sharia at the University of Al-Qarawiyyin in Fes, Morocco and holds a doctorate in Islamic Studies from Mohammed Al-Khamis University.

Tariq Ramadan: Tariq Ramadan is Professor of Contemporary Islamic Studies at the University of Oxford (Oriental Institute, St Antony's College) and also teaches at the Oxford Faculty of Theology. He is Visiting Professor at the Qatar Faculty of Islamic Studies; Senior research Fellow at Doshisha University (Kyoto, Japan); and Director of the research Center of Islamic Legislation and Ethics (CILE) (Doha, Qatar). He holds an M.A. in Philosophy and French literature and Ph.D. in Arabic and Islamic Studies from the University of Geneva. In Cairo, Egypt, he received one-on-one intensive training in classic Islamic scholarship from Al-Azhar University scholars (*ijazat* — authorization to teach — in seven disciplines). Through his writings and lectures Tariq Ramadan has contributed to the debate on the issues of Muslims in the West and Islamic revival in Muslim-majority countries. He is active at academic and grassroots levels, lecturing extensively throughout the world on theology, ethics, social justice, ecology, and interfaith as well intercultural dialogue. He is President of the European think tank European Muslim Network (EMN) in Brussels. His books include *The Arab Awakening: Islam and the New Middle East* (2012), *The Quest for Meaning, Developing a Philosophy of Pluralism* (2010), and *Radical Reform, Islamic Ethics and Liberation* (2008).

Introduction

This volume originated from the proceedings of a three-day seminar organized by the research Center for Islamic Legislation & Ethics (CILE) in Doha, Qatar during the period 5–7 January 2013. Besides Tariq Ramadan as CILE Executive Director, Jasser Auda as the then CILE Deputy Director, and myself as the invited moderator from Leiden University in the Netherlands to which I was affiliated at this time, the seminar hosted eight participants from different backgrounds and specializations. The list of the participants included four Muslim religious scholars, two Muslim physicians, and two bioethicists. The participating Muslim religious scholars were Sheikh Ahmed Raissouni (Morocco), Sheikh Abdul Sattar Abu Ghuddah (Syria) Sheikh Ali Al-Qaradaghi (Qatar) and Sheikh Abdullah Bin Bayyah (Mauritania). The two Muslim physicians were Hassan Chamsi-Pasha (Syria) and Mohammed Ali Al-Bar (Saudi Arabia). The two bioethicists were Tom Beauchamp (USA) and Annelien Bredenoord (the Netherlands). The participants' contributions varied between presenting a paper and/or responding to a paper written by another participant. The only exception here was Sheikh Bin Bayyah, who could write neither a paper nor a response, mainly because of his busy schedule and poor health conditions at that time. In order to enhance the interdisciplinary character of the seminar, we were keen that the author of the paper and the respondent to the authored paper come from different specializations.

In the light of a post-seminar critical evaluation of the proceedings and the submitted papers, some new chapters were added in order to fill in certain gaps. All the chapters included in Part I were written after the seminar, and the same holds true for the chapter written by Annelien Bredenoord included in Part II and the conclusion written by Tariq Ramadan. One of the unique aspects introduced by this volume is incorporating the script of the oral discussions and deliberations that took place among the participants during the seminar. I hereby want to thank the five anonymous reviewers who were positive about the book in general and specifically about this point. They shared with us the conviction that these deliberations would be of added value and would provide a rich source of information for a wide range of the expected readers of this work. However, incorporating these deliberations was a considerably daunting task especially because a substantial deal of the discussions was originally in Arabic and had to be translated. This will lead me to the duty of showing my thankfulness for the great help provided by a great number of people whose input was crucial for the successful completion of this project. To start with, the manuscript has benefitted from the professional work done by many colleagues in the Imperial College Press and World Scientific, and I am indebted to them all.

In the name of CILE, I have to acknowledge the generous financial support given by Qatar Foundation throughout the lifetime of the project starting from organizing the seminar up to this resulting publication. I also feel deeply indebted to the two research assistants whose linguistic skills in both Arabic and English and their hard and dedicated work were indispensable for bringing this publication to a satisfactory end. Sarah el-Nashar exerted laudable efforts during the first phase of preparing this publication. Then Sarah handed her tasks over to Noor Doukmak, who incessantly and meticulously worked on various manuscripts of this publication. She was patient enough to check and double check the grammatical and stylistic correctness of the whole text besides the exhausting work on the diacritics of the Arabic terms.

Since I joined CILE in September 2013, I came to know colleagues whose company did enrich my life experience not only as an academic researcher but as a human being in the first instance. Whenever I needed help during my work on this volume, I found them always helpful and supportive. I am thankful to them all; Beula Haddad, Fatima Azzahrae Chaabani, Mawahib Bakr, Mona Al Emadi, Badih Touiss, Chaoiki Lazhar, Fethi Ahmed, Jasser Auda, Mohamed El-Moctar El-Shinqiti, Mokhtar Lehmar, Muetaz Al Khatib, Ray Jureidini, and Tariq Ramadan.

I keep the final word here for my family, the light of my life, whose dedicated support always helped me overcome serious obstacles and frustrating moments during my work on this project. I am wholeheartedly thankful to my wife Karima, our twin daughters Khadija and Maryam, our son Mustapha, our daughter Aisha, our new family member Hamza — the lovely boy who saw life during this project — and last but not least my mother Fawzia. I want to say to them, "My life is unimaginable without you being the sweetest part of it. Thanks for everything and I hope I can properly fulfill my duties towards you as husband, father, and son".

Mohammed Ghaly
Doha, Qatar
23 February 2016

Part I
Methodological Issues

Deliberations within the Islamic Tradition on Principle-Based Bioethics: An Enduring Task

Mohammed Ghaly

Abstract: This introductory chapter reviews the main attempts to formulate principles of biomedical ethics that are either compatible with the Islamic tradition or directly extracted from this tradition. To my knowledge, this is the first review of available studies on this topic, which is why I tried to make it as comprehensive as possible and to refer to each available study, although some of them may include considerable overlap and sometimes even repetition. The studies reviewed in this chapter were divided into two main groups. The first group addressed a specific set of principles introduced by Western bioethicists and tried to demonstrate its compatibility with the Islamic tradition (Instrumentalist Approach). The other group tried to develop a set of principles emanating from, and rooted in, the Islamic tradition itself (Indigenous Approach).

The discipline of principle-based bioethics or principlism figured prominently in the West during the 1970s and early 1980s. Within this new discipline, specific sets of principles were introduced as frameworks of evaluative assumptions hoping that these principles will give the then embryonic field of bioethics some minimal coherence and uniformity. The four-principle theory (autonomy, beneficence, nonmaleficence, and justice) introduced by the two American philosophers Tom Beauchamp and James Childress in their work *Principles of Biomedical Ethics* remains one of the most widely debated theories in the field of bioethics, with arguments for and against it. One of the central propositions of Beauchamp and Childress is that the four principles have a universal character and are thus compatible with different cultures, traditions, and philosophies of life. This point is already reflected in the title of Beauchamp's contribution to this volume, namely, "The Principles of Biomedical Ethics as Universal Principles." The applicability of these four principles to different cultures, societies, and religious traditions has been examined and debated by a great number of researchers, and the Islamic tradition is no exception in this regard.

Despite the rich discussions within the Islamic tradition on a long array of individual bioethical issues, the attention paid to the question of its overall principles still remains immature. In a bid to fill in this gap and to trigger more in-depth discussions on this topic, the research Center for Islamic Legislation and Ethics (CILE) dedicated the first seminar in its research field "Islam and Biomedical Ethics" to this issue. To put the published proceedings of this seminar in their broader context, this introductory chapter will give an overview of the relevant discussions that pre- or ante-dated the CILE seminar. To keep the systematic character of this overview, the studies will be examined in two separate sections: (i) Instrumentalist Approach and (ii) Indigenous Approach.

The first section will focus on the contributions whose authors tried to show the compatibility of a certain set of principles, usually developed by Western bioethicists, with the Islamic tradition. References in the Qur'an and Sunna and, much less frequently, relevant discussions among religious scholars or key (ethical) concepts in the Islamic tradition, are quoted almost exclusively as an "instrument" in order to justify the compatibility of these principles with the Islamic tradition. Thus, the Islamic tradition is not approached as a source of knowledge but as a possible justifier for already existing assumptions embraced by principle-based bioethics. The second section will examine the contributions whose writers tried to search for and develop a set of principles rooted in the Islamic tradition. The starting point of the theorists of this approach is not the principles developed outside the Islamic tradition; sometimes they are even not aware of them. They try to formulate principles by fathoming out the Islamic scriptures (Qur'an and Sunna) in addition to specific genres in Islamic law (*fiqh*) and Islamic legal theory (*uṣūl al-fiqh*) such as the Islamic legal maxims (*qawāʿid fiqhīyah*).

Before delving into the details of the different studies that fall within either of these two sections, a brief note is due about two specific contributions with relevance to this topic. The term "principles" found its way into contemporary Islamic bioethics already by the beginning of the 1980s when this new field was roughly in its embryonic phase. To my knowledge, one of the earliest examples in this regard was the short paper written by the Turkish Professor of Pediatrics, Yūnus Al-Muftu, entitled *Mabādiʾ al-akhlāq al-ṭibbīyah fī al-Islām* ("Principles of Medical Ethics in Islam"). This paper was presented during the First International Conference on Islamic Medicine held in Kuwait during the period 12–16 January 1981. Despite the interesting title Al-Muftu gave to the paper, he hardly said anything about what these principles are or how to construe them. The paper is considerably concise and gives a simple overview of scattered issues relevant to the history of medical ethics in the Islamic tradition espoused with references to towering figures in the field of medicine throughout Islamic history like Ibn Sīnā (Avicenna).[1] Also the criminologist Muhammad Al-Khani addressed the question of principles in his article "*Al-Mabādiʾ al-akhlāqīyah allatī yajib an yataḥallā bihā al-ṭabīb fī mumārasatih li mihnatih al-ṭibbīyah*" ("The Ethical Principles That a Physician Should Follow in His Medical Profession") published in 1988. Al-Khani reviewed the international efforts to codify "principles of medical ethics" especially as far as combating torture is concerned. He referred to the Declaration of Tokyo issued by the World Medical Association in 1975 and the code of "Principles of Medical Ethics" adopted by the UN General Assembly in 1982. Despite scattered references to the standpoint

[1]Yūnus al-Muftū (1981). Mabādiʾ al-akhlāq al-ṭibbīyah fī al-Islām, *Al-Abḥāth wa aʿmāl al-muʾtamar al-ʿālamī al-awwal ʿan al-ṭibb al-Islāmī*. Kuwait: Ministry of Public Health & National Council for Culture, Arts and Letters: 550–552.

of Muslim religious scholars to specific bioethical issues, Al-Khani was basically interested in the influence of these principles on the codification of law within or outside the Arab world rather than the possible (in)compatibility of these principles with the Islamic tradition.[2]

1. The Instrumentalist Approach

1.1. *The Pioneering Contributions of G. Serour and K. Hasan*

As far as the Instrumentalist Approach is concerned, there are two main pioneers, namely the Egyptian Professor of Obstetrics and Gynecology Gamal Serour (International Islamic Center for Population Studies and Research, Al-Azhar University, Cairo, Egypt) and the Pakistani Professor of Behavioral Sciences K. Zaki Hasan (Baqai Medical College, Karachi, Pakistan). The two professors wrote two separate chapters, respectively entitled "Islam and the Four Principles" and "Islam and the Four Principles: A Pakistani View," which both appeared in the first edition of the edited volume *Principles of Health Care Ethics*, published in 1994.

Serour was quite aware of and was also an advocate of the four principles introduced by Beauchamp and Childress although their book does not appear in Serour's list of references. On the other hand, it seems that Serour was not aware of the contribution of the Syrian religious scholar Abu Ghuddah, which will be examined in the section "Indigenous Approach." The chapter starts with a couple of introductory remarks about the four principles (to which Serour suggested adding a fifth one, namely that the human person should not be subject to commercial exploitation)[3] and about the Islamic tradition, Sharia (defined by the

[2] Muḥammad al-Khānī (1988). Al-Mabādi ʾ al-akhlāqīyah allatī yajib an yataḥallā bihā al-ṭabīb fī mumārasatih li mihnatih al-ṭibbīyah. *Majallat al-Sharīʿah wa al-Qānūn* 2: 129–197.

[3] The standpoint of accepting the four principles, articulated by Beauchamp and Childress, but also suggesting the addition of new principles, thought to be uniquely Islamic, was adopted by other Muslim intellectuals. During a symposium held by Islamic Medical Association of North America (IMANA) on end-of-life issues, the Muslim American physician Shahid Athar gave a presentation on "principles of biomedical ethics." Athar started by enlisting the four principles, and when he addressed the concept of "Islamic Medical Ethics" in particular, he spoke about two principles, namely saving life and seeking a cure (Athar 2011, 140). Strikingly enough, these exact two principles were also named by the Code of Ethics of the Pakistan Medical and Dental Council issued in 2001 (article 7)

author as the set of instructions which regulate everyday activity of life, to be adhered to by good Muslims), and its primary and secondary sources. After these introductory remarks, Serour laid out his bold thesis by saying, "The primary sources of Sharia, namely Qur'an, Sunna and sayings of the Muslim scholars, have stressed the four universally accepted principles of ethics throughout Islamic history. The Islamic Sharia has also given attention to the principle of protection of the human subject against commercial exploitation."[4] The study is replete with extensive quotations from the Qur'an and Sunna (Prophetic traditions) that have been harnessed in order to support this thesis. Other authoritative texts, attributed to both pre-modern and contemporary religious scholars, have also been used for the same purpose, however much less frequently than the Qur'an and Sunna.

A uniform method was adopted throughout Serour's study, namely presenting a simple understanding of a certain principle (autonomy, beneficence, nonmaleficence, or justice) followed by quotations from authoritative texts in the Islamic traditions that, according to Serour, support the respective principle. Because of space limitations, we will only examine here how Serour addressed the principle of autonomy, but it can serve as an illustrative example of how he dealt with the other principles. Autonomy was explained in one short sentence, "The principle of autonomy implies respect for the person."[5] Directly thereafter follows a long list of quotations from the Qur'an (12 Qur'anic verses) and Sunna (five Prophetic traditions) to show how respect for persons has been stressed in different ways. After this, Serour jumps to the bold conclusion, "It is not therefore surprising that Islam, which ordered thinking, learning

---

among the elements that make Islamic bioethics different from Western bioethics. The code is available online via http://www.pmdc.org.pk/Ethics/tabid/101/Default.aspx#7 (retrieved 17 August 2015). A more recent attempt to combine between condoning the four principles (with some reservations on autonomy) and suggesting uniquely Islamic principles was done by the Muslim British physician Yassar Mustafa (Mustafa 2014, 479–483). See Shahid Athar (2011). Principles of biomedical ethics. *Journal of Islamic Medical Association* 43(3): 139–143; Yassar Mustafa (2014). Islam and the four principles of medical ethics. *Journal of Medical Ethics* 40: 479–483.

[4] G. Serour (1994). Islam and the four principles, in Raanan Gillon (ed.) *Principles of Health Care Ethics*, 1st edn. London: John Wiley & Sons Ltd: 78–79.

[5] *Ibid*., 79.

and teaching would maintain autonomy and respect for the person in its beliefs and religion."[6] What is striking here is that no attention is paid to the sophisticated nature of a controversial concept like autonomy and its different theories, as expansively discussed in mainstream Western bioethics. The same holds true for the extensive quotations from the Qur'an and Sunna where no reference is made to the long-standing legacy of Qur'an exegesis and commentaries on Prophetic traditions and how far the interpretation proposed in Serour's study would fit within or relate to this legacy.

As for their relevance to contemporary medical practice, Serour also argued that the four principles have been recently incorporated in the medical oaths of several Islamic countries. He gave different examples of these oaths, but the only one which, according to Serour, included autonomy in specific was the oath accepted by the aforementioned First International Conference on Islamic Medicine held in Kuwait in 1981. The following quotation from Serour's study shows how specific texts are "instrumentalized" to argue for the compatibility of the four principles with the Islamic tradition[7]:

> It [the medical oath] stated that the doctor will respect people's dignity, and their privacy, and will not disclose their secrets (autonomy). The doctor will protect human life in all stages, in all circumstances and conditions, and will do his utmost to rescue it from death, disease, pain, and anxiety (beneficence). The doctor will strive in the pursuit of knowledge and harness it for the benefit of mankind and not for mankind's harm (nonmaleficence). He will extend his medical care to the near and the far, to the virtuous and the sinner and to friend and enemy (justice).

It is to be noted that none of the four principles is mentioned in the original text of the medical oath that Serour is referring to.[8] He just inserted each of the four principles, between brackets, after a certain

---

[6] *Ibid.*

[7] *Ibid.*, 86.

[8] ʿAbd al-Raḥmān al-ʿAwaḍī (1981). *Al-Abḥāth wa aʿmāl al-muʾtamar al-ʿālamī al-awwal ʿan al-ṭibb al-Islāmī*, 2nd edn. Kuwait: Ministry of Public Health & National Council for Culture, Arts and Letters: 700.

sentence that, according to him, should be referring to this principle. Although exploring a great number of the Islamic authoritative texts and searching for their relevance to principlism is a credit for Serour's pioneering study, an in-depth engagement with principle-based bioethics remains missing. In a recent study of his published in 2015, Serour touched again, but this time briefly, upon the four principles. He also made reference to another set of principles, namely those included in the 2005 UNESCO Declaration. "These and almost all the ethical principles in the UNESCO's Declaration of Bioethics and Human Rights are supported in the primary sources of Sharia," Serour reiterated.[9,10]

Like G. Serour, K. Hasan used the four principles developed by Beauchamp and Childress as the starting point. Quotations from authoritative texts in the Islamic tradition or references to key ethical concepts were employed mainly to show the compatibility of these principles with the Islamic tradition. Most of the chapter is dedicated to examining the "responses that Islam, as a metaphysical system based on faith, offers to these four principles,"[11] where each of the four principles was discussed in a separate section. Adopting more or less the same line of thought and reasoning used by Serour, Hasan unequivocally expressed his conviction that these principles can be accommodated within the Islamic tradition, e.g. "There is considerable room for personal autonomy in Islam," "Beneficence (*birr*) is one of the great pillars of the Message of Islam and a clear way to social righteousness," and, "These principles provide a useful analytical framework for practitioners of medicine anywhere."[12] Only in a few places, Hasan referred to the differences between Western societies and those of the Muslim world. For instance, he argued that Western countries, especially those that did not have traditional societies

[9] G. Serour (2015). What is it to practise good medical ethics? A Muslim's perspective. *Journal of Medical Ethics* 41: 122.

[10] The same conclusion was reached by the Egyptian Professor of Philosophy, Bahaa Darwish, when he addressed the principles included in the UNESCO Bioethics Declaration from an Islamic perspective (Darwish 2014, 269–291). See Bahaa Darwish (2014). Arab Perspectives, in Henk ten Have and Bert Gordijn (eds.) *Handbook of Global Bioethics*. Dordrecht, the Netherlands: Springer: 269–291.

[11] K. Zaki Hasan (1994). Islam and the four principles: A Pakistani view, in Raanan Gillon (ed.) *Principles of Health Care Ethics*, 1st edn. London: John Wiley & Sons Ltd: 102.

[12] *Ibid.*, 96, 98, 102.

like the United States and Scandinavian countries, managed to achieve a high level of individual autonomy through a gradual process. However, Hasan added, Islamic countries did not manage to achieve this because the progress towards political autonomy has been extremely low. According to him, such differences would explain the focus on family rather than the individual in the Muslim world, where societies are essentially traditional, and the subsequent different attitudes towards issues like informed consent or communicating bad news to the patients and their families. These differences are not because of inherent variances between the concept of autonomy and the Islamic tradition but because of the "cultural attitudes" prevalent in Muslim countries like Pakistan.[13]

Unlike Serour, Hasan did not heavily depend on quotations from the Qur'an and Sunna. Hasan's references to the Qur'an are much less than those of Serour; he includes only one direct quotation and the remaining references allude to specific concepts in the Qur'an such as beneficence and justice.[14] In order to defend the compatibility of autonomy with Islam, Hasan referred to the phenomenon of the quick spread of Islam throughout the world because it safeguarded individual liberty, which, he argued, often went to great lengths. The Qur'anic concepts of divine lordship (*rubūbīyah*) and human vice-regency (*khilāfa*) were also recalled by Hasan to foster the "Islam-friendly" character of autonomy. "The *Qur'an* says that the spirit of man is the divine spirit itself; if God is free, His essential attribute of freedom is shared by man, being God's vicegerent on earth; hence he too possesses delegated freedom. Adam's first exercise of liberty was in disobedience," Hasan argued. In the same vein, Hasan held that the fact that divine revelation came to an end by the death of the Prophet of Islam and that the development of the legal system is left to be determined by the people in the light of their own reasoning demonstrates that individual autonomy is not alien to the Islamic tradition.[15]

Another striking difference between the study of Serour and that of Hasan is their approach to the role of Muslim religious scholars in the contemporary debates on (bio)medical ethics. For Serour, the involvement

[13] *Ibid.*, 97, 98.
[14] *Ibid.*, 96, 98, 100.
[15] *Ibid.*, 96.

of Muslim religious scholars in these debates was self-evident and positively viewed. He argued that in the absence of relevant references in the Qur'an and Sunna, the opinion of religious scholars would be the reliable reference. He also gave the example of the fruitful collaboration of Muslim religious scholars with a great number of doctors, demographers, lawyers, sociologists, ethicists, policy makers, and representatives of international organizations from all over the world (about 200 in total) during the First International Conference on Bioethics in Human Reproduction Research in the Muslim World, which was held during the period 10–13 December 1991. The deliberations during the conference resulted in a proposed guideline on *Bioethics in Human Reproduction Research in the Muslim World.*[16] However, Hasan commenced his study by speaking about the problem of "the wide gulf that exists in most Islamic — indeed all Third World — countries between the clerical and the professional groups."[17] According to him, this gulf happened because of significant socio-political and cultural changes in society. In the pre-colonial era, Hasan explained, the prevailing traditional medical system in the Indian subcontinent, called *Unani* (lit. Greek), was an eclectic synthesis of more ancient systems, mainly Greek and in a lesser degree Indian and old Persian in addition to a mixture of other exotic and hardly identifiable systems. The practitioners of that system came from the same stratum of society to which religious scholars also belonged. Thus, the teacher, cleric, and healer shared a common role in society and also a common culture. During the colonial era, this traditional system was replaced by the modern Western system, which was adopted by the emerging West-oriented group who became more and more westernized. By time, the practitioners of traditional systems of medicine continued to have more in common with religious scholars, essentially because of a common spiritual content, but got more and more isolated from the professionals who practice modern systems of medicine. Hasan also added an epistemological reason for the supposed gulf between medical professionals and religious scholars. Unlike the Christian clergy, he argued, Muslim clerics did not have state's direct or indirect authority and society changed into groups

[16]Serour (1994), *op. cit.*, 73, 87.
[17]Hasan (1994), *op. cit.*, 93.

of hierarchical families rather than guilds or fraternities with their own codes of honor. This new situation left little room for intellectual dialogue not only between religious scholars and physicians but also between clerics and the various scientific professions.[18]

Hasan's note about the supposed gulf, and absence of dialogue, between religious scholars and physicians triggers critical remarks. First of all, arguing that this gulf does exist not only in the Indian subcontinent, but is also prevalent throughout the Muslim world and even the whole Third World cannot be taken without reservations. In addition to Serour's abovementioned remarks, which counter-argue the veracity of Hasan's claim as far as Egypt is concerned, one can also refer to the series of five International Conferences on Islamic Medicine held during the period 1981–1988 that witnessed a close collaboration between religious scholars and medical professionals. It is to be noted that the fourth conference in this series took place in Karachi, Pakistan during the period 9–13 November 1986 and the then Pakistani Prime Minister, Muhammad Khan Junejo, delivered the inaugural speech. The conference was attended by more than 100 participants including, among others, religious scholars and physicians.[19]

1.2. *The Contributions of the Turkish Researchers S. Aksoy, A. Elmali, and A. Tenik*

The two Turkish researchers at Harran University, Sahin Aksoy (Faculty of Medicine) and Abdurrahman Elmali (Faculty of Theology) presented their study "The Core Concepts of the 'Four Principles' of Bioethics as Found in Islamic Tradition" during the international conference "Medical Law and Ethics in Islam," held in March 2001 at the University of Haifa. The study of Aksoy and Elmali was published in 2002, together with the proceedings of the conference as a thematic issue in the *Journal of*

[18] *Ibid.*, 93, 94.

[19] Sayf al-ʿAlī, Aḥmad al-Jundī and ʿAbd al-Sattār Abū Ghuddah (eds.) (1986). *Al-Abḥāth wa aʿmāl al-muʾtamar al-ʿālamī al-awwal ʿan al-ṭibb al-Islāmī 1*. Kuwait: Islamic Organization for Medical Sciences & Kuwait Institution for the Advancement of Science.

Medicine and Law.[20] Although the authors were well acquainted with the works of the British bioethicist, Raanan Gillon, and had already quoted two of his works in their study, they did not make any reference to the two aforementioned studies written by Serour and Hasan in *Principles of Health Care Ethics* that Gillon edited. Like the other studies in the Instrumentalist Approach, the starting point of Aksoy and Elmali's study is that the four principles articulated by Beauchamp and Childress are compatible with Islam and a relatively big number of quotations from the Qur'an and Sunna (at least six times each) were employed to support this thesis with an average of one Qur'anic verse or Prophetic tradition on every page.[21]

One of the credits of this study is the much more in-depth presentation of the theoretical underpinnings of the four principles. It is worth noting that these two authors are the first to directly quote from the work of Beauchamp and Childress by consulting its fourth edition published in 1994. This helped them give more accurate and nuanced information about the principle-based bioethics. It seems that the educational background of Sahin Aksoy was a key element in this regard. He did his Ph.D. in bioethics at Manchester University, where he studied with the prominent bioethicist, John Harris, for 5 years.[22] Unlike Serour and Hasan who usually inclined to give only a very brief, sometimes insufficient, overview of each of the four principles, Aksoy and Elmali dedicated a substantial deal of their study to the position of the principle-based theory in Western bioethics and to a number of relevant concepts like common morality, coherence theory of justification, reflective equilibrium, and the processes of specification and balancing. The two authors were also keen to stress and explain certain nuances when they presented information about specific principles. For the principle of respect for autonomy, they referred to the distinction made between one's *capacity for self-rule* and another's *reaction to that capacity* and between the autonomy of the patient and that of the physician. Also for the principle of justice, they

[20] Sahin Aksoy and Abdurrahman Elmali (2002). The core concepts of the 'four principles' of bioethics as found in islamic tradition. *Journal of Medicine and Law* 21: 211–224.
[21] *Ibid.*, 216–218, 220–223.
[22] Sahin Aksoy (2010). Some principles of Islamic ethics as found in Harrisian philosophy. *Journal of Medical Ethics* 36: 226.

paid attention to the distinctions to be made between its different categories like distributive justice, rights-based justice, and legal justice and between the different perspectives towards justice that were developed by utilitarian, libertarian, and communitarian theories.[23] Unfortunately, these nuances are missing in the authors' presentation of the Islamic perspective on these principles, which usually took the form of generalizing, sometimes even simplistic statements. For instance, they used one of the Prophetic traditions proscribing force-feeding for patients as evidence that Islam supports the principle of autonomy and that food in the tradition can be read as medication or treatment.[24]

Another significant feature of Aksoy and Elmali's study is their outspoken interest to "make a contribution to the mutual dialogue and understanding between two radically different traditions namely Islamic and Western ones."[25] The claim that we here speak about "two radically different traditions" is hardly proven in their study, which has been trying constantly to show the compatibility of the four principles, presented as a product of the Western tradition, with the Islamic tradition. However, the authors did make a number of references to some (significant) differences between the two traditions concerning ethics in general and bioethics in particular. According to the authors, the four-principle theory belongs to the category of philosophical ethics whose premise is the psychological constitution of man's nature and the obligation laid on him as a social being. On the other hand, the premise of Islamic or theistic ethics in general is God as the Ultimate Unity and the sole Creator of the whole universe and thus it stresses the religious basis of morality. The basic assumption of Islamic ethics, the authors added, starts with faith in God, and morality is the attempt of each individual as well as society to approach Him and be obedient to His ordinances. As for the principle of autonomy in specific, the two authors clarified that Islam sometimes puts limits to one's individual autonomy because acting with knowledge (*'ilm*) has a higher priority than acting according to one's own wishes. Thus, it will be ethically justified from an Islamic perspective, the authors argued,

[23] Aksoy and Elmali (2002), *op. cit.*, 215, 216, 220.
[24] *Ibid.*, 216, 217.
[25] *Ibid.*, 224.

to oblige the patient or authorize the physician to protect the former's health and life once there is a prevailing opinion or a fairly certain presumption based on "knowledge." They gave the example of the religious obligation to eat a necessary amount of food in case of extreme hunger, even if the only available type of food at the time is in normal circumstances religiously forbidden, in order to stay alive. They justified this obligation that may conflict with the principle of respect for autonomy by saying, "Since eating is a treatment itself in those cases, the autonomous decision of the individual is irrelevant as there is a 'prevailing opinion' that failing to act accordingly will harm health and life."[26]

In 2002, Sahin Aksoy collaborated with another Turkish Muslim theologian, Ali Tenik, and published together an article entitled "The 'Four Principles of Bioethics' as Found in 13th century Muslim Scholar Mawlana's Teachings." The motive behind this study aligns with that of the previous study conducted by Aksoy and Elmali. As clearly explained by Aksoy and Tenik, this study is also meant to "make a positive contribution to the mutual dialogue and understanding between two different traditions with common origins (both being 'Abrahamic'), namely Islamic and Western ones."[27] The author made reference to the study of Serour and the study coauthored by Aksoy and Elmali but did not engage in dialogue with these two studies. The authors of this study focused on the works of the Persian mystic and poet Jalāl al-Dīn Rumi (1207–1273).[28] It seems that selecting Rumi in particular was meant to save the main objective of the study, namely nurturing the East–West dialogue. They argued that Rumi has not only influenced the East but also the West, as demonstrated by the writings of the French De Wallenbourg (d. 1806), the Austrian Von

[26] *Ibid.*, 214–216, 218, 219.

[27] Sahin Aksoy and Ali Tenik (2002). The 'four principles of bioethics' as found in 13th century Muslim Scholar Mawlana's Teachings. *BMC Medical Ethics* 3(4): 6.

[28] A similar attempt was also made by two other Turkish researchers, namely H. Ozden and O. Elcioglu. They argued that the four principles articulated by Beauchamp and Childress have already existed in the work of the 11th century Turkish poet Yusuf Khass Hajib, *Kutadgu Bilig* (*Wisdom That Brings Good Fortune*). See H. Ozden and O. Elcioglu (2008). Sample from 11th century: *Kutadgu Bilig* and the four principles of bioethics. *Iranian Journal of Public Health* 37(2): 112–119.

Hammer-Purgtall and the German Friedrich Ruckert, Helmut Ritter, Hans Meinke, and Goethe.[29]

As far as the four principles are concerned, the article did not add anything new to what was mentioned in the previous study conducted by Aksoy and Elmali to the extent that some sentences were even literally repeated. As typical for the Instrumentalist Approach, the works of Rumi were not approached as a sovereign source of information and possible locus for a set of principles relevant to the field of medical ethics. They were rather "instrumentalized" in the sense that they were consulted just to check the compatibility of the four principles introduced by Beauchamp and Childress with Rumi's moral thoughts.

For the principle of respect for autonomy, the two authors elaborated a bit more on the idea raised in Aksoy and Elmali's previous study about the significance of acting on the basis of knowledge (*'ilm*) rather than one's own wishes. According to Rumi, Aksoy and Tenik argued, man is a supreme creature granted with *'ilm* and, therefore, has an inherent right to choose and that man's decision shall be respected once it is taken autonomously with *'ilm.* The authors highlighted another important element for understanding autonomy in Rumi's moral thought, namely the interaction and balance between God's intervention and man's will power in every action. Thus, man wants and God creates, and man's freedom of choice is itself created with God's will, as stated by Rumi. Aksoy and Tenik were aware that this perspective can be interpreted to mean something different than the principle of autonomy as understood in Western bioethical literature. In order to repel this claim, they concluded their discussion for this principle by saying that autonomy in the Rumi's teachings is in fact "a first order autonomy with the 'share' of God in it, and shall be respected, provided that it is done with *'ilm.*"[30]

A great deal of the article was dedicated to the two principles of beneficence and nonmaleficence whose discussion was merged in one rubric. After a short explanation of what these two principles mean in Western bioethical discourse, the authors picked a number of Rumi's thoughts that they saw relevant and supportive for the purport of these two

---

[29] Aksoy and Tenik (2002), *op. cit.*, 6.
[30] Aksoy and Tenik (2002), *op. cit.*, 3.

principles. For instance, they referred to Rumi's *Mathnawi*, in which he held that being helpful to someone who is ill or has some problems is a form of a charity. Also, in Rumi's eyes, the ideal man is the one who overcomes his egoism and commits himself to be beneficial not only to fellow humans but to all creatures of God. Again like the principle of autonomy, the authors had to defend the compatibility of the principle of autonomy with Rumi's teachings and with Islam in general, despite what seems to be contradiction. On one hand, beneficence is usually defined as acting in the interest of others whereas in Islam God promises a generous reward in return for being beneficent. This might imply, the authors explained, that self-interest or egoism is the most important facilitator or motivation of man's altruistic behavior, which is contrary to the abovementioned definition of beneficence. However, the authors argued that while self-interest can be one of the motivations, it is not the major one especially in the mindset of a mature Sufi. Here one easily notices how apologetic the contributions within the Instrumentalist Approach can be in their bid to legitimize the embracement of the four principles, sometimes at the cost of serious engagement with the Islamic tradition. The claim that motivations related to the Hereafter, in this case receiving God's reward for benefiting others, do not play a major role in the Islamic tradition cannot be simply thrown around without in-depth analysis and rigorous argumentation. The general impression here is that specific components of the Islamic tradition are twisted in order to make them fit within the four-principle theory.

In 2010, Sahin Aksoy published his paper "Some Principles of Islamic Ethics as Found in Harrisian Philosophy," whose very title already betrays some of the aforementioned features of the Instrumentalist Approach. Unlike the previous studies that Aksoy coauthored with Elmali and Tenik whose focus was the four-principle theory articulated by Beauchamp and Childress, the main focus of this new study was the positions developed by the British bioethicist John Harrison on a number of key bioethical issues. Speaking about "principles of Islamic ethics" in the title is somehow misleading because it is not the author's intention to construct or to introduce specific "principles" in the technical sense. Rather, the study is meant to highlight the similarities (seen to be greater than the differences) between the Harrisian philosophy and the Islamic ethical tradition.

The paper is divided into six main sections, each of which addressed a specific issue/principle: responsibility; side-effects and double-effects; equality; vicious choice, guilt, and innocence; organ transplantation and property rights; and advance directives. Following more or less the previous studies' line of argumentation, each section starts with the ideas and positions adopted by John Harris on the respective issue then goes on to the justification for why these ideas/positions are compatible with Islam.[31]

One of the main differences between this study and the two previous ones is that the conclusions of this new study about the supposed compatibility between Western bioethics (represented here by John Harris) and the Islamic tradition are much bolder, more controversial, and less grounded. One example should suffice in this respect. In the section on organ transplantation and property rights, Aksoy referred to, according to him, Harris's widely criticized view that the deceased's prior consent for organ removal, although ideal, is not necessary. According to Harris, deceased people cannot be wronged or harmed by the transplant of their organs "against their will" simply because they have no will. Immediately thereafter, Aksoy jumps to the bold conclusion that Harris's controversial suggestion of making cadaver organs available for public benefit is parallel to the opinion of the Muslim religious scholar Ibn Qudama expressed six centuries ago when he permitted the reuse of organs of the deceased! Strikingly enough, Aksoy did not consult the works of Ibn Qudama but based his claim on a secondary source that attributed this opinion to Ibn Qudama. That Ibn Qudama spoke about organ transplantation or organ donation is itself an extremely controversial issue that I have addressed elsewhere.[32] What is far-fetched here is claiming that Ibn Qudama, six centuries ago, adopted the same position as that of John Harris whereas contemporary Muslim religious scholars still strongly debate on the (im)permissibility of organ donation in principle! Also unlike the previous study which touched, albeit briefly, upon the potential bioethical differences between the Western and Islamic traditions, this new study did not elaborate on any possible difference. However, Aksoy noted that once

[31] Aksoy (2010), *op. cit.*, 226–229.

[32] Mohammed Ghaly (2010). *Islam and Disability: Perspectives in Theology and Jurisprudence*. London: Routledge, 127.

we move from the issues of bioethics (should read here principles or theoretical issues) to practical applications, e.g. abortion and euthanasia, one could come across significant and fundamental differences between Harrisian philosophy and Islamic ethical principles. According to Aksoy, this is not surprising because it has here to do with religion-based ethics on one hand and "a materialist, rationalist, utilitarian (may be atheist) 20th century philosopher," on the other hand.[33]

1.3. *The Contributions of the Saudi-based Physicians, M. Al-Bar, H. Chamis-Pasha, and A. Al-Bar*

The two Saudi-based physicians Muhammad Ali Al-Bar (International Medical Center) and Hassan Chamis-Pasha (King Fahd Armed Forces Hospital) have made three important contributions. In 2012, they published *Mawsūʻat akhlāqīyāt mihnat al-ṭibb* (*Encyclopedia of the Ethics of the Medical Profession*), which they coauthored with a third physician, ʻAdnān Al-Bar. The authors dedicated the first chapter of this voluminous work to the main ethical theories, particularly utilitarianism and deontology, and their relevance to the field of (bio)medical ethics. Tom Beauchamp and James Childress were presented as two prominent bioethicists of the modern time, and their work *Principles of Biomedical Ethics* was introduced as an essential textbook for researchers in this field. The authors consulted the fifth edition of the book, which was published in 2001. What is unique about the *Encyclopedia* is that the authors, unlike their predecessors, were not primarily concerned about the possible (in)compatibility of the four principles with the Islamic tradition. Rather, they provided a detailed review of the critical remarks raised by Beauchamp and Childress about the two ethical theories of utilitarianism and deontology. By doing this, they managed to highlight the philosophical background of the principle-based bioethics, which is usually missing in the other writings. However, the authors did not develop an overall Islamic perspective on these two theories nor on the remarks raised by Beauchamp and Childress. They rather gave sporadic comments on specific and concrete issues that they came across while presenting the views of these

[33] Aksoy (2010), *op. cit.*, 229.

two American bioethicists such as honesty towards the patient, confidentiality, and euthanasia.[34]

The authors directed a few critical remarks to Beauchamp and Childress, and we pay attention here to one of them because it was a point of discussion, especially between Beauchamp and Mohammed Al-Bar, during the symposium held by CILE in 2013. The authors spoke about the example of poor African-Americans who suffer from hypertension but cannot be properly treated because they have no health insurance. Guided by the utilitarian approach, some researchers argued that it is not efficient to spend money on examining this group of patients because they have no regular access to medical care anyhow. The authors of the *Encyclopedia* expressed their strong dissatisfaction with this conclusion and lamented these researchers for condoning and even defending the injustice of this deplorable and despicable system instead of criticizing it. Beauchamp and Childress were also criticized for quoting the studies conducted by these researchers without expressing their objection to their conclusions, which would implicitly indicate their agreement with these researchers.[35] During the CILE symposium, this issue was a subject of intensive discussions, and Tom Beauchamp was keen to explain his standpoint and that neither he nor his colleague, James Childress, ever embraced these conclusions. Readers of this volume can follow the detailed discussions about this point especially in the chapter written by Beauchamp and the subsequent deliberations.

The possible compatibility of the four principles with the Islamic tradition was the focus of two other studies conducted by Mohammed Al-Bar and Hassan Chamsi-Pasha, which were published respectively in 2013 and 2015.[36] Al-Bar and Chamsi-Pasha were aware of the previous studies conducted by Serour and those coauthored by Aksoy, Elmali, and Tenik. The study of Aksoy and Elmali was particularly central for Al-Bar's and

[34] Muḥammad ʿAlī al-Bār, ʿAdnān al-Bār and Ḥassān Shamsī Bāshā (2012). *Mawsūʿat akhlāqīyāt mihnat al-ṭibb*. Jeddah, Saudi Arabia: Sheikh Mohammed Hussien Al-Amoudi Chair of Biomedical Practice Ethics.

[35] *Ibid*., 63, 64.

[36] Hassan Chamsi-Pasha and Mohammed Albar (2013). Western and Islamic bioethics: How close is the gap? *Avicenna Journal of Medicine* 3(1): 8–14; Mohammed Ali al-Bar and Hassan Chamsi-Pasha (2015). *Contemporary Bioethics: Islamic Perspective*. Dordrecht, the Netherlands: Springer: 106–152.

Chamsi-Pasha's 2013 study, which inspired them with different ideas, e.g. the difference between secular and religious ethics. It seems that Al-Bar and Chamsi-Pasha were inspired by the very motive behind addressing this issue to the extent that they even used identical phrases to the ones used by Aksoy and Elmali: "It is hoped that this paper will make a contribution to the mutual dialogue and understanding between two radically different traditions namely Islamic and Western ones."[37]

Both studies of Al-Bar and Chamsi-Pasha reflect many of the typical characteristics of the Instrumentalist Approach such as the extensive quotations from the Qur'an and Sunna to reach direct conclusions without serious engagement with the long-standing tradition of related disciplines in the Islamic tradition, including the Qur'an exegesis. The short study published in 2013 included about 18 references to the Qur'an and 20 references to the sayings of Prophet Muhammad, and the long study published in 2015 included more references.[38] These references are usually amassed to strengthen the authors' main argument that the four principles are culturally sensitive, can be easily found in these two scriptural sources and in the teachings of Muslim scholars, and thus are generally compatible with Islam. For instance, the two authors explained the position of William Frankena on the principle of beneficence and its possible division into four general obligations.[39] Thereafter, a Prophetic tradition is quoted, or actually instrumentalized, to show its compatibility with Frankena's ideas. The authors found it amazing that the Prophet of Islam did enjoin Muslims to follow the obligations mentioned by Frankena. In the study published in 2013, they could justify only three of the four obligations mentioned in Frankena's list, but in their study published in 2015 the fourth obligation was also couched in Islamic garb.[40]

It is to be noted, however, that the two authors also stressed the differences between the Islamic tradition and the principle-based bioethics, perhaps more forcefully than any of the previous studies. They differentiated between medicine as a medical profession and medical ethics.

[37] Chamsi-Pasha and Al-Bar (2013), *op. cit.*, 13.
[38] *Ibid.*, 9–12; Al-Bar and Chamsi-Pasha (2015), *op. cit.*, 106–152.
[39] (1) One ought not to inflict evil or harm; (2) One ought to prevent evil or harm; (3) One ought to remove evil or harm; and (4) One ought to do or promote good.
[40] Chamsi-Pasha and Al-Bar (2013), *op. cit.*, 11; Al-Bar and Chamsi-Pasha (2015), *op. cit.*, 121, 122.

Although the practice of medicine now almost everywhere — including in the Muslim world — follows the Western pattern, medical ethics which judges this practice may be different. "This means that the use or non-use of a renowned medical treatment by Muslim doctors will sometimes be guided more by ethics derived from Islamic law than by purely medical considerations," the two authors argued.[41] The stress on the differences was particularly visible when the authors discussed the principle of autonomy. They differentiated between what they called "Western type of autonomy" and "Islamic autonomy." The Western type of autonomy was characterized by a Western attitude of individualism according to which the patient usually decides in disregard of external interventions, including those of one's own family or wider society, and the health provider plays the role of a bystander who just provides data. As far as Islamic autonomy is concerned, the authors explained, the Western attitude of individualism is not accepted. First of all, the patient is not allowed to act as he/she wishes because of the binding rules mentioned in the Qur'an and Sunna that Muslims have to follow. Also familial and social considerations play a role in various decisions to be made by or for the patient. Additionally, Islamic autonomy does not mean that the health provider should have a passive role but on the contrary should play an active role in encouraging the patient to avoid health-related risky behavior and a harmful lifestyle. Within this framework, a patient's autonomy will never entitle the physician to terminate any human life under his/her care.[42]

1.4. *Collective Contributions*

All the abovementioned studies were produced by individual researchers. With the exception of the two Turkish theologians who coauthored the two studies conducted by Sahin Aksoy, all the involved researchers were trained in the field of medicine rather than Islamic studies. Although none of the Islamic institutions dedicated a specific seminar or conference to addressing the issue of principle-based bioethics from an Islamic perspective, they did touch upon this issue within the context of ethical guidelines

[41] Chamsi-Pasha and Al-Bar (2013), *op. cit.*, 8.
[42] *Ibid.*, 10, 11; Al-Bar and Chamsi-Pasha (2015), *op. cit.*, 109, 110.

for conducting research on human subjects. The Islamic Organization for Medical Sciences (IOMS) is known for addressing bioethical questions through a collective approach combining between physicians and religious scholars. During the period 11–14 December 2004, the IOMS held an international symposium whose proceedings were published as *Al-Mīthāq al-Islāmī al-ʻālamī li al-akhlāqīyāt al-ṭibīyah wa al-ṣiḥḥīyah* (*The International Islamic Code for Medical and Health Ethics*), which was released concurrently in both Arabic and English.[43] The second part of the code, which was dedicated to the ethical guidelines for biomedical research involving human subjects, touched upon the question of principles. In its 17th session held during the period 24–26 June 2006 in Jordan, the International Islamic Fiqh Academy (IIFA) endorsed the IOMS ethical guidelines and specifically the principles included therein (http://www.iifa-aifi.org/2223.html).

The whole set of these ethical guidelines, including the principles, were not developed by the participants in the IOMS symposium but were rather imported from the "International Ethical Guidelines For Biomedical Research Involving Human Subjects," a document produced by the Council for International Organizations of Medical Sciences (CIOMS). As far as the principles are concerned, the document did not use the famous set of four principles articulated by Beauchamp and Childress. The CIOMS document adopted the three principles outlined in the well-known Belmont Report that was written by the US National Commission for the Protection of Human Services of Biomedical and Behavioral Research, released in April 1979.[44] The three principles are respect for persons, beneficence, and justice. Within this set of principles, autonomy is included as part of the principle of respect for persons, and beneficence is introduced as a broad principle that conveys the two concepts of beneficence and nonmaleficence that count as two distinct principles in the

[43] ʻAbd al-Raḥmān al-ʻAwaḍī and Aḥmad al-Jundī (2005). *Al-Mīthāq al-Islāmī al-ʻālamī li al-akhlāqīyāt al-ṭibīyah wa al-ṣiḥḥīyah*. Kuwait: Islamic Organization for Medical Sciences; Abdul Rahman al-Awadi and Ahmad Rajai El-Gendy (2005). *The International Islamic Code for Medical and Health Ethics*. Kuwait: Islamic Organization for Medical Sciences.

[44] Jennifer Sims (2010). A brief review of the Belmont Report. *Dimensions of Critical Care Nursing* 29(4): 173–174.

approach of Beauchamp and Childress and their like-minded bioethicists.[45] Tom Beauchamp was member of the US Commission, and he participated in writing the Belmont Report while he was concurrently busy with finalizing the manuscript of the first edition of *Principles of Biomedical Ethics* that was published in 1979 as well. Thus, the two sets of principles are somehow interrelated, although certainly not identical.

The CIOMS document was translated into Arabic and then reviewed by a committee composed of both Muslim religious scholars and biomedical scientists including J. Bryant, who was the CIOMS ex-President and one of the developers of the CIOMS document. The committee was entrusted with the task of providing an Islamic religioethical framework for the document. Thus, the Islamic tradition is not approached as a possible source for certain principles but as a justifying instrument so that it can be eventually argued that these principles are compatible with Islam. It seems that this method goes in line with the aim of the IOMS to produce a code of ethics that has both an international character and also an Islamic tincture, as it appears in the very title of the code. The CIOMS document already had the international character, and the selected committee was asked to add the missing element, namely the Islamic tint. Otherwise, the members of the committee could have worked in a different way and thus would have produced something different. For instance, they could have started from the pioneering study made by the Syrian religious scholar Abdul Sattar Abu Ghudda that set the ground for the Indigenous Approach. Strikingly enough, as we shall see below, Abu Ghudda's study was first introduced in the Second International Conference on Islamic Medicine held in Kuwait in 1982 that was convened by the two key figures who led the IOMS later, namely Abd Al-Rahman Al-ʻAwadi and Ahmad Al-Jundī. Also Abu Ghudda himself was a member of the committee selected by the IOMS for reviewing the CIOMS document.[46]

The whole CIOMS document was reviewed in a uniform way: presenting a selected section of the document followed by the Islamic ethical framing for that section. The three principles of respect for persons, beneficence, and justice were introduced in a separate small section

---

[45] ʻAwaḍī and Jundī (2005), *op. cit.*, 150–152.
[46] *Ibid.*, 20.

(about 300 words in English), exactly as recorded in the CIOMS document. The three principles were introduced as ethical obligations with equal moral force but that could still be expressed differently and given different moral weight in varying circumstances. Each principle was explained in a simple and concise way. Respect for persons entails both respecting the autonomy of those who are capable of deliberation about their personal choices and protecting those with impaired or diminished autonomy. Beneficence is the ethical obligation of maximizing benefits and minimizing harms. It also implies the prohibition of deliberate infliction of harm on persons, sometimes couched in the term *nonmaleficence*, which is counted by some bioethicists like Beauchamp and Childress as a separate principle. Finally, justice means giving each person what is due to him or her and thus refers in this context mainly to distributive justice, which requires the equitable distribution of both the burdens and the benefits although differences can sometimes be justifiable.[47] This is how the question of principles was introduced to the Muslim religious scholars who were tasked with writing an Islamic ethical review. No reference was made to the genealogy of these three principles, the socio-cultural context in which they were born, and their direct link with the Belmont Report. For instance, the authors of the Belmont Report reiterated its own cultural context that influenced the process of choosing these specific three principles. Although "other principles may also be relevant," the authors conceded, "three basic principles, among those generally accepted in our cultural tradition, are particularly relevant to the ethics of research involving human subjects: the principles of respect of persons, beneficence, and justice."[48]

With the simplicity by which the three principles were introduced in a decontextualized way, framing them within the Islamic religioethical tradition seemed unproblematic. To start with, it was boldly stated that the overall CIOMS document including the three principles reflect aspects of a universally shared human nature and common sense whose acceptance

[47] *Ibid.*, 150–152.

[48] National Commission for the Protection of Human Subjects of Biomedical and Behavioral Research (1979). *The Belmont Report: Ethical Principles and Guidelines for the Protection of Human Subjects of Research.* Available online via http://www.hhs.gov/ohrp/humansubjects/guidance/belmont.html (retrieved 10 July 2015), 3–4.

is an Islamic religious obligation. A fourth principle rooted in the Islamic tradition was tentatively suggested, namely *iḥsān* (moral excellence), which entails doing more than what is actually required. This principle did not receive further elaboration in the scholars' religioethical framing, which focused more on the three principles. Each of the three principles was unconditionally endorsed and labeled as one of the established fundamentals in the eyes of Islamic Sharia (*aṣl muqarrar fī al-sharīʿah al-Islāmīyah*). Embracing the three principles in this almost unprecedented way even within the Instrumentalist Approach has, as tentatively explained above, to do with the context in which these principles were introduced to the religious scholars. Here I want to add a few remarks about the significance of the linguistic aspects and their impact on the position adopted by these religious scholars. First of all, they have read an Arabic text in which terms like *manfaʿa*, *maṣlaḥa*, and *ḍarar*, as translation for respectively beneficence, welfare, and harm, popped up more than once. These English terms have specific bioethical connotations, but their Arabic equivalents have their own juristic connotations within the discipline of Islamic law (*fiqh*). The religious scholars who worked on the document approached the Arabic terms as part of the conventional juristic jargon rather than as translations for terms imported from, and loaded with, a different context. Thus, the principle of *manfaʿa* (beneficence) was understood as part of a deeply-rooted objective in Islamic Sharia, namely promoting benefits and warding off harms (*jalb al-maṣāliḥ wa dar' al-mafāsid*). However, the benefits to be promoted and the harms to be averted here, as expounded in the religioethical framing done by the religious scholars, are to be defined and determined by the Sharia itself.[49] This perception is not in tune with the understanding of beneficence in the various works that belong to the genre of bioethics, including the standard reference of the Belmont Report.

The same remarks can be raised about the religious scholars' understanding of the term *autonomy*. It was translated in Arabic as *istiqlālīyah* whose more common English equivalent is *independence* rather than *autonomy*. As it appears in the Arabic text, the paragraph on autonomy speaks about those who can independently (autonomously) take their

[49] ʿAwaḍī and Jundī (2005), *op. cit.*, 158, 160, 161.

decisions and those whose independence (autonomy) is impaired or diminished. This way of presenting autonomy made the religious scholars believe that it has here to do with the juristic concept of legal capacity (*ahlīyah*) according to which people are also categorized as those with complete or incomplete capacity.[50] Although there may be a certain overlap between autonomy and *ahlīyah,* they are definitely not the same thing. The term *ahlīyah* is primarily about the competence to fulfill the religious obligations, which actually can limit the scope of one's autonomy. This is why many of the abovementioned authors whose works fall within the Instrumentalist Approach raised critical remarks about autonomy; they believed that it may conflict with some religious obligations that Muslims are bound to follow. Thus, the religious scholars were more engaged in expounding juristic concepts rooted in the Islamic tradition than engaging in dialogue with principle-based bioethics. This is even more obvious in the resolution adopted by the IIFA, which endorsed the four principles (the three principles in the CIOMS document in addition to the principle of *iḥsān*) mentioned in the IOMS document. The resolution here was referring to a document issued by an Islamic organization, *viz*., the IOMS and not to the CIOMS document.

2. The Indigenous Approach

2.1. *The Pioneering Contribution of the Syrian Religious Scholar Abu Ghudda*

To my knowledge, the earliest study within the Indigenous Approach was introduced during the Second International Conference on Islamic Medicine held in Kuwait during the period 29 March–2 April 1982. During this conference, the Syrian religious scholar Abdul Sattar Abu Ghudda presented a paper entitled *Al-mabādi' al-Shar'īyah li al-taṭbīb wa al-'ilāj* ("Sharia-Based Principles for Practicing the Profession of Medicine and Medical Treatment").[51] The same paper was republished later more

[50] *Ibid.*, 159, 160.

[51] 'Abd al-Sattār Abū Ghuddah (1982). Al-Mabādi' al-shar'īyah li al-taṭbīb wa-al-'ilāj. *Al-Abḥāth wa a'māl al-mu'tamar al-'ālamī al-thānī 'an al-ṭibb al-Islāmī.* Kuwait: Islamic Medicine Organization & Kuwait Foundation for Advancement of Sciences: 780–792.

than once.[52] The content of the paper shows that Abu Ghudda was not aware of the parallel discussions among Western bioethicists, and it seems that the question of the possible universality of the principles he proposed did not preoccupy his mind. As he himself pointed out, Abu Ghudda was clearly motivated by Islamic religious concerns. In order to achieve their mission by preserving health and treating diseases, medical professionals have to employ a number of means, some of which are untraditional and unusual. By legitimizing the profession of medicine in principle, Islam does not necessarily legitimize all of the means that medical professionals are inclined to employ. This is why, Abu Ghudda explained, both physicians and patients should be aware of the (im)permissibility of the means used in healthcare settings from an Islamic religioethical perspective. However, the problem is that having in-depth and specialized knowledge of the Islamic tradition in this field can neither be expected nor required from every physician. On the other hand, general declarations and codes will not avail the physicians when they want to apply these general guidelines to the long list of intricate cases they are routinely confronted with during their work. According to Abu Ghudda, the principle-based approach is the optimal way to help physicians check the (in)compatibility of the means they can make use of in their medical tradition with the Islamic religioethical system without asking too much of them or letting them fall into the trap of superficial, simplistic, and usually erroneous applications of the general codes.[53]

As for terminology, Abu Ghudda clarified that the common term *mabda'* (principle) can be accommodated within the Islamic legal discourse. However, Muslim religious scholars usually prefer the equivalent term *qā'ida* (rule or maxim), which they have been using throughout the history of the Islamic tradition to the extent that one can speak about a distinct genre of Islamic legal maxims (*qawā'id fiqhīyah*). In order to underscore the significance of this genre, Abu Ghudda quoted the prominent Mālikī jurist Shihāb al-Dīn al-Qarāfī (d. 1285) who argued that fundamentals of Sharia can be divided into two main categories, namely

[52] 'Abd al-Sattār Abū Ghuddah (1983). Al-Mabādi' al-shar'īyah li al-taṭbīb wa-al-'ilāj, *Al-Muslim al-Mu'āṣir* 9(35): 105–115; 'Abd al-Sattār Abū Ghuddah (1994). Al-Mabādi al-shar'īyah li al-taṭbīb wa-al-'ilāj. *Majallat Majma' al-Fiqh al-Islāmī al-Dawlī* 8(3): 129–146.
[53] 'Abd al-Sattār Abū Ghuddah (1982), *op. cit.*, 780, 781.

fundamentals of the legal theory (*uṣūl al-fiqh*) and the grand legal maxims (*al-qawāʿid al-fiqhīyah al-kullīyah*). Abu Ghudda composed a list of 23 principles and conceded that the list is by no means comprehensive. His target was to select only those principles with direct relevance to the field of medical ethics. He grouped this long list of principles under five main clusters, namely (i) the concept of benefit or interest (*maṣlaḥa*) which included two principles; (ii) avoiding harms and removing them, which included eight principles; (iii) removing hardship and considering the cases of necessity, which included eight principles; (iv) the right of the other and the necessity of obtaining consent, which included three principles; and (v) cooperation, usefulness, and altruism, which included two principles.[54]

The pioneering study of Abu Ghudda did open important windows for thinking about how to develop a principle-based bioethics rooted in the Islamic tradition. As we shall see in this volume, his approach of employing the genre of Islamic legal maxims (*qawāʿid fiqhīyah*) for developing principles proved to be appealing for various religious scholars who participated in the CILE seminar. However, Abu Ghudda's contribution remained considerably limited in scope by focusing almost exclusively on Islamic law (*fiqh*) and particularly on one branch within *fiqh*, namely the genre of legal maxims. Other disciplines within the Islamic tradition like Islamic theology, higher objectives of Islamic Sharia (*maqāṣid al-sharīʿah*), and their possible contribution to developing a theory of Islamic principle-based biomedical ethics were almost completely missing. Also, a principle-based theory in bioethics cannot be developed by just enlisting a set of principles. It is indispensable to address other interrelated issues like moral theories, moral virtues,[55] and moral status of individuals, which were all missing in Abu Ghudda's study.

2.2. *The Contributions of Abdulaziz Sachedina*

The first encounter between the Instrumentalist and the Indigenous Approaches took place more than a decade after the publication of Serour's

[54] *Ibid.*, 782–791.

[55] For example, Amyn Sajoo (2014). Negotiating virtue: Principlism and *Maslaha* in Muslim bioethics. *Studies in Religion* 43(1): 53–69.

pioneer study. Like its first edition, which included the contributions of Serour and Hasan, the second edition of the edited volume *Principles of Health Care Ethics*, published in 2007, also included a chapter on the Islamic tradition.[56] This chapter was written by Abdulaziz Sachedina, the then Frances Myers Ball Professor of Religious Studies, University of Virginia and now the International Islamic Institute (IIIT) Chair in Islamic Studies, George Mason University. Two years later, Sachedina addressed the same issue in much more detail in his book *Islamic Biomedical Ethics: Principles and Application*. As is clear from its subtitle, the issue of principles represented a focal theme that was recurrently examined throughout the whole book, but it was addressed separately in the longest chapter of the book, "In Search of Principles of Healthcare Ethics in Islam."[57] Because of the substantial overlap between the two studies, I will present Sachedina's ideas as outlined in both works interchangeably and will refer specifically to one of the two studies only when necessary.

Out of all the abovementioned studies, Sachedina was only aware of the two pioneering studies done by Gamal Serour and K. Hasan. He argued that the contributions made by both of them, published in the first edition of *Principles of Health Care Ethics*, failed to provide uniquely Islamic principles of bioethics mainly because of a twofold reason. On one hand, they did not assess the intellectual context, particularly the secular and democratic political philosophy, of the four principles that informs much of the principle-based bioethics in the West.[58] On the other hand, these

---

[56] Abdulaziz Sachedina (2007). Islam and the four principles, in Richard Ashcroft *et al.* (eds.) *Principles of Health Care Ethics*, 2nd edn. London: John Wiley & Sons Ltd: 117–125.

[57] Abdulaziz Sachedina (2009). *Islamic Biomedical Ethics: Principles and Application*. Oxford: Oxford University Press: 25–75.

[58] The proposition that the four principles are essentially the product of secular Western or more particularly American culture rather than having a universal character has been reiterated by various voices within the field of Islamic bioethics (e.g. Atighetchi (2007), 22; Jafarey and Moazam (2010), 353, 360). Some Western physicians, with no Islamic studies background, also expressed their doubts about the supposed cultural neutrality of the four principles (e.g. Westra *et al.* (2009), 1383–1387). See: Dariusch Atighetchi (2007). *Islamic Bioethics: Problems and Perspectives*. Dordrecht, the Netherlands: Springer; Aamir Jafarey and Farhat Moazam (2010). "Indigenizing" bioethics: The first center for bioethics in Pakistan. *Cambridge Quarterly of Healthcare Ethics* 19: 353–362; Anna Westra, Dick Willems and Bert Smit (2009). Communicating with Muslim parents: "The Four Principles" are not as culturally neutral as suggested. *European Journal of Pediatrics* 168: 1383–1387.

contributions did not elaborate on the presuppositions of the Islamic tradition about human action, its ontology, and its ethical evaluation and about the roles of moral reasoning and scriptural sources in addressing practical ethical dilemmas. This happened, Sachedina explained, because the two authors lacked adequate training in the Islamic legal sciences, without which one cannot identify the principles and the rules that Muslim jurists use to justify and assess moral–legal decisions within their own cultural environment.[59]

In order to repair the deficiencies of these two studies, Sachedina dedicated a substantial part of his works to examining a number of methodological issues related to Islamic moral epistemology and ontology. He spoke about the attempts of Muslim religious scholars throughout Islamic history to keep the balance in their ethical reasoning between scripture- and reason-based sources. This balance was required to avoid excessive literal reading of the scriptures that may negatively affect the adaptability of Islamic law to meet the changing needs of society. On the other hand, this balance was also needed to avoid possible arbitrary judgments of reason. Furthermore, Sachedina discussed the problem of situating the credible religious authority empowered to sanction specific modes or conclusions of religioethical reasoning. It did not escape Sachedina in his quest for exploring "distinctly Islamic, and yet cross-culturally communicable, principle-rule based deontological–teleological ethics" to show that the Western-American set of four principles does have some features that can hardly fit within the Islamic tradition. His critique for the principle of autonomy serves as a representative example in this regard. Sachedina said that the highly rated principle of autonomy in the West will not enjoy the same status within the Islamic tradition, which gives higher priority to communitarian ethics when the consequence of a medical decision on the family and community resources should be seriously considered. Thus, Sachedina argued, the dominant principle of autonomy, which is based on liberal individualism, should be substituted by the rule of consultation (*shūrā*), which is an indigenous part of Islamic ethics.[60,61]

---

[59] Sachedina (2007), *op. cit.*, 117; Sachedina (2009), *op. cit.*, 26, 27.

[60] Sachedina (2007), *op. cit.*, 118, 122; Sachedina (2009), *op. cit.*, 30–45.

[61] The Ph.D. dissertation "Beyond Clerics and Clinics: Islamic Bioethics and Assisted Reproductive Technology in Iran" written by Robert Tappan and supervised by Sachedina,

Sachedina introduced two main broad principles, namely common good (*maṣlaḥa*) and "no harm, no harassment" (*la ḍarar wa la ḍirār*). According to him, these two principles are deeply rooted in the Islamic tradition and their ascription to the authoritative Islamic sources is undisputed. On the other hand, Sachedina argued that these two principles are flexible enough to accommodate and address the new ethical issues in the modern field of healthcare. He gave the example of the ethical issues raised by prenatal genetic diagnosis (PGD) and how the principle of common good can help resolve them. He also explained how the principle of "no harm, no harassment" can help addressing some end-of-life ethical issues like (not) using life-support machines for terminally ill patients. According to Sachedina, this principle is at the heart of the ethical deliberations around almost 90 percent of cases confronting people working in the healthcare sector in the Muslim world.[62]

The two contributions of Sachedina, besides the above-mentioned work of Abu Ghudda, demonstrate the appeal of the genre of Islamic legal maxims (*qawāʿid fiqhīyah*) to those who search for principle-based bioethics stemming from the Islamic tradition.[63] Whereas Sachedina introduced two main principles, Abu Ghudda introduced five clusters of principles each of which included a number of subprinciples or legal maxims. Also the UK-based Muslim physician Yassar Mustafa has recently made use of the same genre to articulate five principles (*qaṣd* (intention), *yaqīn* (certainty), *ḍarar* (injury), *ḍarūra* (necessity), and *'urf*

demonstrated the validity of this argument as far as the bioethical deliberations on Assisted Reproductive Technology (ART) in Iran are concerned (Tappan 2011, 38, 71). See Robert Tappan (2011). Beyond Clerics and Clinics: Islamic B ioethics and Assisted Reproductive Technology in Iran. Dissertation presented to the Graduate Faculty of the University of Virginia in Candidacy for the Degree of Doctor of Philosophy.

[62] Sachedina (2007), *op. cit.*, 121–124; Sachedina (2009), *op. cit.*, 49–75.

[63] Aziz Sheikh and Abdul Rashid Gatrad (2001). Medical ethics and Islam: Principles and practices. *Archives of Disease in Childhood* 84: 75; Kamel Ajlouni (2003). Values, qualifications, ethics and legal standards in Arabic (Islamic) medicine. *Saudi Medical Journal* 24(8): 820–821; Aida Al Aqeel (2007). Islamic ethical framework for research into and prevention of genetic diseases. *Nature Genetics* 39(11): 1295–1297; Bagher Larijani and Farzaneh Anaraki (2008). Islamic principles and Decision Making in Bioethics. *Nature Genetics* 40(2): 123; Hamza Yusuf Hanson (2008). In Aziz Sheikh and Abdul Rashid Gatrad (eds.) *Caring for Muslim Patients*. Oxford, NY: Radcliffe: 47–49.

(custom), each of which revolves around a number of legal maxims.[64] Throughout this volume, we will also see that the religious scholars who participated in the CILE seminar advocated this approach, although they did not come to a clear conclusion about which maxims should be selected and which selection criteria should be employed. Thus, making benefit of the genre of Islamic legal maxims seems promising, but a lot of work should still be done. The engagement of these authors with the principle-based approach of bioethics remains minimal. This holds true even to Abdulaziz Sachedina, who is well aware of the four-principle approach developed by Beauchamp and Childress (the latter wrote a foreword for Sachedina's book). Despite his serious efforts to introduce two "distinctly Islamic yet metaculturally communicable" principles, Sachedina said almost nothing about how similar/different these two principles are in comparison with the two principles of beneficence and nonmaleficence.[65] Furthermore, the term *justice* and its derivatives appeared more than 70 times throughout Sachedina's book, and it was sometimes used alongside the principle of common good or public benefit to determine the ethical weight of specific biomedical interventions.[66] However, the author did not explain why justice was not categorized as a distinct bioethical principle.

3. Concluding Remarks: The Unfinished Task

All the studies reviewed in this chapter reflect a kind of consensus among experts in Islamic bioethics about the uncontested benefit of having a set of principles that governs this emerging field in order to secure a certain degree of conformity and coherence. However, these experts have disagreed on how to formulate this set of principles. The diverging opinions on this question were divided in this study into two main approaches, namely Instrumentalist Approach and Indigenous Approach, each of which has its own characteristics, strengths, and weaknesses. By the end of this section, a tentative proposal for a hybrid approach is presented as a possible research agenda for the future.

[64] Yassar Mustafa (2014). Islam and the four principles of medical ethics. *Journal of Medical Ethics* 40: 480.
[65] Sachedina (2009), *op. cit.*, 65, 66.
[66] *Ibid.*, 170.

The Instrumentalist Approach, almost monopolized by biomedical scientists trained in Western academies,[67] proved to be more productive, quantitatively speaking, than the other approach. One of the common convictions shared by the advocates of this approach is that the principles outlined in Western bioethical literature, especially the four principles of Tom Beauchamp and James Childress, are universal and transcultural in nature. Thus, their compatibility with the Islamic tradition is taken by default and all what these advocates have been trying to do is to "reveal" or "unearth" this compatibility for their audiences. Their main instrument for achieving this task is quoting Islamic authoritative texts, especially from the Qur'an and Sunna. The proponents of this approach also showed common interest in building bridges between Islam and the West. In a bid to demonstrate that the Islamic tradition is not always the passive partner that receives what Western bioethics has produced, some of these advocates argued, usually in an apologetic tone, that the principles articulated by contemporary Western bioethicists have already existed for centuries in the works of pre-modern Muslim religious scholars. The principles introduced by Western bioethicists were not equally embraced by all the advocates of this approach. Whereas some of them almost unconditionally accepted all principles, many of them expressed reservations about specific principles. The principle of respect for autonomy seems to be the most controversial one to the extent that some researchers spoke about "Islamic autonomy" versus a "Western type of autonomy" with significant differences between the two versions of autonomy. Also some authors suggested adding some principles, in their view uniquely Islamic in nature, to the list articulated by Western bioethicists.

---

[67] Available studies show that this generalization holds true for physicians with both Sunni and Shīʿī backgrounds. Although most of the contributions reviewed in this study expressed Sunni perspectives, contributions made by physicians with Shīʿī backgrounds echo almost identical thoughts with quotations from figures or sources acclaimed in the Shīʿī tradition. See for example: Kiarash Aramesh (2008). Justice as a principle of Islamic bioethics. *The American Journal of Bioethics* 8(10): 26–27; Shabih Zaidi (2014). *Ethics in Medicine*. Dordrecht, the Netherlands: Springer: 75–99. The work of the Dutch convert Abdulwahid van Bommel, who worked as Muslim chaplain and *imam*, can also be categorized within the Instrumentalist Approach. See A. van Bommel (1999). Medical ethics from the Muslim perspective. *Acta Neurochirurgica Supplements* 74: 18–21.

The main strength of the Instrumentalist Approach is its dependence on a well-structured and coherent theory that managed to gain wide international recognition although its birth was in an exclusively Western or even particularly American context. The feasibility of the principle-based theory to address different bioethical dilemmas has been amply proved. Because of the strong appeal of this theory among biomedical scientists and bioethicists worldwide, its "Islamized" version, the advocates of this approach believe, would do a good service to the Islamic tradition by making their contribution an integral part of the global bioethical discourse. On the other hand, the main weakness of this approach is the lack of sophisticated discourse and sometimes even the use of superficial arguments and hasty conclusions. This holds true for their understanding of, and explanation for, the principle-based theory but becomes more flagrant when they try to demonstrate the compatibility of specific principles with the Islamic tradition. The advocates of this approach also hardly say anything about how these principles can be applied within the religioethical framework of the Islamic tradition. One of the chronic problems of the principle-based theory is the so-called process of "specification" or how to downstream these broad principles and apply them to particular case studies. The principle of beneficence can serve as a good illustrative example here. By adopting this principle, which implies doing all possible efforts to achieve the benefit of the patient, the central question will be: What makes a certain medical intervention a benefit? This used to be the estimation of the physician (Hippocratic paternalistic model), but in contemporary Western bioethical discourse, this should be the patient's discretion and the physician is exclusively entitled to provide the patient with information (informative model). However, in the Islamic religioethical tradition, "benefit" is to be determined in the first instance by God, and what contradicts God's ordinances cannot be considered beneficial even if it is demanded by both the patient and the physician. Thus, endorsing a set of principles will not guarantee uniformity in bioethical reasoning as long as the process of specification is also fine-tuned, and this cannot be done anyhow without a more in-depth understanding of the Islamic tradition.

As for the Indigenous Approach, the pool of its advocates consists mainly of religious scholars and specialists in Islamic studies,[68] and their scholarly output is, quantitatively speaking, still modest. The advocates of this approach share the strong conviction that the Islamic tradition is rich enough to produce a set of indigenous and homegrown principles that can enrich the contemporary field of bioethics. They are also much more concerned about demonstrating the viability of the Islamic tradition in modern times and protecting its identity than building bridges with other traditions. Their engagement and interaction with principle-based theories is minimal, and some of the advocates of this approach are simply unaware of such theories.

The main strength of the Indigenous Approach is the depth of the Islamic religioethical discourse introduced by its advocates, which far exceeds what we come across in the publications of the Instrumentalist Approach. This explains the existence of a common conviction shared by the advocates of this approach that their discourse should be more appealing for Muslim individuals and communities. Thus, unlike the proponents of the Instrumentalist Approach, they do not feel obliged to defend the "Islamic character" of their approach or its compatibility with the Islamic tradition. On the other hand, the main weakness of the Indigenous Approach is that its advocates hardly engage in serious dialogue with the principle-based bioethical discourse developed within the Western tradition. The product of principle-based bioethics or principlism, whose theorists have been working for decades, is not just a list of principles but a full-fledged theory or even a number of related theories. Had they studied these theories properly, the proponents of this approach would have

[68] One of the few exceptions that I am aware of is an article published in 2001 by two Muslim UK-based physicians, namely A. R. Gatrad and A. Sheikh. They both expressed their dissatisfaction with the call for having universal ethical codes and proposed what they called an alternative approach, which focused on the particularity of the Islamic tradition. They included a considerably heterogeneous list of principles drawn from Qur'anic verses, prophetic traditions, Islamic legal maxims, and quotations from the works of Muslim writers. It is clear that the main target of Gatrad and Sheikh was to simplify Islamic bioethics for the non-Muslim physicians working in the UK rather than to develop a principle-based Islamic bioethical discourse (Sheikh and Gatrad 2001, 72–75). See Aziz Sheikh and Abdul Rashid Gatrad (2001). Medical ethics and Islam: Principles and practices. *Archives of Disease in Childhood* 84: 72–75.

been able to go beyond the debate on which list of principles is more compatible with Islam. The sophisticated debates on the methodological and analytical tools of principlism would have helped them produce parallel principle-based theories rooted in the Islamic tradition rather than just a list of principles. Also, the advocates of this approach focused almost exclusively on the genre of Islamic legal maxims (*qawāʿid fiqhīyah*). Although this genre proved promising for producing bioethical principles rooted in the Islamic tradition, future studies should also explore the possible contribution of other genres and disciplines like the higher objectives of Islamic Sharia (*maqāṣid al-sharīʿah*), Islamic theology, and spirituality.

Bearing in mind the characteristics, strengths, and weaknesses of each of these two approaches, this edited volume presents the seed for, and foretells the features of, a hybrid and more elaborated approach whose realization still awaits more research in the future. Below, we highlight the main features of this proposed approach that takes into consideration the positive and negative aspects of the two approaches reviewed in this chapter.

Producing a coherent theory claimed to be rooted in the Islamic tradition necessitates broadening our understanding of what the Islamic tradition actually is. Besides the genre of Islamic legal maxims, the proceedings of the CILE seminar did open new windows for exploring new horizons. For instance, the paper of Sheikh Ahmed Raissouni showed the relevance of the genre of virtues (*faḍāʾil* or *makārim*), the paper of Sheikh Abu Ghudda examined the relevance of the long-standing genre of *adab al-ṭabīb* (practical ethics of the physician), and the paper of Sheikh Ali al-Qaradāghī explored the vast genre of the higher objectives of Sharia and its possible interrelatedness with the genre of legal maxims. All these terrains will need much more research in the future as well.

On the other hand, serious and critical engagement with the principle-based theories articulated by Western bioethicists is indispensable. These theories have found their way to the overwhelming majority of physicians worldwide and, as we have seen in this chapter, those of Muslim background were no exception in this regard. The first ever face-to-face discussions between Tom Beauchamp and Muslim religious scholars during the CILE seminar was a significantly enriching element that surely necessitates many more steps in this direction in the future. However, researchers should be mindful that principle-based bioethics is broader than the works of Beauchamp and Childress. Other contributions made by individuals like the renowned American bioethicist Robert Veatch,[69] by international organizations like UNESCO,[70] and by theologians from religious traditions like Catholicism[71] should also be studied. Furthermore, engagement with principle-based theories should not be confined to checking their compatibility with Islam as if these theories make part of a "Holy Scripture" of Western bioethics. Engagement with these theories should be critical towards these theories as they stand. As an attempt to fill in this gap, this volume includes a chapter written by the Dutch bioethicist, Annelien Bredenoord, on the arguments for and against principlism within the Western bioethical discourse. Muna Ali's chapter in this volume also strongly argues for the point that future bioethical discourse should be critical not only of the religioethical traditions but also to our understanding of the profession of medicine itself.

Finally, no full-fledged theory of bioethics can be realized without paying due attention to metaethics, the branch of ethics that addresses questions about the source of ethics and morals and how they can be justified or reasoned. As the reader will observe, a great deal of the deliberations during the CILE seminar had to do with the role of religion in producing "universal" bioethical principles. Is it possible to produce universal principles with(out) serious engagement with religion? Does a certain set of principles become "Islamic" only when they originate from the Islamic tradition itself or also whenever these principles are in tune with its spirit? To think a bit outside the box, we also need to address questions like: Does the principle-based model represent the optimum model for guaranteeing coherence and consistency in the Islamic bioethical discourse? Is it possible to guarantee similar, or maybe even stronger, levels of coherence and consistency by employing specific

---

[69] Robert Veatch (2012). *Basics of Bioethics*, 3rd edn., Boston: Pearson Education, Inc., 47–143, 164–179.

[70] Henk Ten Have and Michèle Jean (eds.) (2009). *The UNESCO Universal Declaration on Bioethics and Human Rights: Background, Principles and Application.* Paris: United Nations Educational, Scientific and Cultural Organization.

[71] Scaria Kanniyakoni (2007). *The Fundamentals of Bioethics: Legal Perspectives and Ethical Approaches.* Kottayam, India: Oriental Institute of Religious Studies: 268–328.

aspects of the discipline of Islamic legal theory (*uṣūl al-fiqh*), which has been used for centuries to address complicated religioethical issues from an Islamic perspective? This volume is meant to provide researchers with provocative intellectual foodstuff so that they may conduct more research on such questions and their relevance for principle-based bioethics, surely an enduring task for researchers in this emerging field for years to come.

The "Bio" in Biomedicine: Evolution, Assumptions, and Ethical Implications

Muna Ali

Abstract: As biomedicine and its research and technologies globalize, they are accompanied by Principlism, the dominant Western bioethical theory. The Muslim response has roughly taken two tracks: (i) criticism of principlism as a neo-imperialistic attempt to universalize what is specific or (ii) harmonization of principlism with Islam by showing not only that the four principles (autonomy, beneficence, nonmaleficence, and justice) are universal, but that indeed Islam had, long ago, codified them in its ethico-legal tradition. In these debates, medicine and biomedicine are conflated and bioethics is reduced to principlism. This is problematic because biomedicine is but one medical system and principlism is one among several (feminist, religious, narrative, global) theories. This chapter examines some of the relevant critical questions to bring insights from the philosophy, anthropology, and sociology of medicine and of bioethics to bear on the current discussion on Islam and bioethics and the questions posed by the research Center for Islamic Legislation and Ethics (CILE).

Muslim scholars and medical professionals have grappled with pressing ethical issues (abortion, *in-vitro* fertilization, end-of-life issues, and organ donation/transplantation presented by the advances in biomedicine and tried to offer guidance to Muslim practitioners, patients, and policy makers. Their ethico-legal response to these questions and efforts to engage the dominant Western bioethical theory (principlism)[1] have contributed to an "Islam and medical ethics" discourse, though an "Islamic bioethics" theoretical framework is yet to emerge.

As biomedicine and its research and technologies globalize, they are accompanied by the principlism theory of bioethics. The Muslim response has, more or less, taken two tracks: (i) criticism of principlism as a neo-imperialistic attempt to universalize what is specific and rooted in Western philosophical tradition and historical context or (ii) harmonization of principlism with Islam by showing not only that the four principles (autonomy, beneficence, nonmaleficence, and justice) are universal, but that indeed Islam had, long ago, codified them in its ethico-legal tradition. Both positions also reference the "ethics of the physician" to elaborate a framework for Islamic medical ethics. In these debates, medicine and biomedicine are conflated and bioethics is reduced to principlism. This is problematic because biomedicine is but one medical system and principlism is one among several (feminist, religious, narrative, global) theories to address the moral conundrums presented by biomedicine.

The virtues and failings of biomedicine and principlism are more frequently debated within the West itself. It is critical that Muslim religious and medical experts acquire expertise and contribute to these debates in order to adequately address emerging biomedical ethical questions and for Islamic moral reasoning and ethical theory to have any relevance in the contemporary world. To do so, upstream from the urgent biomedical issues or the critique of "Western bioethics," what is needed is a deep reflection and rigorous examination that begins with the critical interrogation of foundational concepts. What is "biomedicine," and what historical trajectory resulted in the prefix "bio"? What does that reveal and conceal about underlying moral positions and values and epistemological and metaphysical assumptions about how we know what we know and what is "real"? How does biomedicine conceptualize the human being, the

[1] Beauchamp and Childress (1979) detail their four principles (autonomy, benevolence, nonmaleficence, and justice) theory in their seminal book *Principles of Biomedical Ethics* (1979). The term Principlism was coined by Clousser and Gert in their 1990 critique of this theory in an article titled "A Critique of Principlism" published in the *Journal of Medicine and Philosophy* 15: 219–236. It has since become a more neutral term and shorthand for Beauchamp and Childress's theory.

body, and the relationship of self with others and with nature? What meanings and understandings of health, illness, life, and death guide the research and practice of biomedicine and biotechnologies? This chapter aims to examine these critical questions and others to bring insights from the philosophy, anthropology, and sociology of medicine and of bioethics to bear on the current discussion on Islam and bioethics and the questions posed by the research Center for Islamic Legislation and Ethics.

1. Biomedicine: A Brief History

Healers (shamans, bonesetters, etc.) attending to human ills have always existed in every culture. Complex medical systems such as Chinese, Ayurvedic, and Unani medicines are still practiced.[2] The Hippocratic Oath remains the foundation of medical ethics today. Medieval Muslim physicians, mastering both religious and medical sciences, made lasting contributions to medicine, and Ibn Sina's (Avicenna) *The Cannon of Medicine* remained the primary textbook at Western universities until the 17th century. Many of his concepts and theories are still present in modern medicine. Today, Muslims engaging the discourse on bioethics invoke this history and the centuries-old code of ethics for physicians developed by Al-Ruhawi and Al-Razi.[3] However, the medicine practiced then is not the biomedicine of today. While traditional medicine maintains the connection of patients with their spiritual, physical, and social realms, biomedicine has not only severed these relationships, but other entities (the state, insurance companies, and medical facilities administrators) now mediate the patient–physician relationship in what has been termed the "medical–industrial complex."[4]

---

[2]Chinese medicine and Ayurvedic Indian medicine are gaining cosmopolitan status as they spread outside China and India. Unani medicine remains mostly in the Middle East and South Asia and links Muslim medicine with Greek medicine and Hippocrates who is referred to as the father of medicine.

[3]Aasim I. Padela (2007). Islamic medical ethics: A primer. *Bioethics* 21(3): 169–178. PBS, Frontline (2001). *Organ Farm*. Available online via http://www.pbs.org/wgbh/pages/frontline/shows/organfarm/ (retrieved 1 July 2013).

[4]Raymond De Vries (2011). The uses and abuses of moral theory in bioethics. *Ethic Theory Moral Practice* 14: 424.

Medicine in the West changed drastically with the advent of the scientific revolution of the 17th century when dissection enabled an "anatomical gaze resulting in the objectification of bodies."[5] By the 19th century, population studies generated statistical data on group-based biological features leading to the development of "norms" to which individual bodies could be compared.[6] With this, a universalized human body emerged: a biological entity responding to disease in the same way everywhere. This launched the development of biomedicine.[7] Often simply called "medicine," the dominant contemporary medical system is variously referred to as "modern medicine," "Western medicine," or "allopathic medicine." Calling it only "medicine" deems other long-established medical systems simply "folk" practices based on "belief" and not on "knowledge."[8,9] Consequently, the term "biomedicine" has been coined to distinguish "the body of knowledge and associated clinical and experimental practices grounded in medical sciences that were gradually consolidated in Europe and North America from the 19th century on."[10] This is a technology-based medical system consisting of an "assemblage of activities" in physicians' offices, hospitals, research centers, and elsewhere which is ever

[5] Margaret Lock and Vinh-Kim Nguyen (2010). *An Anthropology of Biomedicine*. Chichester, West Sussex: Wiley-Blackwell: 27.

[6] As the state embarked on the double task of modernization and imperial expansion, it needed a healthy work force and ways of managing populations at home and in the colony and thus created the infrastructure for the statistical studies of large populations and for ever more complex clinic laboratory work. (Harold Vanderpool (2008). The religious features of scientific medicine. *Kennedy Institute of Ethics Journal* 18(2): 82.)

[7] Lock and Nguyen (2010), *op. cit.*

[8] The study of Biomedicine as one among several medical systems was a later development. Social scientists considered Western medicine the standard medical system, presumably scientific and therefore unbiased and above the effect of culture, against which all else was measured and deemed to be "cultural" or folk healing practices. This not only dismissed any scientific grounding for the other systems but it also "stripped the illness experience of its local semantic content and context" (Gaines and Davis-Floyd (2004), 96). It was only in the past 30 years that closer examination of biomedicine as a Western "ethnomedicine" began to challenge Biomedicine's monopoly over authoritative knowledge. See Atwood Gaines and Robbie Davis-Floyd (2004). Biomedicine, in Melvin Ember and Carol Ember (eds.), *Encyclopedia of Medical Anthropology*, Dordrecht, Netherlands: Kluwer Academic Publishers.

[9] Gaines and Davis-Floyd (2004), *op. cit.*

[10] Lock and Nguyen (2010), *op. cit.*, 365.

more connected with "global capital."[11] The prefix "bio" indexes the centrality of biological and other natural sciences and ontological and epistemological assumptions undergirding this dominant system.

2. The Social Construction of the Body and of Knowledge

Enlightenment ideas about nature, human being, progress, and knowledge shaped the sciences upon which biomedicine is built.[12] The emergence of physics' universal laws that explain how nature works inspired efforts to similarly formulate universal biological laws that govern organisms including the human body and what ails it. The body is assessed through standardized processes and compared to "norms," and the generated knowledge and associated technologies and ways of thinking are to be spread globally.[13] Biological sciences have contributed greatly to our understanding of the human body. The knowledge produced is real, but rather than being "different representations of the same ontological reality — the universal body," these insights are more "snapshots" by "lenses onto a shifting and contingent reality."[14,15] Advances in molecular biology now challenge the assumption of a "normal" biological body against which all differences are measured and deemed "abnormal"[16] and affirm that bodies are products of their physical–social–historical contexts. Likewise, the knowledge about this body emerges from technologies of particular socio-cultural contexts. The questions asked, what is knowable, and how knowledge is interpreted emerge not from a detached observer aiming for universal knowledge, but from a local context and have political implications.[17]

---

[11] *Ibid.*
[12] *Ibid.*
[13] *Ibid.*, 20.
[14] For example, a human fetus is a real entity but, as Barad argues, is one that we come to know through medical imaging technology that renders the mother invisible and represents the fetus as a "self-contained, free floating object under the watchful eye of scientific and medical surveillance" (Lock and Nguyen (2010), *op. cit.*, 94) whose fate and rights are contentiously debated.
[15] Lock and Nguyen (2010), *op. cit.*, 93.
[16] *Ibid.*
[17] *Ibid.*

Biomedicine is unique among other medical systems in its "systematic approach to objectifying, classifying, and quantifying the human body itself assumed to be derived from a universal template."[18] Biomedicine, like modern science, cannot be disentangled from the historical and socio-cultural context from which it emerged. Both are steeped in unexamined assumptions and neither is culture or value neutral.[19] Additionally, technologies are not mere application of knowledge; they also serve as instruments and methods in the production and practice of knowledge.[20] Social scientists and philosophers have illustrated that how we perceive nature in many ways reflects our cultural understandings and worldview. As Gaines and Davis-Floyd pointed out, each medical system has these cosmological understandings and assumptions at its foundation.[21] Claims that biomedicine is unencumbered by belief and cultural values would make it an oddity among medical systems.[22]

[18]Harold Vanderpool (2008). The religious features of scientific medicine. *Kennedy Institute of Ethics Journal* 18(2): 203–234.

[19]No human endeavor is free from the tacit cultural beliefs and values or power relations within which one is immersed, and biomedicine is no exception. Biomedical knowledge and practices reflect cultural norms and inequalities based on gender, class, ethnicity, or race and at times reinforce them by giving them "scientific" cover and medicalization. Additionally, the knowledge and classification of illness (for example, HIV–AIDS) are the products of the socially constructed, contested, and negotiated by diverse players (physicians, scientists, pharmaceutical companies, activists, and policy makers) and not so much the result of "pure" science and research (Conrad (2010)). See Peter Conrad and Kristin K. Barker (2010). The social construction of illness: Key insights and policy implications. *Journal of Health and Social Behavior* 51: S67–S79.

[20]Lock and Nguyen (2010), *op. cit.*

[21]Gaines and Davis-Floyd (2004), *op. cit.*

[22]Biomedicine's values and beliefs include what Gaines and Davis-Floyd (2004) have referred to as "the myth of technocratic transcendence" where technology is believed to be the panacea for all that ails or limits humans physically, cognitively, or even socially. Often religion and sciences are framed in opposition, and religious discourse is assumed to be based on beliefs without critical thinking: "What is interesting here is that those who most decry the alleged moral certitude of religious believers and other strong moral evaluators are themselves awash in unyielding certitude that manifests itself in not taking seriously the arguments of those they oppose" (Elshtain (2008), 167). As much as biomedicine distances itself from religion by privileging empirical knowledge, devaluing intuitive and revealed knowledge, and disregarding patients' religious beliefs, Gordon (1988) pointed out the religious-like features of biomedicine and biomedicine cosmology in its view of nature as neutral, its neglect of human relations, and its bio-reductionist approach to illness. Biomedicine is seen as scientific because it relies on evidence for

Disease and illness are often considered interchangeable notions, and health is understood as a disease-free state. However, one could be ill and unhealthy without having a disease. Disease is a formal category within medical systems while illness captures how disease is experienced and given meaning within a particular socio-cultural context. Health, according to the World Health Organization, is a state of mental, physical, spiritual, and social well-being and not the mere absence of disease.[23] The categorizations and meanings of illness are embedded in local socio-cultural contexts which determine how it is viewed, diagnosed, and treated and what resources are allocated to it. Illness is a social and not merely biological reality. Ethnographic studies have demonstrated the cultural differences in the understanding and experience of pain and of conditions such as HIV and AIDS. There are conditions that are culturally specific (for example, anorexia in the West, Zar in the Middle East, Kuru in Guinea) and classified as "culturally bound syndromes." This social construction of illness becomes most evident in the process of medicalization of behavior (alcoholism, malnutrition, anxiety, hyperactivity, and recently obesity) and of female biological functions (menstruation, pregnancy and childbirth, and

---

diagnosis and treatment, but the practice of biomedicine is not "a science" like physics; though, as noted earlier, many insights from physics have been extended to medicine. This is because even as it purports to "discover" diseases, these are socio-culturally constructed and informed by a societal ethos, economics, and politics (Gordon (1988)). Furthermore, while it rationally and objectively is in counterdistinction to religious belief and subjectivity, it cannot block patients' and practitioners' worldviews from informing the clinical encounter. Its religious-like features include its "promises of rescue and salvation, and its ever-increasing guardianship over human life" (Vanderpool (2008), 224). These features notwithstanding, biomedicine is non-religious and technology-based and has as its central metaphor the body as machine. Consequently, practitioners aim to cure, as in "to fix malfunctions," and not to heal, as in "the long-term beneficial changes in the whole somatic–interpersonal system," which results in neglecting the psycho-spiritual-social-environmental aspect of health (Kirmayer (2004), 46). See Gaines and Davis-Floyd (2004), *op. cit.*; Jean Bethke Elshtain (2008). Why science cannot stand alone. *Theoretical Medicine and Bioethics* 29: 161–169; Deborah, Gordon (1988). Tenacious Assumptions in Western medicine, in M. Lock and D. Gordon, (eds.), *Biomedicine Examined* Dordrecht: Kluwer Academic Publishers; Vanderpool (2008) *op. cit.*; Kirmayer, Laurence J. (2004). The cultural diversity of healing: Meaning, Metaphor and Mechanism. *British Medical Bulletin* 69: 33–48.

[23] World Health Organization definition of health. Available online via http://www.who.int/about/definition/en/print.html (retrieved 20 July 2013).

menopause) which now require monitoring and interventions.[24] Similarly, a growing pursuit of physical enhancements through drugs (Viagra, growth hormone, etc.) and cosmetic surgeries to sculpt the body to fit an idealized body is also indicative of the medicalization process.[25]

Metaphors are also an important aspect of the social construction of illness. Metaphors are not mere linguistic embellishment but are important tools for conceptualization. They are "epistemological device[s], serving to conceptualize the world, define notions of reality, and construct subjectivity."[26] Metaphors do powerful cognitive work by integrating "sensory, affective and motivational levels of representation in ways that can help account for psychophysiological effects of symbolic interventions."[27] Metaphors used to represent an affliction shape how it experienced, how it is viewed by others and how it is diagnosed and managed. They are central to healing, illustrating a mind–body connection often ignored in biomedicine. All medical systems use metaphors. Traditional Chinese, Ayurvedic Indian, and Unani[28] medical systems conceptualize health as a state of balanced energies or substances resulting from a harmony between the body, mind, nature, social, and spiritual realms. Disease indicates an imbalance of energies or substances resulting from disharmony among these realms. The metaphors of imbalance/disharmony inform the interventions aimed at restoring health. The body here is not assumed to be the same everywhere, and any commonalities between patients' experiences of a malady are attributed to similarities in body-type or shared constitution and environment.[29]

---

[24] Technologies focused on female biology and pathologies are among the rapidly evolving ones and include reproductive technologies (contraception and *in vitro* fertilization), childbirth technologies (fetal monitors, hormones to induce birth), screening and hormone therapy (Gaines and Davis-Floyd (2004)). This is because the standard universal machine-like human body created by biological reductionism in medicine is male and a female body is found dysfunctional in as much as it deviate from this male "norm." Feminists have long criticized biomedicine for its "patronizing pathologization of the female" (Gaines and Davis-Floyd (2004), 101).

[25] Lock and Nguyen (2010), *op. cit.*

[26] Deborah Lupton (2003). *Medicine as Culture*. London: Sage: 59.

[27] Laurence J. Kirmayer (2004), *op.cit.*, 37.

[28] Greek based Middle Eastern, medicine that spread to South Asia with the spread of Islam.

[29] Lock and Nguyen (2010), *op. cit.*, 60.

In contrast, biomedicine draws on multiple coexisting metaphors, each emerging at a historical junction in the evolution of biomedicine. A mechanistic metaphor is the dominant one and the earliest to develop arising from industrialization's focus on maintaining a healthy workforce. With the development of microbiology and the germ theory of disease, a military metaphor emerged framing the body as the "scene of total war between ruthless invaders [microbes] and determined defenders."[30] The physician is the commander-in-chief whose orders are to be executed by nurses and therapists without questioning. Other metaphors include "the gift of life" for organ donation and "persistent vegetative state" for comatose patients. Winslow sees these individual metaphors as complementary parts of a system of metaphors in healthcare discourse that "work synergistically both to describe and preserve distinct meanings of health care."[31]

In the dominant mechanistic metaphor, the body consists of progressively smaller parts (systems, organs, tissue, cells, genes, and molecules) shielded by the skin from an outside world poised to invade it. These parts, in biomedical thinking, can malfunction and could be examined separately by various specialists, repaired with chemicals, surgery, or radiation, and replaced with mechanical or biological parts. The patient is the object of examination and the site of interventions in isolation from the psycho-socio-spiritual and physical environment that are implicated in affliction.[32] Where other medical systems see imbalance in energies, substances, or social relations, biomedicine attributes disease to invasion of organisms or malfunction of parts. This is why it is more successful in treating acute conditions than in treating chronic conditions like hypertension, type II diabetes, or heart disease where a patient's behavior,

---

[30] Emily Martin (1990). Toward an anthropology of immunology: The body as nation state. *Medical Anthropology Quarterly* 4(4): 410–426.

[31] G. R. Winslow (1996). Minding our language: Metaphors and biomedical ethics, in E. E. Shelp (ed.), *Secular Bioethics in Theological Perspective,* Dordrecht, the Netherlands: Kluwer Academic Publishers.

[32] More humanistic models based on a "bio-psycho-social" approach and "holistic medicine" that see patients more than a biological entity have gained public attention and some traction in biomedicine, but the machine model remains dominant (Gaines and Davis-Floyd (2004)). Unsatisfied patients seek "complementary" medicine alongside biomedical intervention and are creating a market for these "alternative" interventions.

modes of thinking, and social and physical environments are significant contributing factors.[33]

Because biomedicine and its technologies are based on biological and other natural sciences, it sees itself, and is seen as, representing empirical "scientifically" proven facts and presumed to be an unbiased, culturally-neutral system of knowledge and practices. The claim of unquestioned "objectivity" has been challenged by the early 20th century. Ludwig Fleck argued that "phenomena that scientists work with are the products of technologies, practices, and preconditioned ways of seeing and understanding" and the scientist does not stand external to the world under study.[34] Though biomedicine practitioners are taught to believe their craft is science-based, typically evidence that supports established practices and long held assumptions are adopted, while those challenging them are resisted for decades before they are assimilated into medical education and practice; this leads to an "evidence-practice gap."[35] There is new emphasis on "evidence-based medicine" which is driven by a variety of stakeholders.[36] The "subjective" reporting of the patient is separate and only supplementary to the "objective" findings of physical exams and diagnostic technology upon which the classification of a condition is based. The requirement of and reliance on evidence (usually quantitative, measurable, and reproducible) demand the classification of disease and dysfunction be standardized, categorized, and quantified. This implies reliance on "norms" in which real people's bodies often do not fit, and this forces practitioners to choose between limited options into which to fit their diagnosis and interventions.[37]

---

[33] Lock and Nguyen (2010), *op. cit.*

[34] *Ibid.*, 18.

[35] Gaines and Davis-Floyd (2004), *op. cit.*, 97.

[36] It is championed as much by practitioners as by healthcare insurers who, in order to cover the cost, demand proven evidence of the efficacy for diagnostic and therapeutic interventions.

[37] In the US, there are limited diagnoses and only specific interventions for which a practitioner can get paid for a particular diagnosis. This not only frustrates practitioners who struggle to "fit" the findings and intervention into these limited options, but it also contributes to the evidence-practice lag because practitioners are disincentivized to try new interventions that they will not get paid for.

3. The Globalization of Biomedicine

Biomedicine has spread around the world through a formal medical education system that produces physicians trained in its technologies, practices, ways of thinking and knowing, and its conceptualization of the body. It has also spread among ordinary people who, even when they cannot afford its interventions, cannot fully escape its reach as they encounter its influence on traditional practitioners who are affected by its discourses and appropriate its interventions.[38] Biomedicine, however, is not practiced exactly the same everywhere, and it undergoes a process of appropriation or modification. Unlike the case in European countries, medical practice in the United States is dominated by technology and invasive procedures. In the global South, pharmaceutical drugs are accessible without physicians and are taken along with traditional interventions. Biomedicine's dominance has not eliminated other medical systems. Instead, they are used as "alternative" or "complementary" medicine. In this "medical pluralism," the systems borrow from each other. Nevertheless, biomedicine privileges its status as modern and scientific and discounts traditional medicines' epistemology, demanding from practitioners adherence to biomedicine's practice standards if they are to have a place within the official healthcare delivery system.[39,40] Pluralism creates a hybridity of sorts, but not on equal terms. Biomedicine attempts to restrain competing systems, not only by questioning their efficacy, but also by integrating their knowledge, medicines, and interventions by subjecting them to its research and regulations.[41,42]

---

[38] Lock and Nguyen (2010), *op. cit.*

[39] *Ibid.*

[40] For example, traditional midwives are disabused of "nonscientific" beliefs and "professionalized" by retraining, and pharmaceutical companies engage in bioprospecting by harvesting then patenting indigenous medicines as new drugs on the global market which natives cannot afford (Gaines and Davis-Floyd (2004)).

[41] Lock and Nguyen (2010), *op. cit.*; Claire Wendland (2012). Animating bioemedicine's moral order: The crisis of practice in Malawian medical training. *Current Anthropology* 53(6): 755–788.

[42] For example, when Tibetan healers attempt to tap into the global pharmaceutical market, their interventions must pass the scrutiny of randomized trials and when they do, biomedical providers are able to prescribe these medicines and interventions. Yet, US based Tibetan healers would be prosecuted for practicing medicine without license, if they used

Biomedicine has eradicated some diseases, saved lives, and improved people's health. These achievements are not devalued by criticizing biomedicine's shortcomings or failures. Understanding the nature of biomedicine's social construction is not merely to critique its epistemology and call for alternative ones; such understanding and recognition of the various actors involved raises awareness and calls for vigilance about how all this affects people and policies that have local and global impact. Additionally, when a condition is medicalized, the focus shifts to medical intervention rather than assessing the socio-economic and political factors involved.[43] This critique highlights biomedicine's "deterministic logic,"[44] reveals its hidden assumptions, and opens spaces where action for improvement is possible. How an issue is conceptualized is foundational to how, and whether or not, it is addressed. Gaining this understanding and foregrounding these features of biomedicine enlightens the debates and deliberations of practitioners, scholars of religion, and policy makers. A similar exploration of bioethics would enrich the deliberation.

4. Bioethics: The Birth of a Field

The 40-year-old field of bioethics originated from a history of exploitation of research subjects and patients by the "medical–industrial complex."[45] Bioethics is an academic and applied field as well as a cultural phenomenon.[46] Engelhardt contends that bioethics emerged from dramatic cultural shifts (changes in medicine, moral pluralism, rising individualism, and distrust of tradition) in the United States that created a "moral vacuum" and bioethics promised to provide moral guidance and manage

these interventions once they are appropriated by biomedicine (Seth 2009). See Suman Seth (2009). Putting knowledge in its place: Science, colonialism, and the postcolonial. *Postcolonial Studies* 12(4): 373–388.

[43] Peter Conrad and Kristin K. Barker (2010). The social construction of illness: Key insights and policy implications. *Journal of Health and Social Behavior* 51: S67–S79.

[44] *Ibid.*, S76.

[45] Raymond De Vries (2011). The uses and abuses of moral theory in bioethics. *Ethic Theory Moral Practice* 14: 419–430.

[46] Gaines and Davis-Floyd (2004), *op. cit.*, 103.

diversity with a common language.[47] To do so, the divergent voices and substantial information needed for ethical decision-making were distilled into a few principles that serve as a "commensurable unit" which, as Evans put it, provides a common language and singular method for measuring differing features and simplifying decision-making.[48] This concept of commensuration captures the "lure of calculability and predictability" that principlism promises, making it attractive to philosophers and scientists alike.[49]

Though principlism offers potentially contradictory metric scales as its four principles (autonomy, beneficence, nonmaleficence, and justice) are weighed, the "system of commensuration" still applies because these principles offer a method to strip away the density of real life problems and fit the moral dilemma into the metric.[50] Beauchamp argues that the four principles he coformulated are simply "frameworks of general guidelines that condensed morality to its central elements and gave people from diverse fields an easily grasped set of moral standards."[51] Though its simplicity and common language account for the spread of the principlism approach to bioethics, the state accounts for both its birth through the Belmont Report[52] — the outcome of meetings at the behest of the state — and its institutionalization through regulations and funding policies.[53] Critics of principlism see in its simplicity an oversimplification of complex moral issues. David Callahan criticizes its diminished ability to engage and benefit from the "insights of religion, of cultural observation and social

[47] Tristram Engelhardt (2012). Bioethics after Four Decades: Looking to the Future, Portuguese Association of Bioethics. Oporto, Portugal, 16 March 2012.

[48] John H. Evans (2000). A sociological account of the growth of principlism. *Hastings Center Report* 20(5): 31–38.

[49] *Ibid.*, 32.

[50] *Ibid.*

[51] *Ibid.*, 32, 33.

[52] This is a product of the 1979 National Commission for the Protection of Human Subjects of Biomedical and Behavioral Research. The commission summarized its recommendations in the Belmont Report of Ethical Principles and Guidelines for the Protection of Human Subjects of Research which continues to be the reference for all human related research in all fields. Available online via http://www.hhs.gov/ohrp/humansubjects/guidance/belmont.html (retrieved 20 July 2013).

[53] Evans (2000), *op. cit.*

analysis … and of concepts of human dignity and purpose that had a wider scope than mere autonomy."[54]

Bioethics has become synonymous with Georgetown University's principlism in a process that overshadowed the history of the term and the theoretical diversity in the field. Bioethics as a concept was first coined by van Rensselaer Potter at the University of Wisconsin-Madison. Potter, a research oncologist concerned with the very survival of the human species, envisioned bioethics in broader terms with environmental and social dimensions.[55] Bioethics was to bridge the study of science, particularly biology (bio), and humanities, which examines human values (ethics).[56] For Potter, a defining feature of bioethics was "humility with responsibility" that will remind science it has no monopoly on truth nor can it alone answer the complex questions.[57,58] Potter knew that scientific knowledge could be used to help or harm. He thought bioethics could offer the "wisdom to manage dangerous knowledge" where values guide policy deliberation on the effects of emerging scientific facts.[59]

Around the same time, Helleger and colleagues at Georgetown were considering institutionalizing a new discipline that combines science and social science along with religious and secular ethics — a bioethics project. The Georgetown approach to bioethics concerned Potter who saw how it could confirm and maintain the biomedical field's propensity to focus on treatment and ignore prevention and social and environmental causes of illness. Epistemologically, Potter's and Georgetown's approaches differed in that Potter considered bioethics a "search for wisdom," the actionable knowledge that would equip us to arrive at "good judgment"

[54] *Ibid.*, 37.

[55] Warren Thomas Reich (1994). The word "bioethics": Its birth and the legacies of those who shaped it. *Kennedy Institute of Ethics Journal* 4(4): 319–335.

[56] *Ibid.*

[57] As a scientist, Potter valued science's great material progress and physical health contribution, but he questioned its being a source of wisdom because he saw it disconnected from values. This inspired him to envision a multidisciplinary bioethics field that draws on the contributions of science and the wisdom of human values (Reich (1995)). See Warren Thomas Reich (1995). The word "bioethics": The struggle over its earliest meanings. *Kennedy Institute of Ethics Journal* 5(1): 19–34.

[58] Henk ten Have (2012). Potter's notion of bioethics. *Kennedy Institute of Ethics Journal* 22(1): 61.

[59] *Ibid.*, 64.

regarding what makes for "physical, cultural, and philosophical progress toward a valued survival."[60] The Georgetown approach focused on solving moral dilemmas presented by biomedical research and practice using a standardized framework of common moral principles.

With public concerned about safeguarding individuals and communities from abuses in medicine and research, the simplicity of Georgetown's approach in dealing with pressing questions and Potter's concern with more entrenched environmental and social factors marginalized Potter's model, and principlism dominated.[61] Two decades later, however, Potter proposed a "Global Ethics." Global in three senses: it focuses on issues affecting the world, attends to issues of biomedical and environmental concerns, and expands its ethical sources to include all "relevant values, concepts and modes of reasoning and disciplines."[62,63] Potter's global ethics is now reflected in the United Nations' Universal Declaration on Bioethics and Human Rights, which is concerned with health care, the biosphere, future generations, and social justice.[64]

Though principlism is the most common theory, bioethicists draw on a number of moral theories including casuistry and care ethics.[65] This reliance on moral theory and its ability to "solv[e] puzzles" rather than analyze social structures, De Vries argues, is why bioethics theories focus on quick resolutions to ethical dilemmas and not on investigating the underlying causes. Due to this tendency, some sociologists argue that American bioethics suffers from "cultural myopia" that makes it blind to its own socio-cultural roots and resources[66] and the "ethical dilemmas," it adjudicates, further

[60] Reich (1995), *op. cit.*, 21.

[61] *Ibid.*, 19–34.

[62] *Ibid.*, 21.

[63] Helleger, the cofounder of the Georgetown Kennedy Institute for ethics, was also advocating a global ethics (in all three senses) in his own work and was critical of the institute's more narrow approach though he continued to work there. Reich notes that Helleger's global approach drew on conscience and religion in answering the critical question of "what do we think of the significance of the human?" He wanted bioethics that focused more on "the crisis in values than with applying principles to biomedical dilemmas" (Reich (1995), 28).

[64] ten Have (2012), *op. cit.*

[65] De Vries (2011), *op. cit.*

[66] R Fox and J Swazey (1984). Medical morality is not bioethics — medical ethics in China and the United States. *Perspectives in Biology and Medicine Journal* 27(3): 336–360.

conceal that. What is needed, De Vries argues, is the crucial work of "upstream bioethics" that will examine the social causes of these ethical problems. That is precisely the imperative work for Muslim scholars of the text and context. If that is not done, bioethicists (and religious scholars) function as "the emergency department for ethical crisis" that triages the urgent issues without examining and addressing the root causes of these problems.[67]

As biomedicine globalizes, so does principlism. De Vries and Rott use the metaphor of "missionary work" to describe this movement of bioethics from the West to the Global South. Here the gospel ("the good news") is not the Christian message, but "good clinical practice," the Belmont Report, and the Declaration of Helsinki.[68,69] Benefiting from what Christian missionaries had learned — that "indigenization" is more effective than "exportation" — De Vries notes, Western bioethics institutions are bringing bioethicists from the developing world for training. These "native" bioethicists acquire "the language and logic of Western bioethics" then go back home to "spread the gospel" in linguistically and culturally relevant ways.[70] Both religious missionary and bioethics work have the "noble intent" of sharing what proponents see as the benefit of advancement, but good intentions do not guarantee good results and could instead cause harm. In these training programs, the power differential results in a unidirectional flow of wisdom and values from the West to the rest. Instead of exploring local wisdom and putting it in dialogue with Western bioethics, the participants become competent in bioethics' principles, international regulations, and how to ensure proposed research adheres to these standards.[71] Training participants learn different ethical theories and apply them to issues like reproductive technologies and genetics that are of little relevance to their local situations. The absence of dialogue and

---

[67] De Vries (2011), *op. cit.*, 425.

[68] The Declaration of Helsinki is a set of ethical guidelines developed by the World Medical Association in 1964 and has since had several amendments. The declaration outlines ethical principles to which those conducting medical research must adhere. For details, http://www.who.int/bulletin/archives/79(4)373.pdf (retrieved 20 July 2013).

[69] De Vries (2011), *op. cit.*, 426.

[70] *Ibid.*

[71] *Ibid.*, 419–430.

mutual enrichment impoverishes bioethics both in the global South and in the West. The dialogue could move us away from principlism's contested claims of universality based on a "common morality" which De Vries argues is inappropriate and results in focusing too much on moral theory and not enough on the necessary work of moral philosophy.[72] De Vries' proposed approach would draw on "distributive morality" instead of "common morality." Consequently, wholesale adoption or appropriation of principlism would be replaced by a dialogue between the Western ethical tradition and local moral traditions in a collaborative quest for and proposal of ethical guidelines that are grounded in the local moral and social world.[73]

Bioethics and its dominant theory of principlism are criticized by diverse Western groups who challenge its purported universality and who argue it erases their specificity. These critics contend that they have a particular epistemic position that is shaped by their respective histories and concerns as gender, sexuality, race, and religious-based groups. Each group has contributions to make to bioethics based on its own epistemic vantage point that enables particular insights. Garcia, for example, proposes that an African-American medical ethics perspective would be "anti-majoritarian and anti-utilitarian, anti-situationalist, and distrustful of an 'ethics of trust'."[74] It is an approach "free from the bonds of scientism" and "open to insights from religious faith," one in which the patient is ultimately the decision maker but the role of family and community are recognized without being "romanticiz[ed]."[75] Garcia is not advocating a distinct African-American bioethics but argues for an ethics that is "faithful, informed by, and seriously responsive to important forms of experience characteristic of African-Americans, that is, informed and responsive in its topics (foci), methods, and moral features, or content."[76]

---

[72] *Ibid.*
[73] *Ibid.*
[74] Jorge Garcia (2007). Revising African American perspectives on biomedical ethics: Distinctiveness and other questions, in Edmund Pellegrino and Lawrence Prograis (eds.) *African American Bioethics*: *Culture*, *Race*, *and Identity*, Washington, DC: Georgetown University Press: 3.
[75] Garcia (2007), *op. cit.*, 2.
[76] Garcia (2007), *op. cit.*, 3.

These experiences have been shaped by centuries of oppression, disenfranchisement, and discrimination embodied in lasting health problems (such as diabetes, hypertension, and obesity) that disproportionately affect African-Americans.[77]

Bioethicists speaking from a religious epistemic stance also argue for the value and specificity of their contribution. Engelhardt, a physician bioethicist, contends that bioethics is based on "secular fundamentalism" that came to fill the moral vacuum left by the Enlightenment project and accomplished what the Enlightenment could not, usurping religion's authority to define "good" and "right" and bestowing it on philosophers and ethicists.[78] Principlism's claim to universality is that it derived the four principles from a common morality. These principles are not exhaustive of the shared values and can be made specific by adding context-relevant moral content.[79] Engelhardt, who works both on secular and Christian bioethics, challenges this universalist claim arguing that once culture-specific contents are added, these moral principles diverge too far to be common and bioethics remains challenged by moral plurality.[80] He distinguishes Christian bioethics for its "understand[ing] that the impersonal set of moral principles and goals in secular morality gives a distorted account of the moral life" that is focused on relationship with God.[81]

Religiously-based values persist even in the West and continue to inform medical ethical decision-making[82] because of the existential and

[77] Studies have shown that the prevalence of the low birth weight of African-American children regardless of socio-economic status of the mothers is actually due to adaptive changes in their genes due to the history of oppression and what Nancy Krieger called "biologic expressions of race relations" (Lock and Nguyen (2010), 99).

[78] Judah Goldberg and Alan Jotkowitz (2012). In defense of religious bioethics. *The American Journal of Bioethics* 12(12): 32.

[79] T. Beauchamp and J. Childress (2008). *The Principles of Biomedical Ethics*, 6th edn. New York: Oxford University Press.

[80] Tristram H. Engelhardt (2009). Moral pluralism, the crisis of secular bioethics, and the divisive character of christian bioethics: Taking the culture wars seriously. *Christian Bioethics* 15(3): 234–253.

[81] *Ibid.*, 234.

[82] Social scientists and psychologists have found that, when grappling with these weighty issues, people rely on moral intuition and religious values and not on the calculations of rational secular ethics because questions of meaning are not always answerable by mere deductive reasoning (Goldberg and Jotkowitz (2012), 32).

metaphysical nature of the issues with which bioethics grapples. These issues are not merely about resolving conflicts about distribution of social goods.[83] Advocates of Christian or Jewish bioethics are not arguing for discarding secular bioethics, but like feminists and racial minorities, they are arguing for "epistemological pluralism, in which deductive reasoning is but one of many roads to ethical and moral knowledge. Direct intuition, collective deliberation, and even received tradition — whether rooted in theology or in non-religious culture — are all alternate, and complementary, pathways."[84] This, they posit, recalls bioethics' roots; after all, its founding fathers (Joseph Fletcher, Paul Ramsey, Immanuel Jakobovits, and Richard McCormick) were writing from their respective religious epistemic stances. Furthermore, if bioethics can accommodate its disparate ethical theoretical perspectives, why should religious ones not be part of the sources of bioethics?[85,86]

5. Biomedicine and the Urgent Existential Questions

With mechanical device implantation, organ transplantation, genetic manipulation, and potent pharmaceuticals, medical technology has blurred the boundaries between self and other, life and death, and nation-states have shattered barriers considered natural or cultural and have raised fundamental questions about what is normal or not, what is just and moral and what is not, and what is human or not.[87] Two issues, organ transplantation and human enhancement, exemplify the great potential of biotechnology and the existential ethical questions it raises.

5.1. *"Brain Death" and What Makes us Human*

The definition and meaning of death and what happens after death are ontological and epistemological issues deeply embedded in a socio-cultural

[83] Goldberg and Jotkowitz (2012), *op. cit.*, 32.
[84] *Ibid.*
[85] Daniel Callahan (1990). Religion and the secularization of bioethics. Special supplement: "Theology, Religious Traditions and bioethics. *Hastings Center Report* 20(4): 2–4.
[86] Goldberg and Jotkowitz (2012), *op. cit.*
[87] Lock and Nguyen (2010), *op. cit.*

milieu. Biomedical advances have brought unforeseen social and legal challenges. For example, biotechnology that sustains artificial breathing and/or circulation raises the question of when and if it is ethical to withdraw it, and at which point can death be declared and organs procured? Only a fraction of people with failing organs undergo organ transplantation. The gap between supply and demand necessitated a new and problematic definition of death as "Brain Death." Countries differ on whether the higher brain, brainstem, or whole brain death defines death. In the United States, the definition is "the irreversible cessation of all functions of the entire brain, including the brain stem" (National Conference of Commissioners on Uniform State Laws 1981),[88] and 30 years later the debates are unabated.

Central to the arguments of those in support of "brain death" criteria are two interconnected ideas. One is the understanding that a human being is a person because of the capacity for conscious experience which is irreversibly lost when the brain is catastrophically damaged.[89–91] The other is that the brain serves an integrative role without which a single being ceases to be and becomes a collection of organs. Proponents of brain death argue that the person is dead, but the mechanical assistance to the heart and lungs gives a false impression of life. However, once the mechanical devices are disconnected, the cardiopulmonary function will cease and death will be apparent to all. The assumption is that the organs of such an individual would go to waste if not procured in time and, in light of the number of people on waiting lists, that would be unethical. Some even argue for a preliminary diagnosis of "imminent brain death" for patients

[88] National Conference of Commissioners on Uniform State Laws (1981). *The Uniform Determination of Death Act 1981*. Available online via http://lchc.ucsd.edu/cogn_150/Readings/death_act.pdf (retrieved 6 July 2013).

[89] Dr. David L. Perry (2001). *Ethics and Personhood: Some Issues in Contemporary Neurological Science and Technology*." Avaliable online via http://www.scu.edu/ethics/publications/submitted/Perry/personhood.html (retrieved 6 July 2013).

[90] Robert Truog and Franklin G. Miller (2008). The dead donor rule and organ transplantation. *The New England Journal of Medicine* 359(7): 674–675.

[91] Alan D. Shewmon (2001). The Brain and somatic integration: Insights into the standard biological rationale for equating 'brain death' with death. *Journal of Medicine and Philosophy* 26(5): 457–478.

who have sustained "irreversible catastrophic brain damage of a known origin" so they are recognized early as potential organ donors.[92,93]

Physicians and bioethicists critical of brain death argue that the definition is based on a misunderstanding of death as an event and not a process.[94] The tests of the irreversibility of function, in fact, cannot guarantee this irreversibility; therefore, the definition fails to meet its own requirement. In other words, "'brain death' is not even 'brain death'."[95,96] Shewmon, a pediatric neurologist, challenges the assumption that the brain performs the integrative function for the whole body, arguing that somatic integration is not locatable in one "critical" part. Instead, it is a "holistic phenomenon involving mutual interaction of all the parts"; therefore, "the body without brain function is surely very sick and disabled, but not dead."[97]

These findings have made for very lively debates in bioethics, philosophy, and medical publications. Yet they have not had any practical, legal, or clinical impact and have not reached the public, leading Truog to conclude that "Brain death [is] too flawed to endure, [but] too ingrained to abandon."[98] To resolve this impasse, he proposed a change in the "dead

---

[92] Y. J. de Groot, Jan Bakker, Eelco F. M. Wijdicks and Erwin J. O. Kompanje (2011). Imminent Brain death and brain death are not the same: Reply to serheijde and Rady. *Intensive Care Medicine* 37(1): 174.

[93] De Groot *et al.* argue that this is not an early declaration of death, but "a tool for early recognition of a potential organ donor" (2010, 174).

[94] See Amir Halevy (2001). Beyond brain death? *Journal of Medicine and Philosophy* 26(5): 493–501; Mohamed Rady and Joseph L. Verheijde (2009). Islam and end-of-life organ donation. Asking the Right Questions. *Saudi Medical Journal* 30(7): 882–886; and Alan D. Shewmon (2009). Brain death: Can it be resuscitated? *Hastings Center Report.* 39(2): 18–24.

[95] Critics argue this irreversibility is contradicted by the fact that the procured heart of an individual considered "brain dead" because of suffering an irreversible cardiac arrest has "successfully functioned in the chest of another" (Truog and Miller (2008), 674). This reversi-bility might even occur during the procurement surgery when the artificial circulation intended to preserve organs may resuscitate vital signs of this "brain dead" donor (Rady and Verheijde (2012)). See Truog and Miller (2008), *op. cit.*; Mohamed Y. Rady and Joseph L. Verheijde (2012). Brain-dead patients are not cadavers: The need to revise the definition of death in Muslim communities. *Healthcare Ethics Committee Forum* 25: 25–45.

[96] Halevy (2001), *op. cit.*, 498.

[97] Shewmon (2009), *op. cit.*, 473.

[98] R. D. Truog (2007). Brain death — too flawed to endure, too ingrained to abandon. *Journal of Law, Medicine and Ethics*, 273. Also available online via http://www.ncbi.nlm.nih.gov/pubmed/17518853 (retrieved 1 July 2013).

donor rule" and the "informed consent," which does not fully disclose the controversy around brain death. There have been calls for a moratorium on the practice of cardiocirculatory death diagnosis in the context of organ procurement as well until full public disclosure and a society-wide debate have taken place.[99–101] Shewmon even suggested a footnote in the consent form warning individuals that they may not be dead when their organs are procured.[102,103]

This controversy reveals deep-rooted biological reductionism and underlying body–mind dualism assumptions that raise ontological and epistemological questions. There are those who locate the soul in the brain and brain death is the loss of the "vital and unifying principle ('substantial form') of the body." Others also locate the soul in the brain but see brain death as the "loss-of-personhood," the "thinking substance, in principle dissociable from an animal body the vitality of which is essentially mechanistic."[104] In both positions, the separation and opposition of the body and brain persist. This is because modernity changed meanings of life and death, making them into legal and medical matters rather than metaphysical ones. This secularization of life and death, argued some intellectuals, relegated the divine to the private sphere and replaced the "soul" with a rational "self" — the person — that is lost with "brain death" leaving behind collections of organs that could be used by someone else.[105]

What are we to make of this human being who is in a liminal state of "dead" mind but living body? This is not only confusing for ordinary people who see no visible signs of death (the body is warm, breathing, urinating, and growing) but also to medical practitioners whose biomedical

---

[99] A. Joffe, J. Carcillo, N. Anton, A. deCaen, Y. Han, M. Bell *et al.* (2011). Donation after cardiocirculatory death: A call for a moratorium pending full public disclosure and fully informed consent. *Philosophy, Ethics, and Humanities in Medicine* 6(17): 6–17.

[100] Truog and Miller (2008), *op. cit.*

[101] Rady and Verheijde (2012), *op. cit.*, 25–45.

[102] Shewmon (2009), *op. cit.*

[103] The footnote would say, "Warning: It remains controversial whether you will actually be dead at the time of removal of your organs. This depends on the conceptual validity of 'position two' in the analysis of the determination of death conducted by the President's Council on Bioethics. You should study it carefully and decide for yourself before signing an organ donor card" (Shewmon (2009), 18).

[104] Shewmon (2001), *op. cit.*, 475.

[105] Lock and Nguyen (2010), *op. cit.*

training tells them the person is dead but whose intuition tells them otherwise.[106] The general public is unaware of these doubts and debates. The "gift of life" language of organ donation conceals "the significant scientific and commercial interests that are at play," and the language of rights that dominates bioethics obscures the politics of commerce and corruption and the glaring inequalities that make poor people's bodies serve as spare parts for the well-to-do through medical tourism.[107]

5.2. *Biological "Enhancement" and Transgenetics*

Genetic manipulations of plants and animals had promised disease and decay resistant nutritious food that would solve world hunger. Instead, it has only enriched agribusiness, and we are confronted with unknown risks to humans and non-humans alike. New trans-species genetic manipulations that turn animals and plants into factories for commercial products and pharmaceuticals are emerging.[108] Millions of animal neural cells have been implanted in the brains of patients in clinical trials to address neural dysfunctions.[109] Studies of genetically modified pigs that could produce organs for humans are seen as very promising in addressing the organ donation shortage.[110] These "advances" are great scientific feats that raise critical ethical questions, most importantly about the essence of humans, plants, and animals.

[106] One experienced intensive care physician said that he lies awake wondering if the individual he declared brain dead "was that person really dead? It is irreversible — I know that, and the clinical tests are infallible. My rational mind is sure, but some nagging, irrational doubt seeps in." (Lock and Nguyen (2010), 240).
[107] Lock and Nguyen (2010), *op. cit.*, 222.
[108] The insertion of human gene into goats or chickens to produce antithrombin (blocks blood clot formation) in their milk or eggs and adding a spider gene into goat to produce silk-making proteins are examples of transgenic experiments that are hailed as great scientific advances. R. R. Moura, L. M. Melo, and V. J. D. F. Freitas, (2011). Production of recombinant proteins in milk of transgenic and non-transgenic goats. *Brazilian Archives of Biology and Technology* 54(5): 927–938. A. Lazaris, S. Arcidiacono, Y. Huang, J. F. Zhou, F. Duguay, N. Chretien, and C. N. Karatzas, (2002). Spider silk fibers spun from soluble recombinant silk produced in mammalian cells. *Science* 295(5554): 472–476.
[109] PBS, Frontline (2001). *Organ Farm: Four Patients and Their Clinical Trials*. Available online via http://www.pbs.org/wgbh/pages/frontline/shows/organfarm/ (retrieved 1 July 2013).
[110] *Ibid.*

The possibility of selecting the sex of a child and removing "defective" or "disease causing" genes seemed fictional a few years ago. However, the first is now a reality, the latter is in the works, and both raise ethical questions. Further, physical enhancement through cosmetic surgery, growth hormones, performance enhancing drugs, and cognitive (appetite, mood, concentration, and memory) enhancement through pharmaceuticals are now routine though only accessible to those with material means. These "enchantments" are but the first steps towards making "better people" and what some have called trans-humanism or even post-humanism, where surgery, genetic engineering, and ever smaller technologies inserted into the body ostensibly defy aging and disease and make much "improved" (stronger, smarter, faster, and better communicator) humans.[111,112]

The assumption driving biomedical technology and practice is that genetic determinism fully accounts for health, illness, and who we become. But research in genetics itself (epigenetics) is challenging that paradigm and demonstrating the multiple possibilities for non-DNA based mechanisms at play. But epigenetics too will not be able to answer fully what is human nature or what makes humans who they are.[113] Religious fundamentalism justifiably invokes great fears, but there is also what Elshtain called a "scientific fundamentalism" that reduces who a person is or becomes to their DNA and sees the body as the site of a project of perpetual enhancement.[114] But to what ends, and are there limits?[115]

---

[111] Paul Miller and James Wilsdon (eds.) (2006). *Better Humans? The Politics of Human Enhancement and Life Extension*. Demos. Available online via http://www.nanopodium.nl/CieMDN/content/Demos_Better_humans.pdf (retrieved 1 July 2013).

[112] Michael Hauskeller (2013). Cognitive Enhancement — To What End? *Cognitive Enhancement Trends in Augmentation of Human Performance* 1: 113–123.

[113] Lock and Nguyen (2010), *op. cit.*

[114] Jean Bethke Elshtain (2008). Why science cannot stand alone. *Theoretical Medicine and Bioethics* 29: 161–169.

[115] With all the potential (negative or positive) of bioengineering technology, Watson codiscoverer of DNA and Nobel prize winner, predicted a conflict between those who hail these advances and those who question them on religious or ethical grounds and wondered why would we not make better humans if we can (Lock and Nguyen (2010)). He argued that if early genetic intervention spares individuals and families the "cruel fates" of the "genetic dice" then to do nothing would be indecent because "if we don't play God, who will?" (Watson (1995), 197). See Lock and Nguyen 2010, *op. cit.*; James Watson (1995).

Ethical issues abound. Beyond the health hazards inherent in crossing species boundaries, do other species have rights to exist without being tampered with to "benefit" humans? How do these other beings, now embodied in the self, affect one's sense of self?[116] If you insert parts of other beings (human or otherwise), does that affect "human nature?" Science cannot answer these questions. They are more suited to being tackled by philosophy and religions, but only if they are informed and critically engaged.

6. Muslim Contributions

Muslim scholars of the text and medical practitioners enter the discussion on biomedicine and its technologies in the context of questions about reproductive technologies, cloning, withdrawing care, and organ donation. The specifics of each issue are outlined and scholars of the text are confronted with conflicting medical opinions reflecting debates on these issues within medicine. The two groups deliberate to arrive at consensus on an "Islamic position." The physicians not only offer medical facts but they also engage in interpreting the religious texts from their perspectives using current scientific facts. Physicians assertively defend their interpretations, at times pressuring scholars of the text to adopt certain positions[117]

Values from a Chicago upbringing. DNA: The double Helix perspective and Prospective at 40 Years. *Annals of the New York Academy of Science* 758: 194–197.

[116] Studies have shown the psychological issues that organ recipients of heart transplants have apart from the persistent concerns about their health and survival there were also concerns about acquiring habits, emotions, and thoughts of the donor. Often these reports are dismissed as side-effect from medication or the work of active imagination and "magical" beliefs as Inspector and David (2004) called it. Others argue the medication or coincidence "are likely insufficient to explain the findings. The plausibility of cellular memory, possibly systemic memory, is suggested" (Pearsall *et al.* (2000), 65). See Y. Inspector, I. Kutz and D. David (2004). Another person's heart: Magical and rational thinking in the psychological adaptation to heart transplantation. *Israel Journal of Psychiatry and Related Sciences* 41(3): 161–173; Paul Pearsall, Gary E. R. Schwartz and Linda G. S. Russek (2000). Changes in heart transplant recipients that parallel the personalities of their donors. *Integrative Medicine* 2(2): 65.

[117] Mohammed Ghaly (2012). The beginning of human life: Islamic bioethical perspectives. *Zygon: Journal of Religion and Science* 47(1): 175–213.

or they contest the conclusions of collective *fatāwā* councils[118] or challenge classic understandings about the nature of human beings and call for an updated "completely naturalistic account of human personhood" that is more consistent with biomedicine.[119] Muslim physicians directly accessing the religious texts and *fatāwā* councils' conclusions are shaping an emerging "Islamic bioethics" discourse.

While medical practitioners presumably speak objectively from a "scientific" position, religious scholars, past and present, are frequently faulted for lacking the scientific facts and interpreting texts from a particular epistemic position influenced by their gender, socio-cultural milieu, and school of thought. However, Muslim medical practitioners, their religious adherence notwithstanding, also speak from particular epistemic positions informed, among other things, by the ontological and epistemological systems of biomedicine and science. They interpret religious discourse and debate issues informed by biomedicine's metaphors and conceptualization of the body and mind, illness, and nature and by the triumphant narrative of science, technology, and progress.

Neither physicians nor textual scholars can claim a neutral and "objective" stance; each knows and speaks from a particular epistemic vantage point. If they only deliberate to answer the urgent ethical dilemmas, they become "staff" solving moral puzzles in what De Vries called "the emergency department for ethical crisis."[120] What is needed, instead, is a moral philosophy and the deliberation upstream about the underlying causes of these dilemmas, the unspoken assumption of biomedicine, and the existential questions about what makes us human beings: What is our relationship with nature? What we can know? What ought we to do? What we can hope for? These are not questions that can be "scientifically" answered but ones that can be grappled with collaboratively utilizing diverse ways of knowing including intuitive and revealed knowledge.

Though principlism dominates the bioethics theoretical landscape, it is but a procedural ethics, a rubric for answering pressing clinical and research ethical dilemmas. In answering these questions, however, bioethicists

[118] Rady and Verheijde (2012), *op. cit.*

[119] Omar Sultan Haque (2008). Brain death and its entanglements: A redefinition of personhood for islamic ethics. *Journal of Religious Ethics* 36(1): 13.

[120] De Vries (2011), *op. cit.*

confront existential issues about the nature of human beings and the meaning of life and death. They try not only to understand what it is but also to offer answers and guidance on what ought to be. These existential matters, however, are the domain of religion and philosophy. To be relevant, experts in religion and philosophy must not only be conversant about the current biomedical technology and debates, but also about futuristic possibilities and how those will impact individuals, societies, and nature. This way, scholars not only respond to the actual problems but explore potential ones that are on the verge of being actual and see the spaces between the actual and the potential so as to chart a better future. Dismissing future possibilities as not-worth-the-time conjectures will have serious consequences.

An honest, social debate that seeks the insights of biomedical practitioners, scientists, social scientists, philosophers, religion scholars, and ordinary people about biomedical research and practice, about the psycho-social-spiritual and politico-economic and environmental aspects of health and well-being is imperative. Through it all, we have to consider the historical context that gave rise to biomedicine and its technologies and to bioethics; we need to critically examine their current developments, interests, successes, and failures, and we have to assess the risk and opportunities they present for current and future generations. For Muslims to criticize biomedicine and science as "Godless Western" systems and tools of imperialist ambitions is to deny something of oneself; after all, modern medicine and science stand on the shoulders of the Islamic civilization. Nonetheless, to uncritically embrace these fields on the basis of these past and present contributions or on the premise that Islam "has no problem with reasoning and science" is to assume medicine and science today are those of *Ibn Sina* and *Ibn Rushd* and to abdicate our responsibility. Muslim contributions to ethics are lacking and urgently needed. A starting point is to interrogate all that lies hidden in the space between "bio" and "ethics."

A *Maqāṣid*-Based Approach for New Independent Legal Reasoning (*Ijtihād*)

Jasser Auda

Abstract: This chapter explores how the higher objectives of Sharia (*maqāṣid al-sharī'ah*) could contribute to the application of the Sharia in today's reality, utilizing a few illustrative examples in the area of bioethics. The soundness of Sharia's application and related policies is subject to the degree of universality and flexibility of the Islamic rulings with changing circumstances, discussed from various viewpoints in this chapter. After a survey of the system of values that the higher objectives of Sharia represent, two reasoning (*ijtihād*) methods are explored: (i) differentiating between scriptural texts that are means (*wasā'il*) to higher ends and those that are ends (*ahdāf*) in their own right, and (ii) preferring a multidimensional understanding for the conciliation of opposing juridical evidences, instead of reductionist methods such as abrogation (*naskh*) and giving preference to one opinion over another (*tarjīh*). A number of examples are provided throughout the chapter in order to explain the impact of the proposed methods on contemporary Islamic rulings.

1. Introduction

Applications of the Sharia in any contemporary context or profession require a methodology that represents the Sharia's universality and flexibility with changing circumstances. Without the components of the Sharia that are pertinent to accommodating various environments and cultures, or in other words the dimensions of history and geography of the people, any such application or policy would be counter-productive. This is because it would jeopardize the very well known and absolute system of values and principles of the Sharia itself, e.g. the principles of justice, wisdom, mercy, and common good.

Shamsuddin bin Al-Qayyim (d. 748 AH/1347 CE) summarized these principles with the following strong words:

> Sharia is all about wisdom and achieving people's welfare in this life and the afterlife. It is all about justice, mercy, wisdom, and good. Thus, any ruling that replaces justice with injustice, mercy with its opposite, common good with mischief, or wisdom with nonsense, is a ruling that does not belong to the Sharia, even if it is claimed to be so according to some interpretation.[1]

The higher objectives of Sharia serve as a system of values that could contribute to a desired and sound application of the Sharia. After a section that introduces the system of values and the various theories of *maqāṣid*, this chapter suggests — in three consecutive sections — that it is necessary to determine the following:

(a) Whether a proposed ruling of the Sharia is an absolute and fixed end in its own right, or whether it is in itself a means to an end and thus subject to changing with changing circumstances. This method is expressed in the following maxim: Differentiating between changing means and absolute ends.

(b) Whether the Qur'anic verse or *hadith* under consideration should be understood with another verse(s) or *hadith*(s), all in a unified context,

---

[1] Shamsuddin, Ibn Al-Qayyim (1973). *I'lām al-muwaqqi'īn* (annotated by Taha Saad) vol. 1. Beirut: Dar Al-Jeel: 333.

or whether there is no "opposing evidence" that exists and requires such consideration. This method is expressed in the following maxim: Reconciling "opposing evidences" is better than ignoring some of them.

First, however, this next section will introduce *maqāṣid al-sharīʿah* as a system of values that has several theories, classifications, and viewpoints.

2. The Higher Objectives of Sharia as a System of Values

Maqāṣid al-sharīʿah are the objectives/purposes/intents/ends/principles behind the Islamic rulings,[2] which found expression in the Islamic philosophy/theory/fundamentals of law in various ways, such as public interests (*al-maṣāliḥ al-ʾāmmah*)[3]; "unrestricted interests" (*al-maṣāliḥ al-mursalah*)[4]; the avoidance of mischief (*darʾ al-mafsadah*)[5]; the wisdom behind the scripts (*al-ḥikmah*)[6]; the appropriateness of the juridical analogy (*munāsabat al-qiyās*)[7]; the basis behind juridical preference (*aṣl al-istiḥsān*)[8]; the basis behind the presumption of continuity principle (*aṣl al-istiṣḥāb*)[9]; and a large number of other tools for independent legal reasoning (*ijtihād*).

Recently, a large number of researchers from various backgrounds attempted to explore the theory and application of the higher objectives of

---

[2] Mohamed al-Tahir Ibn ʿAshur (1997). *Maqāṣid al-sharīʿah al-Islāmīyah* (annotated by Mohamed Al-Tahir Al-Mesawi). Kuala Lumpur: Al-Fajr: 183.

[3] Abdul-Malik Al-Juwayni (1400 AH). *Al-burhān fī uṣūl al-fiqh* (annotated by Abdul-Azim al-Deeb). Qatar: Wazarat al-Shu'un al-Diniyah: 183.

[4] Abu Hamid Al-Ghazali (1413 AH). *Al-mustaṣfá fī ʿilm al-uṣūl* (annotated by Mohammed Abdul-Salam Abdul Shafi). vol. 1: Beirut: Dar al-Kutub al-'ilmiyah: 172.

[5] Shihabuddin Al-Qarafi (1994). vol. 5: *Al-dhakhīrah*. Beirut: Dar al-Arab: 478.

[6] Ali Al-Amidi (1404 AH). *Al-iḥkām fī uṣūl al-aḥkām*. vol. 5: Beirut: Dar al-Kitab al-Arabi: 391.

[7] Abdullah Ibn Qudama (1399 AH). *Rawḍat al-nāẓir wa-jannat al-manāẓir* (annotated by Abdul Aziz Abdul Rahman Alsaeed). vol. 3: Riyadh: Muhammed bin Saud University: 42.

[8] Muhammad Al-Sarakhsi (n.d.). *Uṣūl al-Sarakhsī*. vol. 9: Beirut: Dar Alma'rifa: 205.

[9] al-Izz Ibn Abdul-Salam (n.d.). *Qawāʿid al-aḥkām fī maṣāliḥ al-anām*. vol. 1: Beirut: Dar al-Nashr: 23.

Sharia in various fields that belong not only to Islamic jurisprudence but also to the social sciences and humanities.[10]

Purposes or higher objectives (*maqāṣid*) of Islamic law are themselves classified in various ways, according to a number of dimensions. The following are some of these dimensions:

(i) Levels of necessity, which is the traditional classification.
(ii) Scope of the rulings aiming to achieve the purposes.
(iii) Scope of people included in the purposes.
(iv) Level of universality of the purposes.

Traditional classifications of the higher objectives divide them into three "levels of necessity," which are necessities (*ḍarūrīyāt*), needs (*ḥājīyāt*), and luxuries (*taḥsīnīyāt*). Necessities are further classified into what "preserves one's religion, life, wealth, intellect, and offspring." Some jurists added "the preservation of honor" to the above five widely popular necessities. These necessities were considered essential matters for human life itself. There is also a general agreement that the preservation of these necessities is the "objective behind any revealed law," not just Islamic law.

Purposes at the level of needs are less essential for human life. Examples are marriage, trade, and means of transportation. Islam encourages and regulates these needs. However, the lack of any of these needs is not a matter of life and death, especially on an individual basis.

Purposes at the level of luxuries are "beautifying purposes," such as using perfume, wearing stylish clothing, and living in beautiful homes. These are things that Islam encourages, but Islam also asserts that they should take a lower priority in one's life.

The levels in the hierarchy are overlapping and interrelated, as noted by Imam Al-Shatibi (who will be introduced shortly). In addition, each level should serve the level(s) below. Furthermore, the general lack of one item from a certain level moves it to the level above. For example, the decline of trade on a global level during the time of global economic crises

---

[10] Mohammad Kamal Imam (2010). *Al-dalīl al-irshādī ilá maqāṣid al-sharīʻah al-Islāmīyah* (6 vols). London: al-Maqasid Research Centre.

moves "trade" from a "need" into a "life necessity," and so on. This is why some jurists preferred to perceive necessities in terms of "overlapping circles" rather than a strict hierarchy (see Figure 1 below).

Modern scholarship introduced new conceptions and classifications of the higher objectives by giving consideration to new dimensions. First, considering the scope of rulings they cover, contemporary classifications divide *maqāṣid* into three levels[11]:

(i) General higher objectives: These higher objectives are observed throughout the entire body of Islamic law, such as the necessities and needs mentioned above and newly proposed higher objectives, such as "justice" and "facilitation."
(ii) Specific higher objectives: These higher objectives are observed throughout a certain "chapter" of Islamic law, such as the welfare of children in family law, deterring criminals in criminal law, and preventing monopoly in financial transactions law.
(iii) Partial higher objectives: These higher objectives are the "intents" behind specific scripts or rulings, such as the intent of discovering the truth in seeking a certain number of witnesses in certain court cases, the intent of alleviating difficulty in allowing an ill and fasting person to break his/her fasting, and the intent of feeding the poor in banning Muslims from hoarding meat during Eid/festival days.

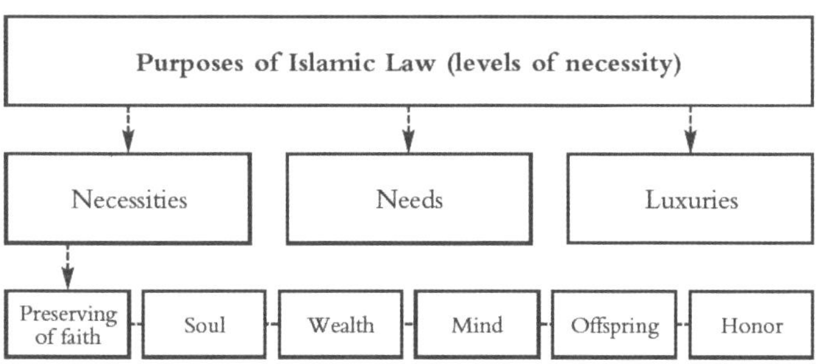

Figure 1. The classification of higher objectives based on their levels of necessity.

[11] Nu'man Jughaym (2002). *Ṭuruq al-kashf 'an maqāṣid al-shar'*. Malaysia: Dar al-Nafa'is: 26–35.

Moreover, the notion of higher objectives has been expanded to include a wider scope of people — the community, nation, or humanity in general. Ibn 'Ashur (also to be introduced shortly), for example, gave higher objectives that are concerned with the "nation" (*ummah*) priority over higher objectives that are concerned with individuals. Rashid Rida, as a second example, included "reform" and "women's rights" in his theory of higher objectives. Yusuf Al-Qaradawi, a third example, included "human dignity and rights" in his theory of the higher objectives. The above expansions of the scope of higher objectives allow them to respond to global issues and concerns and to evolve from "wisdoms behind the rulings" to systems of values and practical plans for reform and renewal.

Contemporary scholarship has also introduced new universal higher objectives that were directly induced from the scripts, rather than from the body of *fiqh* (Islamic law) literature in the schools of Islamic law. This approach, significantly, allowed the higher objectives to overcome the historicity of Islamic law edicts and represent the scripts' higher values and principles. Detailed rulings would, in turn, stem from these universal principles. The following are examples of these new universal higher objectives:

(i) Rashid Ṛida (d. 1935 CE) surveyed the Qur'an to identify its higher objectives, which included "reform of the pillars of faith, and spreading awareness that Islam is the religion of pure natural disposition, reason, knowledge, wisdom, proof, freedom, independence, social, political, economic reform, and women's rights."[12]

(ii) Al-Tahir Ibn 'Ashur (d. 1907 CE) proposed that the universal higher objective of Sharia is to maintain orderliness, equality, freedom, facilitation, and the preservation of pure natural disposition (*fiṭrah*).[13] It is to be noted that the purpose of "freedom" (*ḥurrīyah*), which was proposed by Ibn 'Ashur and several other contemporary scholars, is different from the purpose of "freedom" ('*itq*), which was mentioned by jurists such as Al-Siwasi.[14] '*Itq* is freedom from slavery, not

[12] Mohammad Rashid Rida (n.d.). *Al-waḥī al-Muḥammadī: thubūt al-nubūwah bi-al-Qur'ān*. Cairo: Mu'asasat Izziddin: 100.
[13] Ibn 'Ashur, 1997, *op.cit.*, 183.
[14] Kamaluddin Al-Siwasi (n.d.). *Sharḥ fatḥ al-qadīr*. vol. 4: Beirut: Dar al-Fikr: 513.

"freedom" in the contemporary sense. "Will" (*mashī'ah*), however, is a well-known Islamic term that bears a number of similarities with current conceptions of "freedom" and "free will." For example, "freedom of belief" is expressed in the Qur'an as the "will to believe or disbelieve" (Qur'an 18:29). In terms of terminology, "freedom" (*ḥurrīyah*) is a "newly-coined" purpose in the literature of Islamic law. Ibn 'Ashur, interestingly, accredited his usage of the term *ḥurrīyah* to "literature of the French revolution, which were translated from French to Arabic in the 19th century CE,"[15] even though he elaborated on an Islamic perspective on freedom of thought, belief, expression, and action in the *mashī'ah* sense.[16]

(iii) Muhammad Al-Ghazali (d. 1996 CE) called for "learning lessons from the previous 14 centuries of Islamic history" and therefore included "justice and freedom" as part of the higher objectives at the level of necessities.[17] Al-Ghazali's prime contribution to the knowledge of higher objectives was his critique on the literalist tendencies that many of today's scholars have.[18] A careful look at the contributions of Muhammad Al-Ghazali shows that there were underlying higher objectives on which he based his opinions, such as equality and justice, and on which he based all his famous new opinions in the area of women under Islamic law and other areas.

(iv) Yusuf Al-Qaradawi (1926 CE–) also surveyed the Qur'an and concluded the following universal higher objectives: preserving true faith, maintaining human dignity and rights, calling people to worship God, purifying the soul, restoring moral values, building good families, treating women fairly, building a strong Islamic nation, and calling for a cooperative world. However, Al-Qaradawi explains that proposing a theory in universal higher objectives

[15] Mohamed Al-Tahir Ibn 'Ashur (2001). *Uṣūl al-niẓām al-ijtimā'ī fī al-Islām* (annotated by Mohamed Al-Tahir Mesawi). Amman: Dar al-Nafa'is: 256, 268.
[16] *Ibid.*, 270–281.
[17] Jamal Atiyah (2001). *Naḥw taf'īl maqāṣid al-sharī'ah*. Amman: al-Ma'had al-'Alami lil-Fikr al-Islami: 49.
[18] Mawil Izzi Dien (2004). *Islamic Law: From Historical Foundations to Contemporary Practice*. Edinburgh: Edinburgh University Press: 131–132.

should only happen after developing a level of experience with detailed scripts.[19]

(v) Taha Al-Alwani (1354 AH/1935 CE–) also surveyed the Qur'an to identify its "supreme and prevailing" higher objectives, which are, according to him, "the oneness of God (*tawḥīd*), purification of the soul (*tazkiyah*), and developing civilization on earth (*'umrān*)."[20]

All of the above-cited higher objectives were presented as they appeared in the minds and perceptions of the above jurists. Therefore, the structure of the higher objectives is best described as a "multidimensional" structure, in which levels of necessity, scope of rulings, scope of people, and levels of universality are all valid dimensions that represent valid viewpoints and classifications (see Figure 2 for an illustration of this

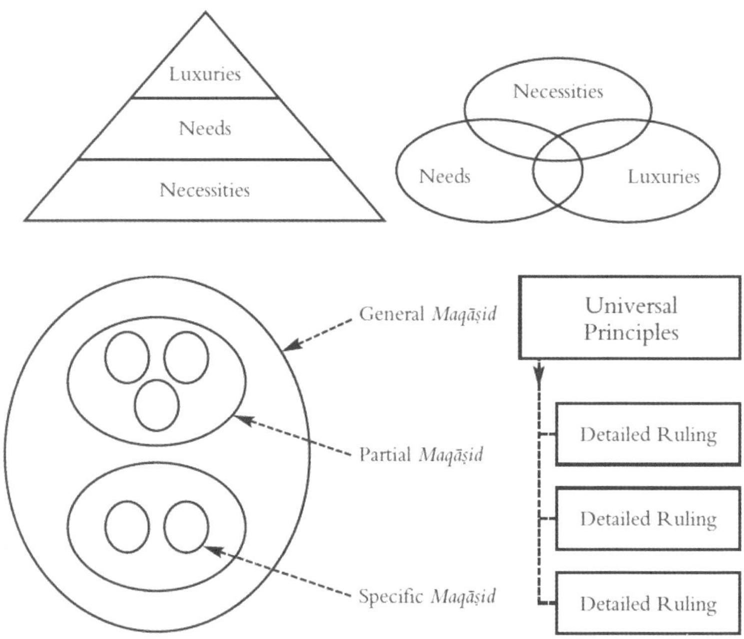

Figure 2. Various dimensions of the theories of *maqāṣid*.

[19] Al-Qaradawi Yusuf (1999). *Kayf nata'āmal ma' al-Qur'ān al-'aẓīm?* Cairo: Dar al-Shuruq.
[20] Taha Jabir Al-Alwani (2001). *Maqāṣid al-sharī'ah*. Beirut: IIIT and Dar al-Hadi: 25.

structure). As explained above, the next three sections explore different ways of utilizing higher objectives towards a much needed contemporary reasoning or independent legal reasoning (*ijtihād*) for the application of the Sharia in new circumstances.

3. Differentiating between Changing Means and Absolute Ends

Some scripts (Qur'anic verses or *hadiths*) are "scripts of means" (*nuṣūṣ wasā'il*) and are not intended to be ends in their own right and hence are not meant to be applied to the letter. A higher objective-based (*maqāṣidī*) understanding of these scripts helps in identifying their true meaning and intent.

For example, God states, "Hence, make ready against them whatever force and horse mounts you are able to muster, so that you might deter thereby the enemies of God, who are your enemies as well..." (Qur'an 8:60). "Horse mounts" are means and not "ends" in their own right that should be literally sought. In fact, the whole concept of "getting ready with force" is a means to the ends of justice and peace, rather than an end in its own right. The late Sheikh Muhammad Al-Ghazali extended this concept by differentiating between means (*al-wasā'il*) and ends (*al-ahdāf*), wherein he argued for the possibility of what he called "expiry" (*intihā'*) of the former and not the latter. Sheikh Al-Ghazali mentioned the whole system of the distribution of the booty of war as one example, despite the fact that it is mentioned explicitly in the Qur'an.[21] God states, "And know that whatever booty you acquire [in war], one-fifth thereof belongs to God and the Apostle, and the near of kin, and the orphans, and the needy, and the wayfarer. This you must observe if you believe in God and in what We bestowed from on high upon Our servant..." (Qur'an 8:41).

The above understanding validates today's policies, in which army personnel are compensated according to a scheme of salaries, ranks, and benefits, which are categorically separate from any economic gains they achieve via warfare.

---

[21] Mohammad al-Ghazali (1996). *Al-sunnah al-nabawīyah bayn ahl al-fiqh wa-ahl al ḥadīth.* Cairo: Dar Al-Shuruq: 161.

Recently, Sheikhs Yusuf Al-Qaradawi and Faisal Mawlawi elaborated on the importance of the "differentiation between means and ends" during the deliberations of the European Council for Fatwa and Research. They both applied the same concept to the visual sighting of Ramadan's new moon (*hilāl*) being mere means for knowing the start of the month rather than being an end in its own right. Hence, they concluded that pure calculations shall be today's means of defining the start of the month. Thus, Ministries of Islamic Affairs, Ministries of Awqaf, and Houses of Fatwa in various countries could correctly base their calendar decisions on official, astronomical reports and findings, instead of a costly contingency plan every month, especially during the seasons of fasting and pilgrimage. Sheikh Al-Qaradawi also applied the same concept to Muslim women's garment (*jilbāb*), amongst other things, which he viewed as mere means for achieving the objective of modesty.[22]

A similar expression is Ayatollah Mahdi Shamsuddin's recommendation for today's jurists to take a "dynamic" approach to the scripts, and "not to look at every script as absolute and universal legislation, open their minds to the possibility of 'relative' legislation for specific circumstances, and not to judge narrations with missing contexts as absolute in the dimensions of time, space, situations, and people." He further clarifies that he is "inclined to this understanding but would not base (any rulings) on it for the time being." Nevertheless, he stresses the need for this approach for rulings related to women, financial matters, and *jihād*.[23] Fathi Osman, as another example, considered the "practical considerations" that rendered a woman's testimony to be less than a man's, as mentioned in Al-Baqarah (Qur'an 2:282). Thus, Osman "re-interpreted" the verse to be a function to these practical considerations, in a way similar to Al-Alwani's approach mentioned above.[24] Sheikh Hassan Al-Turabi holds the same view regarding many rulings related, once again, to women and their daily-life practices and attires.[25]

---

[22] Mohamed el-Awa (ed.) (2006). *Maqāṣid al-sharī'ah al-Islāmīyah: dirāsāt fī qaḍāyā al-manhaj wa-majālāt al-taṭbīq*. London: Al-Maqasid Research Center: 85.

[23] Medhi Shamsuddin (1999). *Al-ijtihād wal-tajdīd fī al-fiqh al-Islāmī*. Beirut: al-Mu'assassah al-Dawliyah: 128–129.

[24] Abdelwahab el-Affendi (ed.) (2001). *Rethinking Islam and Modernity: Essays in Honour of Fathi Osman*. London: Islamic Foundation: 45.

[25] Hassan al-Turabi (2000). *Emancipation of Women: An Islamic Perspective*. London: Muslim Information Center: 29.

To demonstrate the implication of the aforementioned higher objective-based approach to the area of bioethics, the differentiation between means and ends in medicine and medical procedures is important. A number of scholars argue for the significance of "Islamic" or "Prophetic" medicine, by which they mean the remedies and the specific tools that were used during the time of the Prophet (PBUH[26]). The application of the above idea to this context implies that medicine itself and medical procedures as well are changeable means and not fixed ends in their own right. The saying of the Prophet (PBUH) that God did not reveal any ailment without revealing its cure as well, as related in the canonical collection of Bukhari, becomes the absolute end, and all procedures and medicines become means to achieving that end.

4. A Multidimensional Understanding of "Opposing Evidences"

In Islamic juridical theory, there is a differentiation between opposition or disagreement (*ta'āruḍ* or *ikhtilāf*) and contradiction (*tanāquḍ* or *ta'ānuḍ*) of scripts (Qur'anic verses or Prophetic narrations). Contradiction is defined as "a clear and logical conclusion of truth and falsehood in the same aspect" (*taqāsum al-ṣidq wa-al-kadhib*).[27] On the other hand, conflict or disagreement between evidences is defined as an "apparent contradiction between evidences in the mind of the scholar" (*ta'āruḍ fī dhihn al-mujtahid*).[28] This means that two seemingly disagreeing (*muta'āriḍ*) evidences are not necessarily in contradiction. It is the perception of the jurist that they are in contradiction, which can occur as a result of some missing information or dimension regarding the evidence's timing, place, circumstances, or other conditions.[29]

[26]Editor's note: PBUH is an abbreviation of the phrase "Peace and Blessings [of God] be Upon Him" inserted after the name of the Prophet Muhammad (PBUH) in compliance with God's command to invoke peace and blessings upon him whenever his name is mentioned.
[27]Abu Hamid al-Ghazali (1961). *Maqāṣid al-falāsifah*. Cairo: Dar al-Ma'arif: 62.
[28]Ahmad Ibn Taymiyah (n.d.). *Kutub wa-rasā'il wa-fatāwā* (edited by Abdur-Rahman al-Najdi). Riyadh: Maktabat bin Taymiyah: 131.
[29]Abdul-Aziz al-Bukhari (1997). *Kashf al-asrār*. vol. 3: Beirut: Dar al-Kutub al-'Ilmiyah: 77.

On the other hand, true contradiction takes the form of a single episode narrated in truly contradicting ways by the same or different narrators.[30] This kind of discrepancy is obviously due to errors in narration related to the memory and/or intentions of one or more of the narrators.[31] The "logical" conclusion in cases of contradiction is that one or more of the narrations is inaccurate and should be rejected.

For example, Abu Hurayrah narrated, according to Bukhari: "Bad omens are in women, animals, and houses." However, also according to Bukhari, Aisha narrated that the Prophet (PBUH) had said, "People during the Days of Ignorance (*jāhilīyah*) used to say that bad omens are in women, animals, and houses." These two "authentic" narrations are at odds with one another and one of them should be rejected. It is telling that most commentators rejected Aisha's narration, even though other "authentic" narrations support it.[32] Ibn Al'Arabi, for example, commented on Aisha's rejection of the above *hadith* as follows: "This [rejection] cannot be taken seriously (*qawl sāqiṭ*). Aisha is rejecting a clear and authentic narration that is narrated through trusted narrators."[33]

According to various traditional and contemporary studies on the issue of disagreement (*ta'āruḍ*), contradiction, in the above sense, is rare. Most cases of *ta'āruḍ* are disagreements between narrations because of an apparently missing context, rather than being due to logically contradicting accounts of the same episode. There are three main mechanisms that jurists have defined to deal with these types of disagreements in traditional schools of law[34]:

(i) Conciliation (*al-jam'*): This method is based on a fundamental rule stating that, "applying the script is better than disregarding it (*i'māl al-naṣṣ awlá min ihmālih*)." Therefore, a jurist facing two

---

[30] Jasser Auda (2006). *Fiqh al-maqāṣid: ināṭat al-aḥkām al-shar'īyah bi-maqāṣidihā*. Virginia: Al-Ma'had al'Alami lil-Fikr al-Islami: 65–68.

[31] Ali Al-Subki (1983). *Al-ibhāj fī sharḥ al-minhāj*. Beirut: Dar al-Nashr: 218.

[32] Auda (2006), *op.cit.*, 106.

[33] Abu Bakr Ibn al-Arabi (n.d.). *'Āriḍat al-Aḥwadhī*. vol. 10: Cairo: Dar al-Wahy al-Mohammadi: 264.

[34] Badran Badran (1974). *Adillat al-tarjīḥ al-muta'āriḍah wa-wujūh al-tarjīḥ baynahā*. Alexandria: Mu'assasat Shabab al-Jami'ah, Chap. 4.

disagreeing narrations should search for a missing condition or context and attempt to interpret both narrations based on it.

(ii) Abrogation (*al-naskh*): This method suggests that the latter evidence, chronologically speaking, should "abrogate" (juridically annul) the former. This means that when verses disagree, the verse that is (narrated to be) revealed last is considered to be an abrogating evidence (*nāsikh*) and others to be abrogated (*mansūkh*). Similarly, when Prophetic narrations disagree, the narration that has a later date, if dates are known or could be concluded, should abrogate all other narrations. Most scholars do not accept that a *hadith* abrogates a verse of the Qur'an, even if the *hadith* were to be chronologically subsequent.

(iii) The concept of abrogation, in any of the above senses, does not have supporting evidence from the words attributed to the Prophet (PBUH) in traditional collections of *hadith*. Etymologically, abrogation (*naskh*) is derived from the root *na sa kha*. I carried out a survey on this root and all its possible derivations in a large number of today's popular collections of *hadith*, including, Al-Bukhari, Muslim, Al-Tirmidhi, Al-Nasa'i, Abu Dawud, Ibn Majah, Ahmad, Malik, Al-Darami, Al-Mustadrak, Ibn Hibban, Ibn Khuzaymah, Al-Bayhaqi, Al-Darqutni, Ibn Abi Shaybah, and Abd Al-Razzaq. I found no valid *hadith* attributed to the Prophet that contains any of these derivations of the root *na sa kha*. I found about 40 instances of "abrogations" mentioned in the above collections, which were all based on one of the narrators' opinions or commentaries, rather than any of the texts of the *hadith*. Thus, I conclude that the concept of abrogation always appears within the commentaries given by companions or other narrators, commenting on what appears to be in disagreement with their own understanding of the related issues. According to traditional exegeses, the principle of abrogation does have evidence from the Qur'an, although the interpretations of the related verses are subject to a difference of opinion.[35]

(iii) Giving preference (*al-tarjīḥ*): This method suggests giving preference to the narration that is "most authentic" and dropping or eliminating

[35] Muhammad Nada (1996). *Al-naskh fī al-Qur'ān*. Cairo: al-Dar al-Arabiyah lel-Kutub: 25.

other narrations. The "preferred" narration is called *al-riwāyah al-rājiḥah*, which literally means the narration that is "heavier in the scale." According to scholars of *hadith*, a weightier (*rājiḥah*) narration must have, as compared to the other narrations, one or more of the following characteristics: a larger number of other supporting narrations, a shorter chain of narrators, more knowledgeable narrators, narrators more capable of memorization, more trustworthy narrators, first-hand account versus indirect accounts, shorter time between the narration and the narrated incident, narrators able to remember and mention the date of the incident more than others, less ambiguity, and less rhetoric, in addition to a number of other factors.

The Hanafi jurists apply abrogation before any other method, followed by the method of *tarjīḥ*.[36] All other schools of law give priority, theoretically, to the method of conciliation (*al-jam'*). Although most schools of law agree that applying all scripts is better than disregarding any of them, most scholars do not seem to give priority, on a practical level, to the method of conciliation. The methods that are used in most cases of *ta'āruḍ* are abrogation and *tarjīḥ*.[37] Therefore, a large number of evidences are canceled, in one way or another, for no good reason other than that the jurists are failing to understand how they can fit them in a unified perceptual framework. Thus, invalidating these evidences is more or less arbitrary. For example, narrations are invalidated (outweighed) if narrators did not happen to "mention the date of the incident"; the wording related to the Prophet (PBUH) happened to be more "metaphoric"; or a narrator happened to be female — in which case the male's "opposing" narration takes precedence.[38] Therefore, *naskh* and *tarjīḥ* reflect the general feature of binary thinking in fundamental methodology. It is essential that the method of conciliation makes use of the concept of multidimensionality

---

[36] Ibn Amir al-Haj (1996). *Al-taqrīr wa-al-taḥbīr fī 'ilm uṣūl al-fiqh*. vol. 3: Beirut: Dar al-fikr: 4.

[37] Auda (2006), *op.cit.*, 105–110.

[38] Abdul Majeed Al-Sousarah (1997). *Manhaj al-tawfīq wa-al-tarjīḥ bayn mukhtalaf al-ḥadīth wa-atharuh fī al-fiqh al-Islāmī*. Amman: Dar al-Nafa'is: 395.

in overcoming this drawback and considers the dimension of *maqāṣid* in the understanding of the scripts.

One practical consequence of canceling a large number of verses and Prophetic narrations in the name of *naskh* and *tarjīḥ* is a great deal of "inflexibility" in Islamic law, i.e. inability to address various situations adequately. Reflection upon pairs of *muta'āriḍ* or opposing narrations show that their disagreement could be due to a difference in surrounding circumstances, such as war and peace, poverty and wealth, urban and rural life, summer and winter, sickness and health, or young and advanced age. Therefore, the Qur'anic instructions or the Prophet's actions and decisions, as narrated by his observers, are supposed to have differed accordingly. Lack of contextualization limits flexibility. For example, the verse that states, 'But when the forbidden months are past, then slay the pagans wherever you find them, and seize them' (Qur'an 9:5) has come to be named the 'Verse of the Sword' (*āyat al-sayf*) and has been claimed to have abrogated hundreds of verses and *hadith*. One significant *hadith* that was claimed to have been abrogated is "The Scroll of Medina" (*ṣaḥīfat al-madīnah*), in which the Prophet (PBUH) and the Jews of Medina wrote a "covenant" that defined the relationship between Muslims and Jews living in Medina. The scroll stated that "Muslims and Jews are one nation (*ummah*), with Muslims having their own religion and Jews having their own religion."[39] Classic commentators on the *ṣaḥīfah* (Scroll) render it "abrogated," based on the Verse of the Sword and other similar verses.[40] Seeing all the above scripts and narrations in terms of the single dimension of peace versus war might imply a contradiction. This misunderstanding eliminates the profession, ministry, and art of foreign policy altogether!

What augmented the problem is that the number of abrogation claimed by the students of the companions (*tābi'ūn*) is higher than the cases claimed by the companions themselves, a fact I concluded on the basis of the survey mentioned earlier. After the first Islamic century, one could furthermore notice that jurists from the developing schools of thought began claiming many new cases of abrogation that were never

[39] Burhan Zurayq (1996). *Al-ṣaḥīfah: mīthāq al-Rasūl*. Damascus: Dar al-Numair & Dar Ma'ad: 353.
[40] *Ibid.*, 216.

claimed by the *tābiʿūn*. Thus, abrogation became a method of invalidating opinions or narrations endorsed by rival schools of law. Abu Al-Hassan Al-Karkhi (d. 951 CE), for one example, writes, "The fundamental rule is: Every Qur'anic verse that is different from the opinion of the jurists in our school is either taken out of context or abrogated."[41] Therefore, it is not unusual in the *fiqhī* literature to find a certain ruling to be abrogating (*nāsikh*) according to one school and abrogated (*mansūkh*) according to another. This arbitrary use of the method of abrogation has exacerbated the problem of lack of multidimensional interpretations of the evidences.

Multidimensional thinking, introduced by the higher objective-based approach, could offer a solution to the dilemmas of a large number of "opposing" evidences. Two evidences might be "in opposition" in terms of one particular attribute, such as war and peace, order and forbiddance, standing and sitting, men and women, and so on. If we restrict our view to one dimension, we will find no way to reconcile the evidences.[42] However, if we expand the one-dimensional space into two dimensions, the second of which is a higher objective to which both evidences contribute, then we will be able to "resolve" the opposition and understand/interpret the evidences in a unified context based on the purpose/*maqṣūd* of both evidences.

For example, there is a large number of opposing evidences related to different ways of performing "acts of worship" (*ʿibādāt*), all attributed to the Prophet (PBUH). These opposing narrations have frequently caused heated debates and rifts within Muslim communities. However, understanding these narrations within a higher objective of easiness (*taysīr*) entails that the Prophet (PBUH) did carry out these rituals in various ways, suggesting flexibility in such matters.[43] Examples of these acts of worship are the different ways of standing and moving during prayers, concluding prayers (*tashahhud*), performing the compensating prostration (*sujūd al-sahū*), reciting "God is Great" (*takbīr*) during *ʿīd* prayers, making up for breaking one's fasting in Ramadan, performing detailed acts of pilgrimage, and so on.

[41] Al-Alwani (2001), *op.cit.*, 89.
[42] Refer, for example, to: Abdullah Ibn Qutayba (1978). *Ta'wīl mukhtalaf al-ḥadīth*. Cairo: Dar Al-Fikr Al-Arabi.
[43] Auda (2006), *op.cit.*, ch. 3.

To present another example, a number of narrations were classified under cases of abrogation even though they were, according to some jurists, cases of gradual application of rulings. The purpose behind the gradual applications of rulings on a large scale is, "facilitating the change that the law is bringing to society's deep-rooted habits."[44] Thus, "opposing narrations" regarding the prohibition of liquor and usury and the performance of prayers and fasting should be understood in terms of the Prophetic "tradition" and "policy" of the gradual application of high ideals in any given society that is originally far from these ideals.

To apply the above fundamental concept in the area of bioethics, a prominent example is the question of the permissibility of organ transplantation. Despite the fact that the majority of contemporary scholars allow it, a few scholars judged prohibition. In terms of the technicalities of the *fatwá*, there was a perceived "contradiction" between the scriptural evidences as highlighted in the following considerations[45–48]:

(i) There is a well-known maxim — based on a number of evidences — that one cannot offer what one does not own. On the other hand, an analogy was made between offering an organ and offering money.

(ii) The perceived contradiction between the verse, "[Satan said]...I will order them to change God's creation" (Qur'an 4:119) and related narrations, and the other verses and narrations that order reform and doing good.

(iii) The perceived contradiction between the narrations that prohibit any form of mutilation of corpses (such as "breaking the bone of the dead is like breaking the bone of the living," narrated by Ahmad, Dawud, and Ibn Majah), versus the other consideration of common good (*maṣlaḥah*).

---

[44] Mohammad al-Ghazali (2002). *Naẓarāt fī al-Qur'ān*. Cairo: Nahdat Misr: 194.

[45] Abdullah al-Ghummari (1997). *Ta'rīf ahl al-Islām bi-ann naql al-'uḍw ḥarām*. Palestine: Mu'assasat Al-Albayt.

[46] Mustafa al-Dhahabi (1993). *Naql al-a'ḍā 'bayna al-ṭibb wa-al-dīn*. Cairo: Darul-Hadith.

[47] Yusuf al-Qaradawi (w.d.). *Mūjibāt taghayyur al-fatwá*. Doha: International Union of Muslim Scholars.

[48] Yusuf al-Qaradawi (2009). *Zirā'at al-a'ḍā' fī al-sharī'ah al-Islamīyah*. Available online via www.qaradawi.net (retrieved 1 June 2014).

(iv) The perceived contradiction between the narrations that consider organs separated from the living to be "dead" (*maytah*, narrated by Ahmad, Tirmidhi, and others) — and thus prohibited to use because of their impurity (*najāsah*) — versus the other narrations that stated that "a believer could never be impure" (Bukhari and Muslim).

The sound methodology — based on this research — would give prominence to the consideration of higher objectives in all of the above evidences and similar ones, instead of the debates of abrogation and giving preference to just one consideration over all others. Thus, the following *fatwá* issued by the International Islamic Fiqh Academy (*Al-Majma' Al-Fiqhī Al-Islāmī*) in Jeddah represents — in my view — a sound methodology based on all of the above:

> It is permitted to transplant or graft an organ from one part of a person's body to another, so long as one is careful to ascertain that the benefits of this operation outweigh any harm that may result from it, and on the condition that this is done to replace something that has been lost, or to restore its appearance or regular function, or to correct some fault or disfigurement which is causing physical or psychological distress.
>
> It is permitted to transplant an organ from one person's body to another, if it is an organ that can regenerate itself, like skin or blood, on the condition that the donor is mature and understands what he is doing, and that all other pertinent *shar'ī* [Sharia-compliant] conditions are met.
>
> It is permitted to use part of an organ that has been removed because of illness to benefit another person, such as using the cornea of an eye removed because of illness.
>
> It is *ḥarām* [impermissible] to take an organ on which life depends, such as taking a heart from a living person to transplant into another person.
>
> It is *ḥarām* [impermissible] to take an organ from a living person when doing so could impair an essential vital function, even though his life itself may not be under threat, such as removing the corneas of both eyes. However, removing organs which will lead to only partial impairment is a matter which is still under scholarly discussion.
>
> It is permitted to transplant an organ from a dead person to a living person whose life depends on receiving that organ, or whose vital functions are

otherwise impaired, on the condition that permission is given either by the person before his death or by his heirs, or by the leader of the Muslims in cases where the dead person's identity is unknown or he has no heirs.

Care should be taken to ensure that there is proper agreement to the transplant of organs in the cases described above, on the condition that no buying or selling of organs is involved. It is not permitted to trade in human organs under any circumstances. But the question of whether the beneficiary may spend money to obtain an organ he needs, or to show his appreciation, is a matter which is still under scholarly debate.

Anything other than the scenarios described above is still subject to scholarly debate, and requires further detailed research in the light of medical research and *shar'ī* rulings.

6. Conclusion

Before calling for the "application of the Sharia" in Muslim societies or juridical systems, policy and methods have to be based on new *ijtihād* in understanding and applying the evidences of the verses of the Qur'an or the *hadith* of the Prophet (PBUH). In order for this *ijtihād* to meet the needs of Muslims with changing circumstances, this chapter suggested that it should be based on differentiating between changing means and absolute ends. A higher objective-based understanding of these scripts helps in identifying their purposes. Also, a multidimensional understanding of "opposing evidences," which is based on a *maqāṣidī* approach, offers a solution for the dilemma of the large number of "opposing" evidences in our juridical heritage. A higher objective-based approach is able to "resolve" the opposition and understand/interpret the evidences in a unified context based on the purpose/*maqṣūd* of both evidences.

Failing to include the above criteria in that proposed *ijtihād* would create applications (or rather, misapplications) of the Sharia that are reductionist rather than holistic, literal rather than moral, and one-dimensional rather than multidimensional. Thus, the proposed higher objective-based approach lifts the juridical decisions and policies to a higher philosophical grade and hence leads to a methodology that is holistic, ethical, and multidimensional. This methodology achieves a much needed flexibility of the Islamic rulings with the change of time and circumstances, a flexibility that is essential for the universality of Islam and its way of life.

Part II
Principles of Biomedical Ethics

The Principles of Biomedical Ethics as Universal Principles

Tom L. Beauchamp

Abstract: The principal subject of this chapter is the role that principles play in the so-called four-principles approach or principlism.[1] The historical and textual background of the positions I will defend are found in *Principles of Biomedical Ethics*, which I coauthored with James F. Childress and in my recent book *Standing on Principles*. In the first section, I investigate the nature and sources of principles in recent biomedical ethics and provide an analysis of the four-principles framework. The second section is devoted to the central role played in the four-principles account by the theory of common morality, which is comprised not only of principles (and rules), but also of virtues, ideals, and rights. The third section shows how universal principles

[1] This term was coined by K. Danner Clouser and Bernard Gert (1990). A critique of principlism. *Journal of Medicine and Philosophy* 15: 219–236. See later discussions and formulations in Bernard Gert, C. M. Culver and K. Danner Clouser (2006). *Bioethics: A Systematic Approach.* New York: Oxford University Press, chap. 4; Oliver Rauprich (2013). Principlism, *International Encyclopedia of Ethics.* Wiley, online encyclopedia; John H. Evans (2000). A sociological account of the growth of principlism, *Hastings Center Report* 30: 31–38; Michael Quante and Andreas Vieth (2002). Defending principlism well understood. *Journal of Medicine and Philosophy* 27: 621–649; Carson Strong (2000). Specified Principlism. *Journal of Medicine and Philosophy* 25: 285–307; and Bernard Gert, C. M. Culver and K. Danner Clouser, Common morality versus specified principlism: Reply to Richardson. *Journal of Medicine and Philosophy* 25: 308–322.

are fashioned into particular moralities and the circumstances under which moral pluralism is consistent with universal morality. The fourth section shows how general principles are made practical for particular moralities by being made more specific, as suitable for particular circumstances. Finally, in the fifth section, I show the relevance of principles for discussions of human rights, multiculturalism, and cultural imperialism.

1. A Framework of Four Clusters of Principles

1.1. *The Origins of Principles in Recent Biomedical Ethics*

Principles that can be understood with relative ease by the members of various disciplines figured prominently in the early developments in the history of biomedical ethics during the 1970s and early 1980s. Frameworks of general principles were readily understood by people with many different forms of professional training and from all moral traditions. The distilled morality of universal principles gave people in a pluralistic society a shared and serviceable group of norms for the analysis of moral problems.

Two published works were the original sources of interest in principles of biomedical ethics. The first was the *Belmont Report* (and related documents) of the National Commission for the Protection of Human Subjects,[2] and the second was *Principles of Biomedical Ethics*.[3] The goal of the former was a general statement of principles of research ethics, whereas the goal of the latter was to develop a set of general principles suitable for biomedical ethics more broadly so that the principles could be specified for particular ethical problems in medicine, research, and public health. One of our proposals was that medicine's traditional preoccupation

---

[2]National Commission for the Protection of Human Subjects of Biomedical and Behavioral Research, *The Belmont Report: Ethical Principles and Guidelines for the Protection of Human Subjects of Research*. Washington, DC: DHEW Publication. For history and commentary, see also James F. Childress, Eric M. Meslin, Harold T. Shapiro, (eds.) (2005). *Belmont Revisited: Ethical Principles for Research with Human Subjects*. Washington, DC.: Georgetown University Press.

[3]Tom L. Beauchamp and James F. Childress (1979). *Principles of Biomedical Ethics*, 1st edn. New York: Oxford University Press; the book is currently in the 7th edn., New York: Oxford University Press, 2012.

with a beneficence-based model of physician ethics be augmented by a principle of respect for autonomy and by wider concerns for social justice.

1.2. *Principles as Abstract Norms of Obligation*

In principlist theory, a basic principle is an abstract moral norm that is part of a framework of prominent starting-points in the landscape of the moral life. If some principles were dropped from the framework, the demands of the moral life would not be what we know those demands to be, just as a landscape would not be the same landscape if certain rocks, trees, or plants were removed from it. In the absence of any one basic principle there might still be a moral life, but it would be fundamentally different from the one familiar to us. More specific rules for health care ethics can be formulated *by reference to* these general principles, but neither rules nor practical judgments can be straightforwardly *deduced* from the principles.

All principles can, in some contexts, be justifiably overridden by other moral norms with which they come into contingent conflict. For example, we might justifiably not tell the truth in order to prevent someone from killing another person. Principles, duties, and rights are not *absolute* (or unconditional) merely because they are *universally valid.* No principles, duties, or rights are absolute. Often some balance between two or more principles must be found that requires some part of each obligation to be discharged, but in many cases one principle simply overrides the other. This overriding may seem precariously flexible and subjective, as if moral guidelines lack backbone and can be magically waived away as not *real* obligations. In ethics, as in law, there is no escape from an exercise of judgment in using principles in the resolution of moral conflicts. In some limited contexts (for example, in religious ethics and in professional ethics) we may need to develop a highly structured moral system or set of guidelines in which a certain class of rights or principles has a fixed priority over others, but no moral theory or professional code of ethics has successfully presented a system of moral principles free of conflicts and exceptions.

I will discuss this problem further below when addressing the problem of *specification.*

1.3. *A Framework of Principles*

The principles in the framework that Childress and I have defended are grouped under four general categories: (i) respect for autonomy (a principle requiring respect for the decision-making capacities of autonomous persons), (ii) nonmaleficence (a principle requiring the avoidance of causing harm to others), (iii) beneficence (a group of principles requiring both lessening of and prevention of harm as well as provision of benefits to others), and (iv) justice (a group of principles requiring fair distribution of benefits, risks, and costs across all affected parties).

The choice of these four general clusters of moral principles as the framework for moral decision-making in bioethics derives in significant part from professional roles and traditions. In this regard, our framework builds on centuries of tradition in medical ethics. Nonmaleficence and beneficence have always played a fundamental role in the history of medical ethics, whereas respect for autonomy and justice were neglected and have risen to prominence only recently. All four types of principles are needed to provide a comprehensive framework for biomedical ethics, but this framework is abstract and thin in content until it has been further specified — that is, interpreted and adapted for particular circumstances — a task to which I return later.

In this section I will examine only the basic content of each of these four clusters of principles.

(a) *Respect for Autonomy*

The starting point for an account of autonomy is self-rule free of controlling interferences by others and freedom from limitations within the individual that prevent choice. The two basic conditions of autonomy therefore are *liberty* (the absence of controlling influences) and *agency* (self-initiated intentional action). Disagreement exists over how to analyze these two conditions and over whether additional conditions are needed.[4] Each of these notions is indeterminate until further analyzed in a theory of autonomy.

---

[4]See the different conceptual analyses of autonomy and theories of autonomy in Joel Feinberg (1986). *Harm to Self*, vol. 3 in *The Moral Limits of the Criminal Law*. Chaps. 18–19.

To respect an autonomous agent is to recognize with due appreciation person's capacities and perspectives, including his or her right to hold certain views, to make certain kinds of choices, and to take certain actions based on personal values and beliefs. The *principle* of respect for autonomy contains both a negative obligation and a positive obligation.[5] As a negative obligation, autonomous actions should not be subjected to controlling constraints by others. As a positive obligation, this principle requires respectful and appropriate informational exchanges and fitting actions that foster autonomous decision-making. Respect for autonomy obligates professionals in healthcare and research involving human subjects to disclose information, to probe for and ensure understanding and voluntariness, and to foster adequate decision-making. True respect requires more than mere non-interference. It includes, at least in some contexts, building up or maintaining others' capacities for autonomous choice while helping to allay fears and other conditions that destroy or disrupt their autonomous actions. Disrespect, on this account, involves attitudes and actions that ignore, insult, demean, or are inattentive to others' rights of autonomy.

Professional ethics is commonly concerned with such failures to respect a person's autonomy, ranging from manipulative under-disclosure of pertinent information to non-recognition of a refusal of medical interventions. For example, in the debate over whether autonomous, informed patients or their families have the right to refuse medical interventions, the principle of respect for autonomy demands that an autonomous refusal of interventions must be respected.[6]

This truly basic principle has been deeply misrepresented in much of the bioethics literature as a principle of individualism, sometimes

---

New York: Oxford University Press, and Sarah Buss (2008). Personal Autonomy, *Stanford Encyclopedia of Philosophy*. Available online via http://plato.stanford.edu/entries/personal-autonomy/ (retrieved on 9 August 2012).

[5] Editor's note: These two types of obligation, i.e. the negative and positive ones, are very close to the two parallel concepts in the discourse on the higher objectives of Sharia that preserving each of these higher objectives also has two aspects, *al-ḥifẓ al-wujūdī* and *al-ḥifẓ al-'adamī*. The former can be translated as the positive obligation, and the latter can be translated as the negative obligation.

[6] Ruth R. Faden and Tom L. Beauchamp (1986). *A History and Theory of Informed Consent*. New York: Oxford.

curiously said to be an "American individualism." But the principle of respect for autonomy has nothing to do with individualism — the strange idea that an individual has the right to do whatever the individual wishes to do with his or her life and to take whatever actions he or she wishes. Nothing is more antithetical to morality than individualism, and the four-principles approach wholly rejects it.

A related misunderstanding of both the four-principles approach and of the principle of respect for autonomy is that it prioritizes the principle of respect for autonomy over other principles and demands in the moral life. Professor Ali Al-Qaradaghi says in his presentation that "the principlist approach prioritizes the principle of respect for autonomy over other principles and demands in the moral life." This statement is incorrect. We do not prioritize this principle — or any principle. However, I hasten to add that the Professor does have a fundamentally correct understanding of our general view when he says that, in our view, "exercises of autonomy can justifiably be restrained or overridden. In this way, it is clear that this principle is not absolute." Yes, that is exactly the right interpretation. As Childress and I have pointed out, in edition after edition, the principle of respect for autonomy has no priority whatsoever, nor does any other principle in the four-principles approach.

It has also been alleged that our book emphasizes a liberal political philosophy of individual rights, while neglecting solidarity, social responsibility, social justice, health policy priorities, and the like. Given our very substantial emphasis throughout the book on both beneficence and social justice as basic principles, this interpretation seems to pay no serious attention to what Childress and I have been writing for 40 years now. Respect for autonomy in our work is not local to any region, not excessively individualistic, and not an overriding or ranked principle.

Many kinds of competing moral considerations can validly override respect for autonomy under conditions of a contingent conflict of norms. For example, if our choices endanger the public health, potentially harm innocent others, or require a scarce and unfunded resource, exercises of autonomy can justifiably be restrained or overridden. Childress and I also defend a limited paternalism in physician care of the patient.

(b) *Nonmaleficence*

The principle of nonmaleficence is the best example of a centuries-old principle in medical ethics. This principle states that we are obligated to abstain from causing harm to others. It has long been associated in Hippocratic medical ethics with the injunction: "Above all [or first] do no harm." The reason for the esteem — almost reverence — for this traditional principle is perfectly understandable, in my view: Of all the basic principles of biomedical ethics, there is none more basic and none more important than the principle of nonmaleficence.

In a classic source of medical ethics, British physician Thomas Percival maintained that a principle of nonmaleficence fixes the physician's primary obligations and triumphs even over respect for the patient's autonomy in a circumstance of potential harm to patients:

> To a patient … who makes inquiries which, if faithfully answered, might prove fatal to him, it would be a gross and unfeeling wrong to reveal the truth. His right to it is suspended, and even annihilated; because … it would be deeply injurious to himself, to his family, and to the public. And he has the strongest claim, from the trust reposed in his physician, as well as from the common principles of humanity, to be guarded against whatever would be detrimental to him.[7]

The principle of nonmaleficence supports a wide variety of more specific moral rules.[8] Typical examples include:

(i) "Don't kill."
(ii) "Don't cause pain or suffering to others."
(iii) "Don't incapacitate others."

---

[7] Thomas Percival (1803). *Medical Ethics: Or a Code of Institutes and Precepts, Adapted to the Professional Conduct of Physicians and Surgeons.* Manchester: S. Russell: 165–166.

[8] See Beauchamp and Childress (2012), 7th edn.: 154.

Precisely how these rules are supported by the principle of nonmaleficence is not a question I will consider here, but it is addressed in the *Principles of Biomedical Ethics* largely in terms of the theory of specification (as discussed below).

Numerous problems of nonmaleficence are found in health care ethics today, some involving blatant abuses and others involving subtle and unresolved questions. Blatant examples of failures to act nonmaleficently are found in the use of physicians to classify political dissidents as mentally ill, thereafter treating them with harmful drugs and incarcerating them with insane and violent persons.[9] More subtle examples are found in the use of medications for the treatment of aggressive and destructive patients. These common treatment modalities are helpful to many patients, but they can be harmful to others.

When I use the term "harm" in expositing nonmaleficence, I do not mean to imply *wrongful injuring* or *maleficence*. I mean "harm" to refer in a non-judgmental way to a thwarting, defeating, or setting back of the interests of an individual, whether caused intentionally or unintentionally. The word "interest" here refers to that which is in an individual's interest — that is, what is to one's welfare advantage in a given circumstance. A *harmful* invasion by one party of another's interests is not always *wrong*, *maleficent*, or *unjustified*.[10] For example, there can be a justified amputation of a patient's leg, justified punishment of physicians for incompetence or negligence, justified imprisonment, etc. Harming therefore is not necessarily wronging.

(c) *Beneficence*

No moral demand placed on physicians is more important than beneficence in the care of patients. Beneficence is a foundational value — sometimes treated as *the* foundational value[11] — in healthcare ethics. Many specific duties in medicine, nursing, public health, and research are

---

[9] See, for example, Sidney Bloch and Peter Reddaway (1984). *Soviet Psychiatric Abuse: The Shadow over World Psychiatry.* Boulder, Colo.: Westview Press, esp. chap. 1.

[10] Beauchamp and Childress (2012), 7th edn., chap. 5.

[11] Edmund Pellegrino and David Thomasma (1988). *For the Patient's Good: The Restoration of Beneficence in Health Care.* New York: Oxford University Press.

expressed in terms of a positive obligation to come to the assistance of those in need of treatment or in danger of injury.

Principles of beneficence require that we prevent harms from occurring, remove harm-causing conditions that exist, and promote the good of others. The physician who professes to "do no harm" is not usually interpreted as pledging never to cause harm, but rather to strive to create a positive balance of goods over inflicted harms. Those engaged in medical practice, research, and public health know that risks of harm presented by interventions must often be weighed against possible benefits for patients, subjects, and the public.

Rules of beneficence often demand more of us than the principle of nonmaleficence because agents must *act to help*, not merely *refrain from harming*, which is what is demanded by the principle of nonmaleficence. Conflating nonmaleficence and beneficence into a single principle — as some philosophers do — obscures some important distinctions. Obligations not to harm others, such as those prohibiting disablement and killing, are distinct from obligations to help others, for example, those prescribing the provision of benefits and protection of interests. Professor Ali Al-Qaradaghi says in his presentation, in objecting to the sharp distinction I make between beneficence and nonmaleficence, that, "Actually, one can argue that the principle of beneficence implies that of nonmaleficence and preventing harm." In principlist theory, such an implication of one principle by another does not occur. Nonmaleficence requires *not acting* — that is, abstaining from acting so as not to cause harm. Beneficence requires *acting* — in particular acting to benefit others. Here it is apparent that beneficence cannot involve nonmaleficence because they are logically and morally different principles.

Some writers in healthcare ethics suggest that certain duties not to injure others are always more compelling than duties to benefit them. They point out that we do not consider it justifiable to kill a dying patient in order to use the patient's organs to save two others, even though benefits would be maximized, all things considered. The obligation to not injure a patient by abandonment has been said to be stronger than the obligation to prevent injury to a patient who has been abandoned by another (under the assumption that both are moral duties). Despite the intuitive attractiveness of these claims, there is no hierarchical ordering rule that ranks nonmaleficence higher than beneficence; obligations of beneficence do, under many circumstances, outweigh those of nonmaleficence. A harm inflicted by not avoiding causing it may be negligibly small, whereas the harm that beneficence requires we prevent may be substantial. For example, saving a person's life by a blood transfusion clearly justifies the inflicted harm of venipuncture on the blood donor.

Perhaps the major theoretical problem about beneficence is whether the principle generates general moral duties that are incumbent on *everyone* — not because of a professional role, but because morality itself makes a general demand of beneficence. Many analyses of beneficence in ethical theory (most notably in utilitarianism[12]) seem to demand severe sacrifice and extreme generosity in the moral life — for example, giving a kidney for transplantation or donating bone marrow to a stranger. However, such beneficent action generally follows from a moral ideal, not a principle of obligation. The line between what the principle of beneficence requires and does not require is undoubtedly difficult to draw, and drawing a precise line independent of the considerations of specific contexts is an impossible goal.

(d) *Justice*

A person in any society has been treated justly if treated according to what is fair, due, or owed. For example, if equal political rights are for all citizens, then justice is done when those rights are accorded. The narrower concept of *distributive justice* refers to fair distribution in society of primary social goods, such as economic goods and fundamental political rights, but burdens should also be within its scope. Paying for a national health plan of insurance is a distributed burden; grants to do biomedical research are distributed benefits.

A prime example of the need for principles of distributive justice is the need to distribute healthcare and its costs fairly within societies. Some governments, especially the United States, tend to pay for many useless

[12] Peter Singer (1999). Living high and letting die. *Philosophy and Phenomenological Research* 59: 183–187; Peter Singer (1993). *Practical Ethics*, 2nd edn. Cambridge: Cambridge University Press; Shelly Kagan (1989). *The Limits of Morality*. Oxford: Clarendon Press.

procedures — a waste of resources that deprives others in society of adequate healthcare. Various governments have concluded that their resources are so limited that little money can be spent on either public health or healthcare. A basic ethical problem in every society is how to structure a principled system such that burdens and benefits are fairly and efficiently distributed and a threshold condition of equitable levels of health and access to healthcare is in place. These ethical objectives are intertwined in the formation of health policy, both internationally and in the policies of individual nations. Moral assessment of the justice of the principles used in these systems is one of the major priorities in contemporary bioethics.

It is easy to get lost in the complications of theories of justice, and this can easily cause a misunderstanding of what Childress and I are arguing in the book. Dr. Al-Bar has a misunderstanding of our book when he says that

> Beauchamp and Childress in "Principles of Biomedical Ethics" stressed the fact that Afro Americans without medical insurance and found to suffer from hypertension … should not be treated, as many researchers found that such poor patients, will not be able to continue medication or follow up.… In fact, without saying it, they agree to let them suffer and die with their hypertension and its sequelae e.g. strokes, heart attacks, heart failure, and kidney failure.… Instead of attacking this unjust system which excludes 50 million citizens from the right of being treated, they make quasi scientific research that claims it is useless to treat such patients.

There are several mistaken understandings here. First, we argue repeatedly that African-Americans must be treated equally; in the passage on hypertension we are criticizing theories that have a utilitarian rationale that we do not accept. The theory under discussion in this passage is not our theory; we are criticizing a theory presented by Professors Milton Weinstein and William B. Stason.[13] We call their theory a "problematic"

[13] Milton Weinstein and William B. Stason (1977). *Hypertension.* Cambridge, MA: Harvard University Press. Public health rounds at the Harvard School of Public Health: Allocating of resources to manage hypertension. *New England Journal of Medicine* 296: 732–739; and (1977). Allocation resources: The case of hypertension. *Hastings Center Report* 7 (October): 24–29.

distribution scheme.[14] Dr. Al-Bar says that we should be "attacking this unjust system," but this is exactly what we do — attack it. We critique all such views at great length in our chapter on justice, where we spend some 50 pages in the book attacking precisely this unjust system. Dr. Al-Bar says, "It's amazing to find these two eminent philosophers of bioethics try to find excuses for not treating the Afro Americans." But we had just spent numerous pages trying to criticize and restructure the system of healthcare in the United States that gave rise to this problem. Our arguments consistently attack discrimination against African-Americans.

Professor Ali Al-Qaradaghi has a similar misunderstanding. He says, "[T]hey [Beauchamp and Childress] did not include equal treatment of all patients in the biomedical ethics. This is an important principle that requires equality and fair treatment without discrimination based on wealth, race, etc." But the claim here is the exact opposite of what we say. We insist on equal treatment of all patients and on the fundamental importance in the biomedical ethics of the principle that requires equality and fair treatment. In fact, we claim even more since we insist on a principle of fair opportunity.

In reading our account of justice, it is important not to look at passages in isolation from the larger theory. Our account of justice is fundamentally that of the moral necessity of creating a just system of healthcare using a suitable model of egalitarian social justice, for both national and international systems of distribution of public health services and healthcare goods.

There is no single principle of justice in the four-principles approach because no single moral principle is capable of addressing all problems of justice. Childress and I have largely defended a group of principles arising from egalitarian theory — for example, the fair opportunity principle, which requires that social institutions affecting healthcare distribution should be arranged, as far as possible, to allow each person to achieve a fair share of the normal range of opportunities present in that society. The fair opportunity principle demands that individuals not receive social benefits on the basis of undeserved advantageous properties

[14] Beauchamp and Childress, *Principles of Biomedical Ethics*, 5th edn.: 347 as used by Dr. Al-Bar.

and should not be denied social benefits on the basis of undeserved disadvantageous properties, because they are not responsible for these properties.[15] I am also influenced by principles of justice that require social support of essential core dimensions of well-being, such as health. These principles require that a decent level of health care be distributed either equally to all citizens or as needed for citizens to achieve a basic level of well-being.[16]

Childress and I take account of the fact that philosophers have developed diverse theories of justice that provide sometimes conflicting principles of justice. We try to show that some merit is found in egalitarian, libertarian, utilitarian, and other theories; and we defend a mixed use of principles drawn from these theories.[17]

2. The Central Place of the Common Morality

An important part of the four-principles approach to biomedical ethics is what Childress and I call *common morality theory*.[18] From centuries of experience we have learned that the human condition tends to deteriorate into misery, confusion, violence, and distrust unless certain principles are enforced through a public system of norms. Everyone living a moral life

---

[15]The fair-opportunity principle descends from John Rawls' principles of justice in *A Theory of Justice*. Cambridge, MA: Harvard University Press: 1971; rev. ed., 1999: 60–67, 302–303 (1999: 52–58). Rawls (2001) later instructively restated, and partially reordered, these principles, giving reasons for their revision, in Erin Kelly (ed.) *Justice as Fairness: A Restatement*. Cambridge, MA: Harvard University Press: 42–43.

[16]This general principle is developed in Madison Powers and Ruth Faden (2006). *Social Justice: The Moral Foundations of Public Health and Health Policy*. New York: Oxford University Press.

[17]For diverse accounts of justice connected to biomedical ethics, see Norman Daniels (2007). *Just Health: Meeting Health Needs Fairly*. New York: Cambridge University Press; Madison Powers and Ruth Faden (2006). *Social Justice: The Moral Foundations of Public Health and Health Policy*. New York: Oxford University Press; Amartya K. Sen (2009). *The Idea of Justice*. London: Allen Lane.

[18]Although there is only one universal common morality, there are various theories of the common morality. For a diverse group of recent theories, see Alan Donagan (1977). *The Theory of Morality*. Chicago: University of Chicago Press; Bernard Gert (2007). *Common Morality: Deciding What to Do*. New York: Oxford University Press; Bernard Gert, Charles M. Culver and K. Danner Çlouser (1997). *Bioethics: A Return to Fundamentals*, 2nd edn. New York: Oxford University Press.

in any society is aware of the fundamental importance of moral standards such as not lying, not stealing others' property, keeping promises, respecting the rights of others, and not killing or causing harm to others. When complied with, these shared norms lessen human misery and foster cooperation. These norms may not be necessary for the *survival* of a society, as some have maintained,[19] but it is not too much to claim that these norms are necessary to ameliorate or counteract the tendency for the quality of people's lives to worsen or for social relationships to disintegrate.[20] The common morality is comprises full set of universal moral norms shared by all persons committed to a moral way of life.[21] Principlism is constructed from this understanding of our common morality.

Some critics think that Childress and I hold that the four principles themselves alone constitute the full set of universal norms. However, we claim far less. We claim only that these principles we have identified and put in the form of a framework for biomedical ethics are a part of universal morality. We selectively draw these principles from the common morality in order to construct a normative framework *for biomedical ethics*. We have not sought a catalogue of universal morality's contents — a vast undertaking. The common morality we hold is consists of *principles (and rules)*, *virtues*, *ideals*, and *rights* — four critical types of norms for understanding the common morality. I will now briefly discuss each of these types.

---

[19]See the sources referenced in Sissela Bok (1995). *Common Values*. Columbia, MO: University of Missouri Press: 13–23, 50–59 (citing influential writers on the subject).

[20]G. J. Warnock (1971). *The Object of Morality*. London; Methuen & Co. esp. 15–26; John Mackie (1977). *Ethics: Inventing Right and Wrong*. London: Penguin: 107ff.

[21]For useful critical assessments of principlist views about common morality theory and its role; see Oliver Rauprich (2008). Common morality: Comment on Beauchamp and Childress. *Theoretical Medicine and Bioethics* 29: 43–71, at 68; K. A. Wallace (2009). Common morality and moral reform. *Theoretical Medicine and Bioethics* 30: 55–68; and Ronald A. Lindsay (2005). Slaves, embryos, and non-human animals: Moral status and the limitations of common morality theory. *Kennedy Institute of Ethics Journal* 15 (December): 323–346.

2.1. *Universal Principles and Rules of Obligation*

I start with a few instances (not a complete catalogue) of universal *principles* and *rules* of obligation in the common morality. The following examples are more concrete rules than the four abstract principles in the framework presented above, but they still are parts of the common morality: (i) Do not kill; (ii) Do not cause pain or suffering to others; (iii) Prevent evil or harm from occurring; (iv) Rescue persons in danger; (v) Tell the truth; (vi) Nurture the young and dependent; (vii) Keep your promises; (viii) Do not steal; (ix) Do not punish the innocent; and (x) Obey the law. These norms have been justified in various ways by various philosophical theories, but I will not treat this problem of justification here.

2.2. *Universal Virtues*

The common morality also contains standards that are *moral character traits,* or *virtues*. Examples are: (i) Honesty; (ii) Integrity; (iii) Nonmalevolence; (iv) Conscientiousness; (v) Trustworthiness; (vi) Fidelity; (vii) Gratitude; (viii) Truthfulness; (ix) Lovingness; and (x) Kindness. The virtues are universally admired traits,[22] and a person is deficient in moral character if he or she lacks these traits. Negative traits amounting to the opposite of the virtues are *vices* (malevolence, dishonesty, lack of integrity, cruelty, etc.). They are substantial moral defects, universally recognized as such by persons committed to morality.

A number of scholars have criticized principlism on the grounds that it neglects the virtues and virtue ethics, thus making principles the sole prominent feature in the landscape of bioethics. This is a mis-assessment:

[22] See Martha Nussbaum's (1988) assessment that, in Aristotelian philosophy, certain "non-relative virtues" are objective and universal: Non-relative virtues: An Aristotelian approach, in Peter French *et al.* (eds.) *Ethical Theory, Character, and Virtue.* Notre Dame, Ind.: University of Notre Dame Press: 32–53, especially 33–34, 46–50.

Childress and I allocate a large segment of our analysis to the role of the virtues in biomedical ethics.[23]

2.3. *Universally Praised Ideals*

In addition to principles of obligation and virtues, moral ideals such as charitable goals, community service, dedication to one's job that exceeds obligatory levels, and service to the poor are also a part of the common morality. These aspirations are not *required* of persons, but they are universally *admired* and *praised* in persons who accept and act on them.[24] Here are four examples that can be interpreted both as ideals of virtuous character and ideals of action: (i) Exceptional forgiveness; (ii) Exceptional generosity; (iii) Exceptional compassion; and (iv) Exceptional thoughtfulness.

2.4. *Universal Rights*

Finally, human rights form an important dimension of universal morality. Rights are justified claims to something that individuals or groups can legitimately assert against other individuals or groups. Human rights, in particular, are those that all humans possess.[25] Human rights language easily crosses national and cultural boundaries and supports international law and policy statements by international agencies and associations. Although human rights are, for this reason, often interpreted as legal rights, this interpretation does not properly capture their status. They are universally valid moral claims, and they have been understood as such at

---

[23] When we published the first edition of *Principles of Biomedical Ethics*, no one in bioethics was then publishing on virtue ethics. We thought this type of theory was an important and unduly neglected subject needing to be brought into the field, especially in light of the history of medical ethics, where the virtues were once prominent in various codes and writings.

[24] See Gert (2007), *op. cit.*, 20–26, 76–77; Richard B. Brandt (1992). Morality and Its Critics, in his *Morality, Utilitarianism, and Rights*. Cambridge: Cambridge University Press: chap. 5.

[25] Cf. Joel Feinberg (1980). *Rights, Justice, and the Bounds of Liberty*. Princeton, NJ: Princeton University Press: esp. 139–141, 149–155, 159–160, 187; See also Alan Gewirth (1996). *The Community of Rights*. Chicago: University of Chicago Press: 8–9.

least since early modern theories of rights were developed in the 17th century.

I defend a strict version of the thesis that rights and obligations are correlative. The correlativity thesis asserts that in all contexts of rights — moral and legal — a system of norms imposes an obligation to act or to refrain from acting so that relevant parties are enabled either to perform some action or to have some good or service provided to them. The language of rights is thus always translatable into the language of obligations: A right entails an obligation, and an obligation entails a right. Obligations without fail imply corresponding rights if they are *bona fide* moral obligations, in contrast to merely self-assumed obligations or personal moral ideals, such as "obligations" of charitable giving.[26] If, for example, a society has an obligation to provide goods such as health care to needy citizens, then any citizen who meets the relevant criteria of need has a right to the available healthcare. All universal principles in this way entail universally valid rights claims. I will return to the connection between principles and moral rights in a later section.

3. Particular Moralities, Moral Pluralism, and Moral Relativism

A persistent question from critics of my views about principles has been concerned with whether the four principles are truly universal. Perhaps they are merely local — e.g. western or American. My emphasis on universal morality also might lead one to think that I do not allow for any form of moral pluralism or for local moral viewpoints — as if morality were a monolithic whole that does not permit disagreements and differences of approach. However, this is a misunderstanding of the connection between universal morality and the moral norms that are particular to cultures, groups, and individuals. Unlike the common morality, with its abstract and content-thin norms, particular moralities present concrete, non-universal, and content-rich norms.

[26] So-called imperfect obligations are moral ideals that allow for discretion in my account. Cf. the somewhat similar conclusions in Feinberg (1980), *op. cit.*, 138–139, 143–144, 148–149.

Particular moralities include the many responsibilities, ideals, attitudes, and sensitivities found in, for example, cultural traditions, religious ethics, and professional guidelines. The reason why norms in particular moralities, including customary moralities, often differ is that the universal starting points in the common morality — its basic principles — can be legitimately developed and specified in different ways to create different guidelines and procedures.

Nonetheless — and this is a key matter in understanding why a moral relativism of principles is an unacceptable theory — *all justified particular moralities share the norms of the common morality with all other justified particular moralities*. That is, all justified particular moralities, without exception, share universal morality. Moral pluralists sometimes seem to claim that there are multiple concepts of morality in the normative sense, and therefore that there are multiple normative moralities. There are, of course, multiple moralities in the descriptive sense of "morality."[27] In the descriptive sense, "morality" refers to groups' codes of conduct. This descriptive sense has no implications for how *all* persons *should* behave. Moralities can differ extensively in the content of their beliefs and in their practice standards. One society might heavily emphasize the liberty of individuals, another, the sanctity of human and animal life over liberty. One society may have established rituals disavowed in another. What is unacceptable in one society might be condoned in another. To let a seriously ill individual die when that person requests shutting down a respirator that sustains the person's life is unacceptable in some societies or institutions, while judged acceptable in others.

In the normative sense of "morality," by contrast, empirical claims about moral belief are not the subject matter. Rather, principles or judgments state what is morally correct under the concept of morality. As stated by Philippa Foot regarding this view, "A moral system [has normative] … starting-points … fixed by the concept of morality.… They belong to the concept of morality — to *the* definition and not to some definition which a man can choose for himself."[28] Moral pluralism, then, is a

[27] On this distinction see Bernard Gert (2002). The Definition of Morality. *The Stanford Encyclopedia of Philosophy*. Available online via http://plato.stanford.edu/entries/morality-definition/(retrieved on 11 February 2008).

[28] Philippa Foot (2002). *Moral Dilemmas*. Oxford: Oxford University Press: 6–7. Peter Herissone-Kelly guided me to this passage.

group-relative notion best interpreted as a version of "morality" in the descriptive sense — that is, as a sociological report on particular moralities. It would be incoherent to formulate the *normative meaning* of the term *morality* as consisting of the norms of multiple moralities with conflicting rules, because morality would, thus, give contradictory advice.

I also caution against an undue emphasis on differences among moral theories that seem to amount to a pluralism *of theory*. Disagreements in theory are usually about the theoretical foundations of morality. Hence, they may mask an underlying and abiding agreement about central considered moral judgments and basic principles. Theoreticians tend to assume, rather than disagree about our deepest moral principles (e.g. prohibiting the breaking of promises, requiring that we not cause harm to others, requiring respect for autonomous choice, etc.). Put another way, many philosophers with different conceptions of the theoretical justification of universal morality do not significantly disagree on the substantive principles, rules, ideals, and virtues that comprise the common morality.

4. The Specification of Norms and the Preservation of Moral Coherence

To say that moral principles have their origins in and find support in the common morality is not to say that their appearance in a well-developed system of biomedical ethics is identical to the norms of the common morality. Principles underdetermine the content of moral judgments because abstract principles have too little content to determine all needed rules and practical judgments. All abstract norms must be carefully defined and then tailored to give specific guidance regarding, for example, how much information must be disclosed, how to maintain confidentiality, when and how to obtain an informed consent, and the like.

General principles must be made specific if they are to become practical. The same is true of laws: If a law is too general, then it will not be a practical instrument. Further legislation would be needed.[29] Specification in morals is a process of adding action-guiding content to general principles.

---

[29] For an excellent study of how the four-principles approach can and should be used as a practical instrument; see John-Stewart Gordon, Oliver Rauprich and Jochen Vollman (2011). Applying the four-principle approach. *Bioethics* 25: 293–300, with a reply by Tom

Specification is not a process of either producing or defending general principles such as those in the common morality. Specification starts only after they are available. Specifying the norms with which one starts, whether those in the common morality or norms that were previously specified, is accomplished by *narrowing the scope* of the norms, not by explaining what the general norms *mean*.[30] As Henry Richardson puts it, specification occurs by "spelling out where, when, why, how, by what means, to whom, or by whom the action is to be done or avoided."[31]

For example, a possible specification of "respect the autonomy of persons" is "respect the autonomy of competent patients when they become incompetent by following their advance directives." This specification works well in some medical contexts but will not be adequate in others, which leaves a need for additional specification. Progressive specification may need to be continued indefinitely, gradually reducing the conflicts of norms that abstract principles themselves cannot resolve. To qualify all along the way as a specification, a transparent connection must continuously be maintained to the initial norm that gives moral authority to the resulting string of specified norms.

More than one line of specification of principles is commonly available when confronting practical problems and moral disagreements. Different persons or groups may justifiably offer conflicting specifications. It is an inescapable part of the moral life that different persons and groups will offer different, sometimes conflicting, specifications, thus potentially creating multiple particular moralities. On deeply problematic

---

Beauchamp (2011). Making principlism practical: A commentary on Gordon, Rauprich, and Vollmann. *Bioethics* 25: 301–303.

[30] Henry S. Richardson (1990). Specifying norms as a way to resolve concrete ethical problems. *Philosophy and Public Affairs* 19: 279–310; and Specifying, balancing, and interpreting bioethical principles, in James F. Childress, Eric M. Meslin, and Harold T. Shapiro (eds.). *Belmont Revisited: Ethical Principles for Research with Human Subjects*. Washington, DC: Georgetown University Press: 205–227; David DeGrazia (1992). Moving forward in bioethical theory: Theories, cases, and specified principlism. *Journal of Medicine and Philosophy* 17: 511–539; and David DeGrazia and Tom L. Beauchamp (2001). Philosophical foundations and philosophical methods, in D. Sulmasy and J. Sugarman (eds.). *Methods of Bioethics*. Washington, DC: Georgetown University Press: esp. 33–36.

[31] Richardson (2005), *op. cit.*, 289.

issues such as abortion, animal research, aid in disaster relief, health inequities, and euthanasia, competing specifications will be offered even by reasonable and fair-minded parties committed to the common morality.

4.1. *Examples of Particular Moralities and Their Specifications*

Professional moralities such as those in biomedical research, medical practice, nursing practice, and veterinary practice are good examples of particular moralities that contain at least some specifications not found in other particular moralities. Medical moral codes, declarations, and standards of practice often *legitimately vary* from other medical moralities in the ways they handle justice in access to healthcare, human rights, justified waivers of informed consent, government oversight of research involving human subjects, privacy provisions, and the like. Both approaches can be justified if they coherently specify universal morality — that is, if they specify the universal principles that form the core of the common morality.

Other examples of particular moralities that contain differing specifications are *religious moralities*. Religious traditions may have multiple moralities within the spread of a single religious faith. So-called Protestant Christianity is an example. Each sect of Protestant Christianity (Lutherans, Presbyterians, Methodists, Episcopalians, etc.) can deviate in the specification of its own code of ethics. They share the common morality, but they do not share whatever makes each one distinctively the religious group it is in its moral outlooks. As with any particular morality distinctive to a tradition, a religious group will state what is permissible and impermissible and what is obligatory and non-obligatory.

A distinctive religious morality, being a particular morality, often has no capacity to reach out into a public arena of discussion in a pluralistic society; that is, public policy cannot in a pluralistic context be fixed purely by appeal to the norms of a particular religious morality. For example, if this morality requires prayers before all public meetings, it cannot expect that this rule is suitable to govern those in society who do not share this belief and practice. This limitation could be considered a disadvantage inherent in particular moralities as they operate in pluralistic societies.

However, I want to be emphatic about the point that very significant advantages are found in a well-specified religious morality. The common morality — being general and only general — does not have and cannot have the same richness and specificity that a particular morality does. Moreover, a particular morality does not forego universal morality; it retains and is governed by universal morality. These are great advantages for particular moralities.

An interesting example of specification is found in some comments made by Professor Ali Al-Qaradaghi when he discusses patient's permission for a necessary medical intervention. He mentions that, "The patient's permission of the treatment is essential if the patient is in full legal capacity to give it. If he is not, the permission of his (or her) legal guardian shall be sought according to the order of guardianship in *Sharia*." The "in *Sharia*" specification is noteworthy. The points he makes about both required permission and guardian authority is in effect a universally observed rule today in biomedical ethics, just as informed consent is. What the language of "in *Sharia*" adds here is how, *in a particular morality, the guardianship matter is to be determined.* Those who follow Sharia law know, as a result of this specification, how it is determined who will be the guardian in any given case. This specification is a guardianship-selection rule. Every particular medical morality will have such a rule of guardianship specification, and quite legitimately so, even though the connected rules of permission and guardianship are universal.

A second rule mentioned in this same context of discussion by the Professor is, "In emergency cases, when the life of the victim is in danger, medical treatment shall not depend on permission." This is a *de facto* universal rule in clinical ethics that is not placed in a context of a particular morality. All medical moralities now accept this principle.

4.2. *Justifying Specifications Using a Method of Coherence*

Since there can be numerous specifications, the question arises of what justifies some specifications and does not justify others. A specification is justified, in my account, if and only if it is consistent with (does not violate) the norms of common morality and maximizes the coherence of the overall set of relevant, justified beliefs of the party doing the specification.

These beliefs could include empirically justified beliefs, justified basic moral beliefs, and previously justified specifications. This position is a version of the philosophical account of method, justification, and theory-construction in ethics known as wide reflective equilibrium.[32] This theory holds that justification in ethics occurs through a reflective testing of moral beliefs, moral principles, and theoretical postulates with the goal of making them as coherent as possible. The goal of any given specification is to achieve an equilibrium while also resolving a contingent conflict of principles.

This method demands assessment of the strengths and weaknesses of the full body of all relevant and impartially formulated judgments, principles, theories, and facts (hence the "wide" scope of the account). Moral views to be included are beliefs about particular cases, about rules and principles, about virtue and character, about consequentialist and non-consequentialist forms of justification, about the role of moral sentiments, and so forth. The resultant moral and political norms can then be tested in a variety of previously unexamined circumstances to see if incoherent results emerge. If incoherence arises, conflicting norms must be adjusted to the point of coherence.

Achieving a state of reflective equilibrium in which all beliefs fit together coherently, with no residual conflicts or incoherence, is an ideal that will not be comprehensively realized by anyone. A stable equilibrium in the full set of one's moral and political beliefs is an unrealistic goal. We can only expect conscientious approximation of the ideal. There is no reason to expect that the process of rendering norms coherent by specification will ever come to an end or be perfected. However, this ideal is not a utopian theory toward which no progress can be made. Particular moralities (of individuals and groups) are, from this perspective, works

---

[32] Norman Daniels (1996). Wide reflective equilibrium in practice, in L.W. Sumner and J. Boyle (eds.). *Philosophical Perspectives on Bioethics*. Toronto: University of Toronto Press: 96–114; John D. Arras (2007). The way we reason now: Reflective equilibrium in bioethics, in Bonnie Steinbock, (ed.). *The Oxford Handbook of Bioethics*. Oxford: Oxford University Press: 46–71; Carson Strong (2010). Theoretical and practical problems with wide reflective equilibrium in bioethics. *Theoretical Medicine and Bioethics* 31: 123–140; Norman Daniels (1996). *Justice and Justification: Reflective Equilibrium in Theory and Practice*. New York: Cambridge University Press; Norman Daniels (2003). Reflective Equilibrium, *Stanford Encyclopedia of Philosophy* (retrieved 24 August 2007).

continuously in progress, a process of improvement rather than a finished product. Moralities can be rendered coherent in more than one way through the process of specification.

To take an example from the ethics of the distribution of organs for transplantation, imagine that an institution has used and continues to be attracted to two policies, each of which rests on a basic rule: (i) distribute organs by expected number of years of survival (to maximize the beneficial outcome of the procedure), and (ii) distribute organs by using a waiting list (to give every candidate an equal opportunity). These two distributive principles are inconsistent and need to be brought into equilibrium in the institution's policies. Both can be retained in a system of fair distribution if coherent limits are placed on the norms. For example, organs could be distributed by expected years of survival to persons 65 years of age and older, and organs could be distributed by a waiting list for 64 years of age and younger. Proponents of such a policy would need to justify and render, as specifically as possible, their reasons for these two different commitments. Such proposals need to be made internally coherent in the system of distribution and also need to be made coherent with all other principles and rules pertaining to distribution, such as norms regarding discrimination against the elderly and fair payment schemes for expensive medical procedures.

5. Human Rights and Multiculturalism

Confusion continues to be plentiful regarding differences in Eastern and Western cultures and about the role, if any, that universal principles play in making judgments about moral claims made in different moral traditions. In my view, little supports the commonly reported thesis that the East — that is, Asia — has fundamentally different moral traditions of liberty, rights, respect for autonomy, and respect for families from those in the West — that is, Europe and the Americas. I will concentrate in my comments on the universal norms of morality, and in particular on human rights.

5.1. *Human Rights and Universal Principles*

The view that I take of cultural differences and basic principles is notably similar to Amartya Sen's in his monograph on "Human Rights and Asian

Values."[33] Sen is, of course, from India, and so his personal history of moral beliefs presumably descends from an Eastern culture. But Sen wholly rejects the way Eastern views are commonly presented, in parts of both the East and the West, especially regarding freedom and human rights. He points out that "no quintessential [moral] values … *differentiate* Asians as a group from people in the rest of the world." He finds that the major constituent components of universally valid ideas of liberty and basic rights of liberty, especially political liberty, are found in both Eastern and Western traditions, even though the idea of human rights is relatively new to *all* parts of the world. The claim that these ideas are friendly to Western tradition and alien to Eastern traditions he finds "hard to make any sense of." I completely agree.

I do not mean that a principle such as respect for individual autonomy is given precisely the same status and prized to the same extent in Eastern traditions as it might be in some Western cultures. Many populations in the East may legitimately prioritize community and relationships over individual autonomy and cultural independence to *a higher degree* than do many populations in the West. But this thesis does not entail that Eastern populations deprecate or reject human rights of individual autonomy or that they disvalue political liberty. Nor does it indicate that Western populations deprecate community and relationships. These claims are fundamentally myths about differences between the East and the West.

Research ethics is an interesting area in which the universal reach of some principles is now globally acknowledged. Around 40 years ago there were no universally accepted principles of research ethics, but today we see a vast similarity, in countries on every continent, in codes, laws, and regulations governing research with human subjects. There are some understandable and justifiable differences from country to country, but the differences pale in comparison to the similarities in the shared moral principles and legal norms governing how biomedical research can and cannot be conducted. Rules of informed consent — which were only a few years ago deeply questioned or simply not discussed in various cultures — are now universally accepted. Here are a few steeply abridged examples of

[33] Amartya Sen (1997). *Human Rights and Asian Values.* New York: Carnegie Council, with an Introduction by Joel H. Rosenthal, esp. 10, 13, 17, 27, 30.

the principles of research ethics that are globally accepted (and violations of them universally condemned):

- Disclose all material information to subjects of research.
- Obtain a voluntary, informed consent to medical interventions.
- Maintain secure safeguards for keeping personal information about subjects private and confidential.
- Receive surrogate consent from a legally authorized representative for incompetent subjects.
- Ethics review committees must scrutinize and approve research protocols.
- Research cannot be conducted unless its risks and intended benefits are reasonably balanced, and risks must be reduced to avoid excessive risk.
- Special justification is required if proposed research subjects are vulnerable persons.

These norms of the obligations of researchers and sponsors all have correlative human rights that protect research subjects.[34]

A Final Point about Universal Morality

Professor Ali Al-Qaradaghi comments that in using the language of "biomedical ethics,"

> [Beauchamp] refers here to the beginning of those four principles as a structured framework and the appearance of writings that focused on interpreting and explaining them. Actually the history of ethics, including medical ethics, is quite old and they are extracted from the ethical values taught by the heavenly religions; namely Judaism, Christianity, and Islam.

---

[34] See, as examples of international documents that can easily be so interpreted, the World Medical Association's *Declaration of Helsinki*, 2008 revision, "Declaration of Helsinki: Ethical Principles for Medical Research Involving Human Subjects," Part B, "Basic Principles for all Medical Research" (first adopted 1964 and currently under revision); Council for International Organization of Medical Science (CIOMS), in collaboration with the World Health Organization (WHO), *International Ethical Guidelines for Biomedical Research Involving Human Subjects* (Geneva: CIOMS 2002) (currently under revision).

The Professor is both right and wrong here. *Biomedical* ethics did not exist until its origins in roughly the last half of the 20th century. The ancient traditions were all about *medical — not biomedical* ethics. Ancient views of medical ethics were literally from a different world lacking medical science. Also, I was not referring to "the beginning of th[e] four principles." I meant only to refer to changes that occurred in the 20th century that led us away from an outmoded Hippocratic medical ethics to a biomedical ethics.

However — and this is an important point to me — when I use the language of the *common morality* I *do* mean to include ancient moral traditions, including what the Professor refers to as "the heavenly religions." These anciently formed traditions do not represent *biomedical* ethics; but they are excellent representatives of the common morality. Likewise, the four principles I defend are part of the common morality. These four principles are not inherently created for biomedical ethics; they must be made suitable for that context and specified. That is, that they are not biomedical principles until they are specifically embedded in a biomedical context is what Childress and I have tried to show.

5.2. *Multiculturalism as a Theory of Universal Principles*

I return now to my earlier observations about particular moralities, pluralism, and relativism. It is an undisputed fact that multiple cultures have constructed unique, particular moralities. This fact suggests to some writers in bioethics that we live in a multicultural world in which diverse particular moral cultures can live together peacefully, without need for the notion of universal, basic principles. However, this characterization has matters upside down. Multiculturalism is not a pluralism or a relativism. It is a theory of universal principles to the effect that particular moralities are owed respect because morality demands it. The term "multicultural world" has been hijacked by some writers in bioethics to suggest the reverse and especially to suggest that there is no commonly held morality.[35]

[35] Examples are H. Tristram Engelhardt Jr. (1996). *The Foundations of Bioethics*, 2nd edn. New York: Oxford University Press; Robert Baker (1998). A theory of international

"Multiculturalism," properly used, refers to a type of theory that supports the moral principle that cultural or group traditions, institutions, perspectives, and practices should be respected and should not be violated or oppressed as long as they do not themselves violate the standards of universal morality. The objective of multiculturalism is to provide a theory of the norms that suitably protect vulnerable groups when they are threatened with marginalization and oppression caused by one or more dominant cultures. Resistance to forceful dominance and cultural oppression are the motivating forces of multiculturalist theory, which holds that respect is owed to people of dissimilar but peaceful cultural traditions *because* it is unjust and disrespectful to marginalize, oppress, or dominate persons merely because they are of an unlike culture or subculture. The moral notions at work in multicultural theory are universal-principle driven theses about rights, justice, respect, and non-oppression.[36] Without universal norms of toleration, respect, restraint, and the like, a multiculturalist could neither explain nor justify multiculturalism.

5.3. *Are Principles a Disguised Form of Cultural Imperialism?*

Some may think that my support of transcendent, universal moral standards is merely a disguised form of cultural imperialism. Persons outside of a given culture who press for recognition within that culture of the human rights of women, minorities, children, the ill, the disabled, the oppressed, the marginalized, the economically disadvantaged, and other vulnerable groups have often been denounced as cultural imperialists who incorporate their own values, which are uncritically assumed to be universally valid, but that — beneath the veneer of fairness, equity, and respect — camouflage the continuance of some form of dominance.

---

bioethics: Multiculturalism, postmodernism, and the bankruptcy of fundamentalism. *Kennedy Institute of Ethics Journal* 8: 201–231; Leigh Turner (2003). Bioethics in a multicultural world: Medicine and morality in pluralistic settings. *Health Care Analysis* 11: 99–117.

[36]Compare the essays in Robert K. Fullinwider (ed.) (1996). *Public Education in a Multicultural Society.* Cambridge: Cambridge University Press; and Amy Gutmann (ed.) (1992). *Multiculturalism and "The Politics of Recognition"*. Princeton NJ: Princeton University Press.

The real problem here is that virtually every region of the world has experienced a horrid history of imperialistic control extending from one people to another, whether from west to east, within regions, or within the borders of a single nation. Numerous cultural traditions, past and present, and in all parts of the world, have held that their values are universal values to which everyone must conform. They all deserve condemnation.

6. Conclusion

I have argued in defense of the four-principles approach to biomedical ethics, now increasingly called principlism. My arguments move to the conclusion that a universal set of moral principles comprises the common morality and that the four clusters of principles of biomedical ethics are part of, but not the whole of, the common morality that all morally committed persons share. Although the content of these norms is thin, owing to their abstractness, they create a wall of moral standards that cannot justifiably be violated in any culture or by any group or individual. They give us our moral compass and are our ultimate bulwark against a descent into relativism.

Response by Ali Al-Qaradaghi to Tom Beauchamp's Paper

Ali Al-Qaradaghi

This chapter is a response to the research presented by Tom Beauchamp regarding The Four Principles of Biomedical Ethics. The methodology adopted by the chapter will be an examination of these principles so as to determine their legal foundation, historical background, and the extent to which they can be considered comprehensive principles. This examination will be framed within an objective, constructive discussion aiming to achieve the goals of benefit and excellence as outlined by the research Center for Islamic Legislation and Ethics (CILE).

The four principles of biomedical ethics according to Beauchamp are:

(a) *Respect for Autonomy*

This principle is concerned with the patient. It is defined as a person's free will and freedom of choice without any interference from other persons. Beauchamp outlines two conditions for autonomy: "liberty (the absence of controlling influences)" and "agency (self-initiated intentional action)."[1] It means that the patient is free to accept or refuse certain medication and

[1] Tom Beauchamp (2016). *The Principles of Biomedical Ethics as Universal Principles*, included in this volume. Singapore: World Scientific.

requires that a physician respects the requests made by the patient, if he is able to, or by his family on his behalf. Despite the ethical issues that arise in situations where a patient refuses a necessary medical intervention, the principlist approach prioritizes respect for autonomy over other ethical principles. However, Beauchamp states that this prioritization may be dismissed in certain cases. He explains, "Many kinds of competing moral considerations can validly override respect for autonomy under conditions of a contingent conflict of norms. For example, if our choices endanger the public health, potentially harm innocent others, or require a scarce and unfunded resource, exercises of autonomy can justifiably be restrained or overridden."[2]

Given this clarification, it becomes clear that this is not an absolute principle and is not applicable in all cases. Rather, it is more of a general rule that is susceptible to exceptions that also require clearly defined guidelines. The guidelines for these exceptional cases were outlined by the International Islamic Fiqh Academy (IIFA), affiliated with the Organization of Islamic Cooperation (OIC), in its resolution no. 69/5/7. The exceptional cases as identified by the resolution are: infectious diseases, caesarian operations for saving the life of a newborn baby even if the mother and her husband refuse the operation, and accidents during which a patient has lost consciousness.[3]

(b) *Nonmaleficence*

This principle refers to the prevention of harm and injury and is associated with the Hippocratic medical ethics according to the mandate, "Above all [or first] do no harm." This principle is also included in the Hippocratic Oath. The principle of nonmaleficence establishes a variety of specific ethical rules, among which are:

(i) "Don't kill."
(ii) "Don't cause pain or suffering to others."
(iii) "Don't incapacitate others."

---

[2] *Ibid.*
[3] See *International Islamic Fiqh Academy* 3(7): 731–733.

In this regard, Beauchamp quotes the British physician Thomas Percival, who asserted that, "a principle of nonmaleficence fixes the physician's primary obligations and triumphs even over respect for the patient's autonomy in a circumstance of potential harm to patients."[4]

(c) *Beneficence*

This principle refers to the promotion of good. Beauchamp acknowledges that the line between that which is demanded under the principle of beneficence and that which is not is undoubtedly difficult to draw. In fact, it is deemed impossible to draw a precise line under this principle without considering the particulars of different contexts.[5] There have been many contentious debates arguing for the sufficiency of the principle of nonmaleficence and the possibility of it replacing the principle of beneficence. However, Beauchamp rejects this proposition, arguing that a physician's commitment to preventing harm cannot be merged with his commitment to providing them with care. An example of the first would be preventing murder or disablement while the latter involves advancing the interests of people.[6] On the other hand, one can argue that the principle of beneficence implies that of nonmaleficence and preventing harm, as will be discussed later.

(d) *Justice*

Justice in this context refers to the fair distribution of health care and its costs within societies. It also refers to the fair opportunity principle.[7] Given this understanding, this principle primarily addresses governments rather than physicians.

After reviewing each of these points, I can honestly say that this is a very well-written research paper serving to elaborate on the four principles of biomedical ethics as developed by Tom Beauchamp and James

---

[4] See Beauchamp (2016), *op. cit.*
[5] *Ibid.*
[6] *Ibid.*
[7] *Ibid.*

Childress since 1976 and to this day. There is no exaggeration in stating that it is invaluable research. Therefore, I merely have a few clarifying points to add with the purpose of providing an Islamic foundation to these principles which, as outlined in my distinct chapter, will lead to the development of a comprehensive theory that is compatible with Islamic values and principles.

1. A Historical Perspective

In introducing the origin of biomedical ethics, Dr. Beauchamp states, "Principles that can be understood with relative ease by the members of various disciplines figured prominently in the early developments in the history of biomedical ethics during the 1970s and early 1980s."[8] In this regard, I believe Dr. Beauchamp is referring specifically to the emergence of these four principles as a structured framework and the appearance of writings that focused on interpreting, explaining, and connecting them. However, the history of ethics (including medical ethics) is rather ancient and can be traced back to the ethical values taught by the heavenly religions, namely Judaism, Christianity, and Islam, notwithstanding slight discrepancies in details, foundations, and terminology. Moreover, the presence of general ethical principles can be found across several ancient civilizations, such as the Pharaonic Civilization, Hamurabi's Code of Laws, ancient Greek philosophy, and Buddhist and Hindu civilizations.

For example, in the Ancient Egyptian civilization, the *Book of the Dead* mentions that a dead person is brought to stand in front of the God Osiris. The dead person then justifies his actions saying, "I come to you my lord in submission to witness your magnificence; I come bearing truth and abandoning dishonesty, for I have never been unjust towards another and have avoided the path of those gone astray." He then accounts that he was never disobedient, nor a liar, nor harmful to others, nor committed or assisted with murder, nor a thief, nor committed adultery or embezzlement, nor violated the sanctity of death, nor cheated in trade. He then states, "I am pure, I am pure, I am pure, and as long as I am innocent of

[8] *Ibid.*

sin, place me amongst the victorious my Lord."[9] Other similar examples include Hamurabi's Code of Law, the Hippocratic Oath and the Islamic Oath.[10]

2. The Source and Authority of Ethics

The argument for the importance of ethics in general, and that of medical ethics in particular, is eloquently presented by Dr. Beauchamp. He explains, "If some principles were dropped from the framework, the demands of the moral life would not be what we know those demands to be, just as a landscape would not be the same landscape if certain rocks, trees, or plants were removed from it."[11] He also adds,

> From centuries of experience we have learned that the human condition tends to deteriorate into misery, confusion, violence, and distrust unless certain principles are enforced through a public system of norms. Everyone living a moral life in any society is aware of the fundamental importance of moral standards such as not lying, not stealing others' property, keeping promises, respecting the rights of others, and not killing or causing harm to others. When complied with, these shared norms lessen human misery and foster cooperation. These norms may not be necessary for the *survival* of a society, as some have maintained, but it is not too much to claim that these norms are necessary to ameliorate or counteract the tendency for the quality of people's lives to worsen or for social relationships to disintegrate.[12]

While Dr. Beauchamp emphasized the importance of ethics as well as the four principles, he considered ethics to be the source from which

---

[9] See Mohammed Ali Al-Bar (2010). *Ethics: Its Religious Fundamentals and Its Philosophical Roots* (*Al-akhlāq: uṣūluhā al-dīnīyah wa-judhūruhā al-falsafīyah*). Kunuz Al-Ma'arif: 62.

[10] See *Encyclopedia Britannica* (1982), 15th edn. vol. 4, 878; Ibn Abi Usaybi'ah (1995). *The Best Accounts of the Biographies of Physicians* (*'Uyūn Al-anbā' Fīṭabaqāt Al-aṭibbā'*) Beirut: Maktabat Al-Hayat, 1965: 45.

[11] Beauchamp (2016), *op. cit.*

[12] *Ibid.*

adherence to the four principles emerges. In this regard he wrote, "All principles can in some contexts be justifiably overridden by other moral norms with which they come into contingent conflict."[13] I argue that the practice and impact of morality will be undermined if commitment to moral principles is contingent merely on ethical obligation. In fact, the foundational commitment to these principles as presented in Beauchamp's paper appears weak and fragile. The reason for this lies in the fact that Beauchamp, as well as other moral philosophers, founded their moral theory on utilitarianism without taking religious aspects into consideration. This means that in situations where ethics conflict with certain economic interests prohibited by Islam and other religions (such as alcohol), priority is given to those interests over religion despite their negative social impact outweighing their benefits. As God explains, "They ask you about wine and gambling. Say, 'In them is great sin and [yet, some] benefit for people. But their sin is greater than their benefit'..." (Qur'an 2:219).

It is well known that the most resolute commitments arise from religious obligation and legislation. Otherwise, we would have to rely on the integrity of a person's conscience, which can be rather volatile. All in all, if a person is not driven by a fear of God and hope for His reward, he will easily be tempted to pursue his own personal interests and will most likely prioritize his own interests above others. It is quite likely that he will surrender to his whims, desires, and individualistic perspective, which, as often seen, has led to the strangest outcomes due to people's lack of piety, fear of God, and negligence of the Day of Judgment.

2.1. *Violations Associated with the "Active Conscience" Slogan*

Below is an example demonstrating that conscience alone is insufficient to ensure moral commitment and that strong religious endorsement and legislation is necessary.

Beauchamp and Childress emphasize in their book *Principles of Biomedical Ethics* the fact that African-Americans suffering from hypertension should not be treated in a hospital's Casualty Department if they do not have medical insurance. They argue that several researchers have

---

[13] *Ibid.*

found that poor patients with such circumstances will be unable to continue or follow-up their medication due to the absence of a family physician or their lack of medical insurance. Hence, they consider treating them to be a waste of time, effort and money.[14] As stated by Dr. Mohammed Ali Al-Bar, both Beauchamp and Childress agree, without explicitly stating so, that these patients should be left to suffer and die from their hypertension or its sequelae e.g. strokes, heart attacks, heart failure, and kidney failure.

If this is the view supported by the authors of *Principles of Biomedical Ethics*, what is to be expected from those who do not concern themselves with writing about ethics? Rather, what was expected from these two ethicists was a criticism of the unjust American healthcare system that excludes 50 million citizens from the right to medical treatment, especially given that America was not suffering from a financial crisis at that time and, in fact, was one of the world's richest countries. It is truly intriguing, on the other hand, to find that Cuba, America's poorer neighbor, provides free medical insurance not only to its citizens, but also to those visiting Cuba.[15] In addition, great deals of serious ethical violations have been taking place since 1915 and to this day, indicating a prevalent lack of morality in experiments conducted by hospitals, pharmaceutical companies, and other institutions.[16]

Sincere belief (*īmān*), on the other hand, establishes God-consciousness (*taqwá*), fear of God, a desire for His reward, and constant awareness of God's watchfulness in all situations. This belief serves as a genuine internal incentive for a person to observe good deeds and avoid harming others. It is described as a state of *iḥsān*, which follows the stages of *īmān* (sincere belief) and Islam. As explained by the Prophet — may the peace and blessings of God be upon him (PBUH) — in the authentic tradition, "*Iḥsān* is to worship God as if you see Him, and if you do not achieve this state of devotion, then (take it for granted that) God sees you."[17]

---

[14] Tom Beauchamp and James Childress (1979). *Principles of Biomedical Ethics*. Oxford: Oxford University Press: 347–348, footnote 8.
[15] *Ibid.*
[16] *Ibid.*
[17] Taken from a *hadith* reported by Bukhari, Book of Iman, no. 4777 and Muslim, Book of Iman, no. 9 on the authority of Abu Hurayrah.

3. Are The Four Principles All-inclusive and Restrictive?

The four principles of biomedical ethics are not representative of all common morality and not based on complete induction. Rather, they form a part of a larger moral framework. Beauchamp acknowledges this (as does Childress in their coauthored book), stating in his research, "Some critics think that Childress and I hold that the four principles constitute the full set of universal norms. However, we claim far less. We claim only that these principles we have identified and put in the form of a framework for biomedical ethics are a part of universal morality. We selectively draw these principles from the common morality in order to construct a normative framework *for biomedical ethics*."[18]

Therefore, these principles are neither comprehensive nor precursory. Instead, they are founded on this larger framework whose very structure is debatable. For instance, whereas justice is included as one of the four principles, the question arises as to why equal treatment of all patients is not included as a principle. Equality is arguably just as significant a principle serving to prevent discrimination based on aspects such as wealth, race, etc. Likewise, there are countless other ethical principles that may be considered worthy of inclusion in the framework of biomedical principles. These include principles such as loyalty towards a physician's teachers and mentors — as included in the Hippocratic and Islamic Oath — and honesty, transparency, keeping promises, and upholding contracts.

It is worth noting that, as acknowledged by both Beauchamp and Childress, these principles are merely an attempt at constructing a normative framework for biomedical ethics and are not intended to encompass all morals, values, and ideals. Nonetheless, these are truly admirable efforts leading to a positive attempt, although there remains a need for further discussion and critique.

3.1. *The Distinction between Principles and Common Morality*

Prior to discussing this topic, it must be noted that Beauchamp differentiates between the four principles and common morality. He defines the

[18] Beauchamp (2016), *op. cit.*

four principles as the normative framework for biomedical ethics and common morality as that which encompasses several other rules and values such as: "(i) Do not kill; (ii) Do not cause pain or suffering to others; (iii) Prevent evil or harm from occurring; (iv) Rescue persons in danger; (v) Tell the truth; (vi) Nurture the young and dependent; (vii) Keep your promises; (viii) Do not steal; (ix) Do not punish the innocent; and (x) Obey the law."[19] Given this distinction, we can confidently say that the four principles do not cover the range of morals, values, and religious and human ideals. In fact, the method through which certain ethics are categorized as principles while others are not is in itself debatable and subject to ongoing discussion.

On a different note, it may be acceptable to conflate nonmaleficence and beneficence under the single principle of beneficence, which is defined as promoting good. This definition implies one's avoidance of causing harm to others. In regards to this issue, some scholars of Islamic jurisprudence have indeed categorized preventing harm under the principle of interests (*maṣlaḥah*) since this prevention is in itself a benefit and seeks to advance interests. In turn, the two principles are considered synonymous.

4. Physician's Internal Morality

The four principles afford little attention to the development of the physician's internal morality. As demonstrated earlier, their concern is primarily with external actions and behaviors. Needless to say, it is the physician in particular, and people in general, around which all these principles and actions revolve and through which they come to fruition. Therefore, in order to ensure the practice of these principles, it is necessary that morals and values be ingrained within all individuals in the field of medicine, ranging from the physician to the custodian. It is a known fact that the process of moral development begins from early childhood and continues on through higher education taking place at home and in other institutions. However, this moral development can only be firmly ingrained through associating it with God-consciousness and a belief in God and the Day of

---

[19] *Ibid.*

Judgment. It is perhaps this negligence of the element of faith, which started during the Renaissance era, that has resulted in today's European and Western reality. In my opinion, this argument is one that is perhaps embraced by all individuals who believe in God and the Last Day, whether they are Jewish, Christian, or Muslim or belong to any other religion that is based on the belief in a person's accountability to an Omniscient God.

The connection between morality and faith is a central issue in Islam and is pervasive throughout its creed, worship practices, and rituals, all of which are intended to affect a person's actions and behavior. For example, a person who, believes that God sees him in all situations will be wary of disobeying God's commandments or committing any sins. He believes that God is Omnipotent over His creation. In turn, he holds a firm conviction that if he commits any injustice, harm, or betrayal towards another person or practices any other type of wrongdoing and does not suffer consequences in this world, he will undoubtedly be held accountable for these actions and will suffer due punishment on the Day of Judgment. On the other hand, if he obeys God's orders and maintains positive conduct, he will be rewarded accordingly and will enter Paradise in the Hereafter.

As with belief, Islam emphasizes a strong connection between worship practices and their impact on a person's behavior. For instance, in regards to prayer, God says, "... Indeed, prayer prohibits immorality and wrongdoing ..." (Qur'an 29:45). In regards to fasting, God says, "O you who have believed, decreed upon you is fasting as it was decreed upon those before you that you may attain *taqwá*" (Qur'an 2:183). Similarly, in reference to almsgiving (*zakāh*), God says, "Take, [O, Muhammad], from their wealth a charity by which you purify them and cause them increase, and invoke [God's blessings] upon them. Indeed, your invocations are reassurance for them. And God is Hearing and Knowing" (Qur'an 9:103). In other words, it is intended to purify their hearts from greed, selfishness, and other evils of the heart and simultaneously enable them to rise to noble character. In fact, prior to prayer, God described good moral behavior and noble character as a form of worship in His saying, "And the servants of the Most Merciful are those who walk upon the earth easily, and when the ignorant address them [harshly], they say [words of] peace" (Qur'an 25:63).

Indeed, all religions founded on the belief in God and the Last Day have a profound effect on their followers and establish a strong commitment to ethics and moral behavior. This element of faith should not be neglected, especially within environments characterized with a strong religious aspect. For those societies that lack this religious element, morality should be nurtured in accordance with the natural disposition (*fiṭrah*) that all humans are born with.

A final issue that I would like to address is the correlation between the principles of beneficence and utilitarianism. There has been a great deal of controversy around this issue by those critics doubting the applicability of beneficence as a foundation for making ethical decisions. In her paper "Applying the Four Principles," Professor R. Macklin describes a study that was designed to determine the economic and health impacts of selling a kidney. The study's participants comprised 305 individuals from Chennai, India who had sold their kidneys. According to the results of the study, 96 percent of the participants had sold their kidneys to pay off debts, and the average price of a kidney was $1,070. Most of the money received was spent on debts, food, and clothing. The study also revealed that the effects of undergoing a nephrectomy included a one-third decrease in the average family income of participants, and 86 percent of participants reported deterioration in their health. Further, 97 percent of the participants did not recommend for others to sell their kidneys.

Although this is one study that took place in one country, it nonetheless highlights a critical issue that remains contentious to this day. That is, how can the negative social, economic, and health impacts be balanced with the benefits received by those who purchase the kidneys?[20] Macklin also referred to another anthropological study that found that the predominant reason behind people selling kidneys was their need to pay off high interest debts to local moneylenders. In addition, it found that most

[20] See Ruth Macklin (2003). Applying the four principles. *Journal of Medical Ethics* 29(5): 275–280.

of the money from selling a kidney ended up with organ brokers, while only a small portion was paid to the sellers themselves.

References Used for this Response

(1) Some Islamic sources including the Qur'an, books of exegesis, books of *hadith*, and books tackling the issue of morality and self-purification such as: Al-Ghazali, M.: *Iḥyā' 'ulūm al-dīn* and books of Ibn Al-Qayyim on ethics and self-purification.
(2) I referred to some books on medicine and medical ethics, such as books of Dr. Mohammed Al-Bar, Dr. Hassan Hathout, etc.
(3) I made use of websites of medicine and medical ethics and some translated journals.
(4) I referred to the following books:

(A) Ali Al-Muhammadi and Ali Al-Qaradaghi (2005). *Fiqh al-qaḍāyā al-ṭibbīyah al-mu'āṣirah*. Beirut: Dar Al-Basha'ir Al-Islamiyah.
(B) Nahidah Al-Baqsami (1993). *Al-handasah al-wirāthīyah wa-al-akhlāq*, 'Alam Al-Ma'rifah series. Kuwait: National Council for Culture and Art.
(C) David B. Resnik (1998). *The Ethics of Science*: *An Introduction*. London: Routledge.
(D) Zuhayr Al-Karmi (1978). *Al-'ilm wa-mushkilāt al-insān al-mu'āṣir*, 'Alam Al-Ma'rifah series. Kuwait: National Council for Culture and Art.

The Principles of Biomedical Ethics Revisited

Annelien L. Bredenoord

Abstract: The four-principles approach became widely used in Western healthcare and academia. However, ever since its introduction, this approach has also evoked debate. How should the principles be interpreted? Is there a hierarchy between the four principles? To whom do they apply, i.e. to whom do we owe these moral obligations and who should be included within the moral circle? How can concrete action-guides be derived from the abstract principles? Are the principles indeed universal, as proponents argue? Are these general principles sufficiently sophisticated to function as a bioethical theory — pejoratively called "principlism"? In this chapter, I examine first the premise and challenges of each principle. Subsequently, I identify three debates regarding principlism as a bioethical theory and method: (i) whether a pluralist or eclectic approach is an appropriate one and if so, whether general principles are sufficiently sophisticated to function as a bioethical theory; (ii) whether there is a hierarchy in the principles; and (iii) how to arrive at concrete moral judgments from general ethical principles. I conclude with some future directions for the four-principles approach.

1. Introduction

Bioethics has become a field of scholarly enquiry in which it is widely accepted to analyze ethical issues from diverse ethical perspectives, using arguments derived from several ethical theories including utilitarianism, deontology, virtue ethics, ethics of care, and contract-based theories. One of the most prominent among such an eclectic or pluralist approach as regards ethical theory is the "four-principles approach," developed in the 1970s by the philosophers Tom Beauchamp and James Childress in their seminal textbook *Principles of Biomedical Ethics*. During these years, the use of a principle-based approach became established in the context of the United States National Commission for the Protection of Human Subjects of Biomedical and Behavioral Research, the first committee in the US to shape bioethics policy and make recommendations for ethical principles in biomedical and behavioral research involving human research participants. The Belmont Report,[1] probably the committee's most well-known document, advanced three principles underlying biomedical research ethics: respect for persons, beneficence, and justice.

Beauchamp (who served as a member of this committee) and Childress offer a principle-based ethical framework, based on four "prima facie" moral commitments: respect for autonomy, beneficence, nonmaleficence, and justice. A "prima facie" or "conditional" duty means that a principle must be fulfilled unless it conflicts with an equal or stronger principle. The approach, however, does not provide a method for choosing, meaning there is no "algorithm" to prioritize a principle and derive the moral answer.[2] Unlike the Belmont Report, Beauchamp and Childress did not select three but four ethical principles, hence, "the four-principles approach." The principles are ranked below ethical theories but above particular rules.[3] Although these principles do not provide action guides

[1]The National Commission for the Protection of Human Subjects of Biomedical and Behavioral Research (1979). *The Belmont Report: Ethical Principles and Guidelines for Protection of Human Subjects of Biomedical and Behavioral Research*. Available online via http://www.hhs.gov/ohrp/humansubjects/guidance/belmont.html (retrieved 15 February 2016).

[2]Raanan Gillon R. (1994). Medical ethics: Four principles attention to scope. *British Medical Journal* 309:184.

[3]K. D. Clouser and B. Gert (1990). A critique of principlism. *Journal of Medicine and Philosophy* 15: 219–236.

and need derivative rules and specification in concrete cases, they aim to help physicians and other healthcare workers make moral decisions in medical practice.[4] They aim to provide a common moral language, compatible with most intellectual, cultural and religious beliefs. This universal claim of the four-principles approach may fit in an intercultural bioethical dialogue that avoids ethical relativism. In that sense, they can be defined as a variant of the Rawlsian "overlapping consensus": essentials we should all agree upon in order to make a society possible.[5]

The four-principles approach became widely used in Western healthcare and academia. However, ever since its introduction, this approach has also evoked debate. How should the principles be interpreted? Is there a hierarchy between the four principles? To whom do they apply, i.e. to whom do we owe these moral obligations and who should be included within the moral circle? How can concrete action-guides be derived from the abstract principles? Are the principles indeed universal, as proponents argue? Are these general principles sufficiently sophisticated to function as a bioethical theory — pejoratively called "principlism"?

In this chapter, I will closely examine the four-principles approach. The premise and challenges of each principle will first be discussed. Subsequently, I will identify three debates regarding principlism as a bioethical theory and method: (i) whether a pluralist or eclectic approach is an appropriate one and if so; whether general principles are sufficiently sophisticated to function as a bioethical theory; (ii) whether there is a hierarchy in the principles; and (iii) how to arrive at concrete moral judgments from general ethical principles. I will conclude with some future directions for the four-principles approach.

2. The Four Principles: General Overview

2.1. *Respect for Autonomy*

The term "autonomy" originally stems from the self-governance of the independent Greek city-states and has subsequently been extended to individuals. There are different understandings of and justifications for

---

[4] Gillon (1994), *op. cit.*

[5] John Rawls (1993). *Political Liberalism.* New York: Columbia University Press.

the concept of autonomy, but individual (or personal) autonomy is generally understood to refer to the capacity to be one's own person, to live one's life according to reasons and motives that are taken as one's own and not the product of manipulative or distorting external forces.[6] Two developments underlie the rise of the principle of respect for autonomy in bioethics in the 1960s: the rapid developments in biomedical technologies and a growing concern about the power exercised by physicians and researchers. Autonomy became a central value in Western (bio) ethics, mainly supported by deontological and utilitarian ethical theories.

I consider the principle of respect for autonomy to be significant for various reasons. First, in a pluralistic world, where people have different conceptions of the good life, the presumption should be that people are given the liberty to make their own decisions and live according to their values and beliefs, or in other words, that people are granted the liberty to act in accordance with their autonomy.[7] This is even more important when it concerns personal and identity determining decisions, which is often the case in healthcare. Second, human flourishing is constituted to a considerable extent in the exercise of one's autonomy.[8] After all, a person may flourish and lead a good life when she is able to formulate and pursue human ends.[9] In healthcare, the principle of respect for autonomy has many implications. The most well-known duty derived from autonomy is the requirement to obtain informed consent (or informed refusal), which can be defined as the autonomous authorization (or refusal) from a patient or research participant for a specific intervention.[10] Medical confidentiality and privacy are other implications of respecting people's autonomy.[11]

[6] J. Christman (2011). Autonomy in moral and political philosophy, in Edward N. Zalta (ed.), *The Stanford Encyclopedia of Philosophy*. Available online via http://plato.stanford.edu/archives/spr2011/entries/autonomy-moral/ (retrieved 15 February 2016).

[7] J. Coggon and J. Miola (2011). Autonomy, liberty, and medical decision-making. *The Cambridge Law Journal* 70(3): 523–547.

[8] R. Gillon (1985). Autonomy and the principle of respect for autonomy. *British Medical Journal* 290: 1806–1808.

[9] P. Gardiner (2003). A virtue ethics approach to moral dilemmas in medicine. *Journal of Medical Ethics* 29(5): 297–302.

[10] J. W. Berg, P. S. Appelbaum, C. W. Lidz and L. S. Parker (2001). *Informed Consent*. Oxford: Oxford University Press, 2nd edition.

[11] Gillon (1994), *op. cit.*

Despite its significance, the precise meaning and interpretation of autonomy has been the subject of ongoing discussion. Consequently, the principle of respect for autonomy also became a widely contested and debated concept — probably the most contested principle in the four-principles approach.

One of the main criticisms in regards to the principle of respect for autonomy has been that the emphasis on autonomy is superficial and eventually degenerates into indifference and a right to rot. Communitarian,[12] feminist, and care ethics approaches,[13] in particular, have specifically criticized the principle of respect for autonomy for being too individualistic, emphasizing that autonomy cannot exist independent of relationships. I think this criticism is partly due to a mistaken and excessively one-dimensional interpretation of the concept. It is important to make a distinction between the negative and the positive aspects of autonomy.[14] Autonomy in its negative (or thin) sense means the right to make one's own decisions without interference or coercion from others. It is "freedom from" and closely associated with the political concept of "liberty" — and sometimes even equaled with the concept of liberty.[15] This account of autonomy is a necessary though insufficient condition for human freedom. Autonomy in its positive sense entails the ability to take control over one's life and to live according to one's values and beliefs. It is more closely associated with concepts such as authenticity, self-expression, and self-governance. Since not everyone will have the same abilities and opportunities to make one's own autonomous decisions and "to be one's own person," we sometimes need others to facilitate and foster our autonomy.[16] People often face several difficulties with unrestricted decision making and in fully exercising their autonomy. These difficulties may comprise internal and external impediments for autonomous decision making, e.g. people's inability to

---

[12] D. Callahan (2003). Principlism and communitarianism. *Journal of Medical Ethics* 29: 287–291.

[13] C. MacKenzie and N. Stoljar (eds.) (2000). *Relational Autonomy: Feminist Perspectives on Autonomy, Agency, and the Social Self.* Oxford: Oxford University Press.

[14] I. Berlin (1969). *Four Essays on Liberty*. Oxford: Oxford University Press.

[15] Coggon and Miola (2011), *op. cit.*

[16] J. Feinberg (1987). *Harm to Self. The Moral Limits of the Criminal Law*, Vol. 3. Oxford: Oxford University Press.

comprehend the information provided, individual difficulties with making complex decisions, people's ambiguity regarding their own values and preferences, a lack of realistic alternatives, the psychological and emotional pressures of making a decision, etc. This is, for example, shown when patients face difficult decisions when undergoing next generation DNA sequencing. The quantity, significance and ambiguity of genetic findings will make any reasonable choice beforehand highly complex.[17] Autonomy is a gradual concept, an ideal, not an absolute reality. As Feinberg[18] has put it: it is an ideal that should be facilitated and fostered. Therefore, I embrace a much more substantial, thick interpretation of autonomy, where both the negative and positive aspects are acknowledged.

A second, related point of discussion concerns the scope of the principle of respect for autonomy. Some individuals are temporarily or permanently considered non-autonomous agents, such as children, the mentally ill, individuals in a permanent vegetative state, comatose individuals, or unconscious individuals. However, there are many shades of grey in this regard. Whereas an unconscious person would not be able to exercise her autonomy, there are many young children and mentally disabled individuals who may be able to make some decisions and express some preferences. Their decision-making capacity fluctuates. It is therefore important to realize that the capacity for autonomy is a gradual concept. Even though children, for example, are not yet able to fully exercise their autonomy, showing respect for children's future autonomy can still be warranted by postponing decisions that unnecessarily restrict their future options in life.[19] In addition, their current rights can be respected by obtaining their assent and engaging them in the decision-making process.[20] Similarly,

---

[17] A. L. Bredenoord, N. C. Onland-Moret and J.J. M. Van Delden (2011). Feedback of individual genetic results to research participants: In favour of a qualified disclosure policy. *Human Mutation* 32: 861–867; A. L. Bredenoord, R. Bijlsma, J. J. M. Van Delden (2015). Next generation DNA sequencing: Always allow an opt out. *American Journal of Bioethics* 15(7): 28–30.

[18] *Ibid.*

[19] A. L. Bredenoord, M. C. De Vries and J. J. M. Van Delden (2013). Next generation sequencing: Does the next generation still have a right to an open future? *Nature Reviews Genetics* 14: 306 doi:10.1038/nrg3459.

[20] N. A. A. Giesbertz, A. L. Bredenoord, and J. J. M. Van Delden (2014). Clarifying assent in pediatric research. *European Journal of Human Genetics* 22(2): 266–229.

psychiatric patients with reduced decision-making capacity can still be involved by means of supportive measures.[21]

A third criticism of the principle of respect for autonomy concerns placing excessive emphasis on the centrality of autonomy, leaving little room for competing societal interests. Indeed, at the macro level, the major shortcoming of autonomy is what Hardin[22] coined the "Tragedy of the Commons." This is the dilemma arising from a lack of coordination among individuals who rely on a shared resource, resulting in the situation in which multiple individuals, acting independently and rationally consulting their own self-interest, will ultimately deplete a shared, limited resource (or shared values) even when it is clear that it is not in anyone's long-term interest for this to happen. For example, all individual, well-informed decisions to abort female fetuses may in the end have a negative net effect on society at large, or all individual decisions to opt out of bio-banking research will ultimately result in impediments in research and healthcare. Actually, respect for autonomy is the moral obligation to respect the autonomy of others "in so far as such respect is compatible with equal respect for the autonomy of all potentially affected."[23] This implies that autonomy "is an important moral limit but also limited."[24]

Just as Beauchamp and Childress have never defended an unfettered, unrestricted place for individual autonomy, I would embrace a much more substantial, thick interpretation of autonomy, where both the negative and positive interpretations are acknowledged. Such a thick account of autonomy is more relational, more in line with human shortcomings, more sensitive to competing societal interests and less prone to the alleged "right to rot" criticism. This view can be positioned in current liberal thinking that can be described as "social liberalism" (or "progressive liberalism"), as opposed to the classical or neo-liberal point of view. Classical

---

[21] F. H. Van der Baan, R. Bernabe, A. L. Bredenoord, J. G. Gregoor, G. Meynen and G. J. M. W. van Thiel (2012). Consent in psychiatric biobanks for pharmacogenetic research. *International Journal of Neuropsychopharmacology* 21:1–6.

[22] G. Hardin (1968). The tragedy of the commons. *Science* 162: 1243–1248.

[23] Gillon (1994), *op. cit.*

[24] J. F. Childress (1990). The place of autonomy in bioethics. *Hasting Center Report* 20(1): 12–17.

and social liberalism differ in their view on mankind, in their interpretation of liberty and autonomy, and in the role they see for the state.[25]

2.2. *Nonmaleficence and Beneficence*

Whereas the principles of autonomy and justice were only introduced in bioethics in the 1960s, the principles of nonmaleficence and beneficence stem from the old Hippocratic tradition in medical ethics. These two principles are the classical "physician" principles, directed at the doctor–patient relationship (contrary to the "novel" principles of autonomy and justice that focus on the individual and society).

The principle of nonmaleficence, or "first, do not harm," requires the avoidance, whenever possible, of causing harm to others. Harm is defined as a setting back of the interests of an individual.[26] Among the four principles, nonmaleficence probably is the least contested principle — as far as we are aware, no authors have criticized this obligation not to harm patients and research participants. One possible criticism could be that the demarcation between nonmaleficence and beneficence is difficult to draw, particularly when, for example, the withholding of a proven beneficial treatment is included in the principle of nonmaleficence. Although withholding a treatment is an omission rather than an action, it represents a decision and could therefore be perceived as an action.[27] This same action, however, could arguably also be allocated to the principle of beneficence.

The principle of beneficence is, in fact, a group of principles. It requires three elements: that we prevent harm from occurring, that we remove harmful conditions that exist, and that we promote the good of the other.[28] I identify three challenges with this principle.

First, if used without restrictions and if not balanced with other principles, it may lead to paternalism, as the physician may use this principle as a justification to endlessly intervene for the sake of the patient. Hence,

[25] A. Van Witteloostuijn, M. Sanders, D. Hessling and C. Hendriks (2012). *Governing Governance. A Liberal–Democratic View on Governance by Relationships, Bureaucracies and Markets in the 21st Century*. Brussels: European Liberal Forum.
[26] T. L. Beauchamp and J. F. Childress (2013). *Principles of Biomedical Ethics*. New York/Oxford: Oxford University Press, 7th edn.
[27] R.Macklin (2003). Applying the Four Principles. *Journal of Medical Ethics* 29: 275–280.
[28] Beauchamp and Childress (2013), *op. cit.*

one must continuously be aware of the thin line between justified and unjustified paternalism. Moreover, we sometimes need to ask individuals what is in their best interest, which is the reason that autonomy is a natural counterpart to this principle.

Second, there is debate regarding the scope and limits of beneficence. Beneficence is a maximizing principle. If taken without restrictions, how much effort could be asked and should be exerted in promoting the interests of others? Here one arrives at the so-called demandingness debate, a debate in philosophy that discusses what individuals may reasonably ask of each other. The physicians' and researchers' protective duties are generally clear and strong. However, physicians' and researchers' duties to promote the best interests of others need more elucidation. The principle of beneficence therefore requires clear demarcations that take into consideration issues such as proportionality, feasibility, and the principle of autonomy.

Finally, some have argued that beneficence, understood as the moral ideal of helping each other, should not be considered a duty, as it is not morally required but rather an ideal that is praiseworthy or even supererogatory and heroic.[29]

2.3. *Justice*

The principle of justice also concerns a group of principles requiring fair distribution of benefits, risks, and costs across all parties in a society. Justice regulates cooperation. However, this principle alone is rather "hollow" and must be supplemented by a theory of justice. Twentieth century political philosophy has exerted considerable efforts to do so.

Equality is regarded by many as being at the heart of justice. Justice, however, is more than mere equality, given that people may be treated unjustly even if they are treated equally,[30] and not all inequalities are necessarily injustices.[31] Moreover, to treat everyone equally is purely impossible. A refinement could therefore be made in that equals receive equal treatment (horizontal equity) while unequals receive unequal treatment in proportion to their morally relevant inequalities (vertical equity).[32]

[29] Clouser and Gert (1990), *op. cit.*
[30] Gillon (1994), *op. cit.*
[31] M. Powers and R. Faden (2006). *Social Justice*. Oxford: Oxford University Press.
[32] Gillon (1994), *op. cit.*

Needless to say, what the phrase "morally relevant inequalities" exactly entails has been the subject of ongoing debate.

A distinction can be made between formal theories of justice and material theories of justice. A formal (also known as procedural) theory of justice defines the procedure for treating each other fairly, usually in reference to the condition espoused by Aristotle: equals must be treated equally, and unequals must be treated unequally. More recent examples constitute theories in "fair process" (or accountability for reasonableness), where the outcomes of fair procedures should count as fair when we cannot agree on more substantive principles for resolving disputes on justice and when specific conditions in such a procedure are satisfied, e.g. that decision-makers are accountable for the reasonableness of their decisions.[33] Such a theory is formal because it identifies no particular respects in which equals should be treated equally and provides no criteria for determining whether two or more individuals are in fact equal. Such a formal principle lacks substance and, in turn, fails to provide a criterion with which to differentiate between individuals. Who is equal and who is unequal? When is differentiation permitted? Which inequalities matter most?[34] For example, if there is a job vacancy, candidates will differ in gender, race, merit, capacities, age, and skills. What basis for differentiation is justified and what is not? Similarly, in situations where organs are limited (e.g. kidneys) and there are several suffering individuals on a waiting list, how can we make a justifiable distinction and whom should be included in the moral circle — are there people to whom we owe more by virtue of special relationships, proximity, or roles? Further, should we include only those who suffer from organ failure due to external circumstances or also include those who became ill due to their own unhealthy behavior?

To answer these questions, one needs a material principle of justice. Traditional (material) theories of justice include utilitarian theories, libertarian theories, egalitarian theories, and communitarian theories in addition to more recent theories of justice which include the capability approach as well as several other well-being theories. Each theory of justice formulates some relevant property on the basis of which burdens and benefits should

[33] N. Daniels (2008). *Just Health*. Cambridge: Cambridge University Press.
[34] Powers and Faden (2006), *op. cit.*

be distributed, e.g. (i) to each person an equal share, (ii) to each person according to individual need, (iii) to each person according to individual effort, (iv) to each person according to societal contribution, and (v) to each person according to merit.[35] Clearly, the principle of justice is only a starting point, but it is a "hollow" concept as such. The real moral work is in choosing and justifying a theory of justice and subsequently arguing for what constitutes morally justified discrimination.

3. Principlism as a Method in Bioethics

Broadly speaking, three (strongly related) debates regarding principlism as a bioethical theory and method can be identified: first, whether a pluralist or eclectic approach is an appropriate one and if so, whether general principles are sufficiently sophisticated to function as a bioethical theory; second, whether there is a hierarchy in the principles; and third, how to arrive from general ethical principles to concrete moral judgments.

3.1. *Pluralism or Monism*

A first topic of ongoing debate has been whether a pluralist or eclectic approach is an appropriate one in bioethics and if so, whether general principles are sufficiently sophisticated to function as a bioethical theory. The general, content-thin character of the four principles has been considered as both an asset and a drawback. It has been applauded for its clarity and simplicity, for being a straightforward method of general (perhaps even universal) principles. Many perceive it as a great educational tool and an attractive and applicable framework for the analysis of everyday bioethical issues. It has particularly been mentioned as a useful checklist approach for clinicians, non-philosophers, and those new to the field.[36]

The four-principles approach, on the other hand, has also been criticized for being simplistic, a kind of ethical reductionism that would

---

[35] Belmont Report (1979), *op. cit.*

[36] Gardiner (2003), *op. cit.*; R. Gillon (2003). Ethics needs principles — four can encompass the rest — and respect for autonomy should be "first among equals". *Journal of Medical Ethics* 29: 307–312; J. Harris (2003). In praise of unprincipled ethics. *Journal of Medical Ethics* 29: 303–306.

ignore the complexity of life and the ambiguity of ethical dilemmas. It would lead to sterility and uniformity of approach.[37] Moreover, some have more profoundly argued that any principlist approach misconceives both ethical theory and practice, for principles neither function as adequate surrogates for moral theories nor as directives or guides for determining the morally right action.[38] Whereas in classical ethical theories the leading principle embodies the ethical theory, principlism offers several often competing principles, without offering a method for choosing and balancing these principles. Principlism would provide a number of conflicting principles and then tell one "to pick whatever combination we like."[39] Since there is no single moral theory that ties the four principles together, it has been criticized for having no action guide that generates clear and coherent rules for action or justifications for those rules.[40]

This kind of criticism touches on underlying epistemological debates in ethics, with differing conceptions of what moral theory is or should be.[41] Whereas foundationalists expect an ethical theory to be well-developed and a clear directive for the morally right action, principlists are less demanding as regards ethical theory and are more willing to accept a loose framework for normative deliberation.[42] Beauchamp and Childress clearly adopt the latter position when they admit that ethics thus far did not find principles that are self-evident or self-justifying: there is an infinite regress, "a never-ending demand for final justification — because each level of appeal to a covering precept requires further general level to justify that precept."[43]

Should the ethicist commit herself to one ethical theory, or is a pluralist or eclectic approach acceptable? I think good reasons exist to steer a middle course here. Whereas it may not be possible and desirable to remain completely neutral with regards to ethical theory, much is to be said for pluralism as a general approach, especially in applied ethics. After all,

[37] Callahan (2003), *op. cit.*; Harris (2003), *op. cit.*
[38] Clouser and Gert (1990), *op. cit.*
[39] *Ibid.*
[40] *Ibid.*
[41] R. B. Davis (1995). The principlism debate: A critical overview. *Journal of Medical and Philosophy* 20: 85–105.
[42] *Ibid.*
[43] Beauchamp and Childress (2013), *op. cit.*, 393.

those dedicated to one particular ethical theory will only convince people who believe in the truth of this ethical theory. In addition, one can doubt the prospect of success of using one single ethical theory to tackle the complex ethical quandaries in modern medicine and life sciences. Moreover, a suitable model to integrate principles, intuitions, morally relevant facts, and different relevant background theories into a coherent moral view is available: "wide reflective equilibrium" (RE).[44] The general idea behind RE is that dealing with moral questions requires an argumentative process of seeking equilibrium between beliefs stemming from practice (morally relevant facts and moral intuitions) and those stemming from theory (principles and background theory). The term RE is used for both the process and the result of moral reasoning.[45] This reasoning process in RE can be characterized as "going back and forth" between beliefs stemming from practice and from theory.[46] From the perspective of RE, ethical reasoning is analogous to methods in science: in a continuous process we test hypotheses, modify them, and refine them or reject them through experiments and experimental thinking.[47] In the ethical analysis, the applied ethicists can use a variety of theories and arguments stemming from various ethical approaches and various disciplines, including methods stemming from the social sciences. RE is therefore particularly suitable as a method for the "empirical turn" in bioethics, where bioethics accommodates empirical research in her analysis.[48] Such a pluralist approach that makes use of RE asks special skills from the ethicist: she should on the one hand be sufficiently "embedded" so as to have knowledge of the relevant facts, considerations, and theories, but she should on

[44] J. Rawls (1971). *A Theory of Justice*, revised edn. Cambridge: The Belknap Press of Harvard University Press.

[45] G. J. M. W. Van Thiel and J. J. M. Van Delden (2008). The justificatory power of moral experience. *Journal of Medical Ethics* 35: 234–237.

[46] J. J. M. van Delden and G. van Thiel (1998). Reflective equilibrium as a normative empirical model in bioethics, in W. Van Der Burg and T. van Willigenburg (eds.). *Reflective Equilibrium*. Deventer, Kluwer: 251–259; Rawls (1971), *op. cit.*; W. Van der Burg and T. van Willigenburg (1998). Introduction, in W. Van Der Burg and T. van Willigenburg (eds.). *Reflective Equilibrium*. Deventer: Kluwer: 1–25.

[47] Beauchamp and Childress (2013), *op. cit.*

[48] P. Borry, P. Schotsmans, and C. Dierickx (2005). The birth of the empirical turn in bioethics. *Bioethics* 19(1): 49–71.

the other hand be sufficiently remote so as to make a critical, ethical assessment. The ultimate aim in bioethics is to reach moral justification, or, in other words, to establish one's case by presenting sufficient and coherent grounds for it, which does not necessarily imply that these grounds should be derived from one single ethical theory. When and under what conditions moral justification is reached (and the limitations therein) is discussed below.

3.2. *Hierarchy*

Ever since the principles were introduced, a second point of debate has revolved around how the principles (should) relate to each other,[49] whether there is a hierarchy in the principles, and whether autonomy would (and should) be given priority. As Davis[50] has highlighted, it is not entirely clear how the four principles systematically relate to one another. Moreover, it is unclear whether they *should* require systematic relation — Beauchamp and Childress seem to adopt the position that this should not necessarily be the case.[51] In addition, the theorists behind the four-principles approach did not prioritize any particular principle. They have repeatedly emphasized that no single principle overrides all other moral considerations: "it is a mistake in biomedical ethics to assign priority to any basic principle over other basic principles — as if morality must be hierarchically structured or as if we must cherish one moral norm over another without consideration of particular circumstances."[52]

This position has been challenged from two directions: some have argued that principlism should prioritize a principle and more specifically that autonomy should be "first among equals,"[53] and others have argued that principlism perhaps not in theory but at least in practice prioritizes autonomy. As one commentator put it: it became "a kind of one note theory with a few underlying supportive melodies."[54]

[49] Davis (1995), *op. cit.*
[50] *Ibid.*
[51] *Ibid.*; Beauchamp and Childress (2013), *op. cit.*
[52] Beauchamp and Childress (2013), *op. cit.*, ix.
[53] Gillon (2003), *op. cit.*
[54] Callahan (2003), *op. cit.*, 289.

I think some good reasons exist to assign a special place to the principle of respect for autonomy, but in that case only autonomy as described above: in a thick account. First, respect for autonomy is the only principle that directly relates to and limits the other three principles; it is the "alpha and omega" of any principle-based approach. For example, to not harm another person, i.e. nonmaleficence, is also to show respect for that person's autonomy. In addition, autonomy forms the natural counterpart of beneficence in order to avoid acting "in the sake of the patient, but without the patient." Even an obviously beneficial treatment can be refused — provided the patient is competent. Promoting someone's interest also requires us to know what constitutes one's interests, which leads to the requirement to obtain informed consent (or refusal) if possible. Finally, respect for people's autonomy must be an integral component of any conception of justice, albeit formal or material theories. Combined with the ethical, religious, and cultural pluralism of modern societies, respect for autonomy can be considered a core concept. Political liberalism assumes that a plurality of reasonable but often incompatible comprehensive doctrines is an essential characteristic of modern democratic regimes.[55] In such a pluralist world, where people have different conceptions of the good life, the presumption should be that a person's autonomy is at least respected and where possible also promoted — with all the caveats and restrictions mentioned above.

3.3. *Specification*

A third topic of ongoing debate is how to arrive from general ethical principles to concrete moral judgments. As discussed above, the general, content-thin character of the four principles has been considered as both an asset and a drawback. Principlism has been attacked for being on the one hand a much too rigid system that would deductively lead to simplistic moral solutions for complex ethical dilemmas and on the other hand for not providing sufficient tools to arrive at concrete moral judgments.[56] Indeed, general principles require further interpretation and application to

[55] Rawls (1993), *op. cit.*
[56] Macklin (2003), *op. cit.*

real-world bioethical problems. To have genuine impact and relevance, bioethics should not only seek to locate the realm of moral issues but also to decide on them.[57] How do general principles relate to particular moral judgments in concrete situations?

Moral problems need conceptual and normative clarification with adequate knowledge of the medical facts, as the particulars of a specific case may give general considerations a special salience. Whereas general principles are content thin, particular moral judgments are content rich.[58] Three ways to bridge principles to concrete, particular judgments can be identified.[59]

(i) **Application:** the right course of action is deduced from general principles and rules.
(ii) **Balancing:** conflicting principles are weighed in order to determine which has priority in the specific situation.
(iii) **Specification:** the process of qualitatively tailoring our norms to cases by spelling out where, when, why, how, by what means, to whom, or by whom the action is to be done or avoided.

Beauchamp and Childress are committed mostly to the process of specification, defined as "a process of reducing the indeterminateness of general norms to give them increased action guiding capacity, while retaining the moral commitments in the original norm."[60] However, problems may lurk when applying principles to specific cases.[61] The challenge of specification has been illustrated by Toulmin when he wrote about his experience as a member (1975–1978) of the United States National Commission for the Protection of Human Subjects of Biomedical

[57] S. Toulmin (1982). How medicine saved the life of ethics. *Perspectives in Biology and Medicine* 25: 736–750.
[58] T. L. Beauchamp (2003). Methods and principles in biomedical ethics. *Journal of Medical Ethics* 29: 269–274.
[59] H. Richardson (1990). Specifying norms as a way to resolve concrete ethical problems. *Philosophy and Public Affairs* 19: 279–320; J. F. Childress (2001). A principle-based approach. In H. Kuhse and P. Singer (eds.). *A Companion to Bioethics*. Blackwell Companions to Philosophy: 61–79.
[60] Beauchamp (2003), *op. cit.*
[61] Macklin (2003), *op. cit.*

and Behavioral Research: "I was struck to the extent by which the commissioners were able to reach agreement in making recommendations about ethical issues of great complexity and delicacy. If the earlier theorists had been right, and ethical considerations really depended on variable cultural attitudes or labile personal feelings, one would have expected 11 people of such different backgrounds as the members of the commission to be far more divided over such moral questions than they ever proved to be in actual fact (....) The problems that had to be argued through at length arose, not on the level of the principles themselves, but at the point of applying them."[62] Whereas very general moral principles could be embraced by all persons, specified moral judgments are "works in progress" or "provisional fixed points" that can legitimately vary between persons and that require continuous refinement and adjustment when relevant data would give cause to do so.[63]

When is a specified moral judgment justified? Beauchamp considers a specification justified if it is (a) consistent with (does not violate) the norms of common morality and (b) internally coherent with the overall set of relevant, justified beliefs of the party doing the specification.[64] Although RE is a suitable model to integrate principles, intuitions, morally relevant facts, and different relevant background theories into a coherent moral view, no accepted account on what constitutes common morality thus far exists. Gert[65] has defined common morality as the moral system that most thoughtful people implicitly use in arriving at moral judgments. Anyone who accepts common morality makes a universal, anti-relativist claim that a morality exists that is compatible with most intellectual, cultural, and religious beliefs. The challenge of course is finding and defining this morality and formulating it in such a language that it can be accepted by people from diverse intellectual, cultural, religious, and professional backgrounds. Beauchamp and Childress "did not attempt to construct a comprehensive theory of the common morality,"[66] but they

[62] Toulmin (1982), *op. cit.*, xx.
[63] Beauchamp (2003), *op. cit.*; Rawls (1971), *op. cit.*
[64] Beauchamp (2013), *op. cit.*
[65] Bernard Gert (2004). *Common Morality: Deciding What to Do*. Oxford: Oxford University Press.
[66] Beauchamp and Childress (2013), *op. cit.*, 396.

do claim that the four principles are *drawn* from the common morality. Whether the four principles will be broadly accepted outside the Western world, by people for example in Islamic, Buddhist, Confucian, and other traditions is not only a theoretical or normative question, but also an empirical one — which would be an interesting field to further explore empirically. An important theoretical issue for future research is to systematically develop an account on common morality and to elaborate on how the principles are positioned in the common morality.

3.4. *Future directions*

In many Western hospitals and universities, (medical) students are taught the four principles of bioethics. Principlism became influential and widely used, but also vigorously debated. Both the content of the principles and the strengths and weaknesses of principlism as a bioethical theory and method have been topics of ongoing discussion. I consider the four-principles approach an attractive and applicable framework for an in-depth analysis of ethical dilemmas in biomedicine as well as a great educational tool to help physicians and other healthcare workers to make moral decisions in medical practice. Due to the general, content-thin character of the principles, principlism may have a wide appeal amongst different professions, cultures, and nationalities and thereby provide a common moral language. However, this also means that the translation of abstract ethical principles in concrete moral judgments requires an elaborate and continuous scholarly process of fine-tuning and extensive argument. The quality of a specification, therefore, shows "the art and experience of the ethicist."

Just as science and ethics are works in progress, resulting in provisional fixed points that require continuous refinement and adjustment, so also does the four-principles approach require continuous maintenance. At least two themes should be on the agenda for future research. First, I think a pluralist approach is an appropriate one, particularly in bioethics. Although I follow Beauchamp and Childress in their position that there is no hierarchy in the principles (if there were a hierarchy, one endorses monism instead of pluralism), at the same time some good reasons exist to assign a special place to the principle of respect for autonomy — based on the thick account, where both the negative and positive interpretations are acknowledged. How the principles should be positioned towards each other and how the (thick account of the) principle of autonomy fits in is an important topic for further research. Second, the four-principles approach leans heavily on the existence of a common morality. Another important theoretical issue for future research is therefore to systematically develop an account on common morality and to elaborate on how the principles are positioned in the common morality. This is of special importance for the purpose of this book, aimed at exploring whether universal principles in bioethics do exist. Just as "medicine saved the life of ethics,"[67] contemporary bioethics could be a fruitful avenue for initiating an intercultural, bioethical dialogue that avoids ethical relativism.

[67] Toulmin (1982), *op. cit.*

Script of Oral Discussions (Day 1, Session 3)

Mohammed Ghaly

In our discussions we will be focusing on two main questions:

(i) What are the Islamic principles in bioethics?
(ii) Are the four principles of bioethics, as defined in the West, universal?

Currently in the field of medical ethics, there is not just a theory or two, but rather a vast domain of science and research related to the establishment of universal principles of medical ethics. We have two well-renowned scholars from the West who wrote and published in this field and whose books are considered the most important resources on biomedical ethics. One of them joins us during the seminar. They defined the four principles and their theory has not only impacted the Western world but has also expanded into the Muslim world. For example, Dr. Al-Bar is busy now writing a book in which he discusses the four principles. What we are hoping to achieve through our discussions is to review these principles from an Islamic perspective and ask questions such as, are these four principles compatible with Islam, its heritage, and its legacy? Are there any adjustments, additions, or deletions that need to be made? We are also asking the central question of whether these ethics are associated with general morals. If so, how can these morals be determined, and more specifically, which of them pertain to the field of medicine?

After **Tom Beauchamp** presented his paper and **Ali Al-Qaradaghi** presented his response paper, the following discussion took place.

Tariq Ramadan

After reading your book and listening to your comments today, Dr. Beauchamp, I have three questions. My first question, especially after our discussion earlier about ethics, medical sciences, and biomedicine, is: Why did you have to come up with these four principles? In fact, why do we need such principles when it comes to ethics? The perception we have while reading and contemplating what you call "common morality" is that we need more ethics because there is less religion. So, do we need to rely on common rationality because we do not have a common reference in terms of religion? Is this the rationale?

The second question that was raised earlier, by Sheikh Raissouni, is: How are these four principles (autonomy, nonmaleficence, beneficence, and justice) specific to medicine or bioethics? For instance, justice could be used as a principle for everything. Nonmaleficence could also be applied to everything. So it is wide, and at the end, what are the specificities that we have with these four principles when it comes to bioethics?

The last question, arising from Sheikh Al-Qaradaghi's last comments, is: How can we be sure when depending only on rationality and common morality that at the end, when we have two contradicting values or ethics, we will not follow the utilitarian process? How can we be sure that we have in fact a method through which we can decide between two conflicting values based on an ethical choice rather than a utilitarian choice within the society?

Tom Beauchamp

One question was: Why did we come to the four principles, and the question was also about the comprehensiveness of the principles. Let me go back and make a distinction that I take to be very important. First of all, we came to these four principles in particular and not many other principles that we could have discussed because we wanted an adequate set of principles *for* biomedical ethics, in a circumstance in which we simply did not have an adequate set of principles. One might say that this religion or that culture or whatever did have an adequate set of principles. However, what we wanted is an adequate set of principles so that all people can talk to all other people. That is to say, one that was universal in character. A part of the question, I believe, has to do with the role of religion. There was a statement that I was not sure I quite understood. It was something to the effect that you need more ethics because of less religion or something of that sort. That is not a view that we take. We think it is simply very critical to have a common morality. You do not get a common morality out of having many different religions, which is the *de facto* situation we have in the world today. We have many different religious faiths with many different kinds of commitments. So, in order for us to talk to one another, we need a common morality that has the values that are shared by all of these religious traditions. I might add, for those of you who do not know, that both my coauthor James Childress, who is a Protestant theologian of the Quaker faith, and I have graduate educations in theology, and we of course have the utmost respect for theological approaches. What we want to say is that the theological approaches in particular traditions will not give you universal principles. What they give you, precisely, is a particular religious tradition.

Another question was concerning what is specific to biomedical ethics. Quite simply, everything in our book is specific to biomedical ethics and not specific to something else. For example, it is not a book of general ethics, and it is not a book about business ethics. It is a book about biomedical ethics. I believe that is the simple answer.

I missed the point about contradictory values and not following utilitarian choices. I am not sure I entirely understand this question, but let me reconstruct it a bit. In modern society, particularly the way national governments work, it is very easy to fall into a kind of utilitarian way of thinking. That is to say, you simply balance risks and benefits across society and you make a decision based purely on what maximizes values. That is a utilitarian position that is easy to fall into. However, there is no reason to think that you have to fall into that. In fact, a great deal of what Childress and I are doing is trying to give you many kinds of options and alternatives precisely so that this does not happen. This is my general answer to what I understand to be the line of questions.

Mohammed Ghaly

Dr. Ramadan asked a question about the reason you chose these four principles and not other principles. He also asked about the methodology you adopted in selecting these four principles only and exclusively.

Tom Beauchamp

The idea is to have all the principles that you need to begin the process of specification to more specific rules. That does not mean that you have all of the values that you need. For example, as I said in my talk, we have a lengthy discussion about virtues. I do not think we can get all virtues out of these four principles. Simply saying that you have four principles that are orienting and guiding parts of your system does not mean that it governs all the values. Clearly, in fact, it does not. For example, I mentioned the moral ideals. Moral ideals do not conform perfectly to the four principles.

You might ask, what then do the four principles give you? They give you a coherent, reasonably approachable structure — in other words, everybody can approach it — body of principles that can be put to work in biomedical ethics to construct much more specific rules, policies, and the like. That is the reason.

One additional principle that some people have tried to advance is the principle of community. If it turns out that we need a principle of community because our account of justice and beneficence does not cover this aspect adequately, then we would have to add a principle of community. I am unconvinced, however, based on many discussions over this year that we need to add or subtract anything.

Mohammed Ghaly

Sheikh Raissouni is asking a question about the fact that the four principles are not specific to medicine and medical practice. Rather, they are broad and applicable to other fields such as economics, politics, education, and so on. He deems it more appropriate that when outlining medical principles, we focus on the doctor–patient relationship and not on these broad principles that can be applied to all aspects of life.

Ahmed Raissouni

As has been mentioned before, it would be appropriate if we could provide these principles to governments as they develop their policies, in all fields. They could even be included as constitutional principles. They could also be a means for educating society about general morality and how it can be applied in daily life. What I mean to say is that they are not more specific to medicine than they are to economics, the stock market, journalism, family matters, or education. From my perspective, they seem to be chosen arbitrarily from scores of principles and, although the authors claim that they are applicable to medicine and medical ethics, they in fact apply to all aspects of life.

In my opinion, if one were to choose principles for the field of medicine, one must research issues that are more directly related to medicine and/or principles that are more relevant to medical practice than to other fields. However, Dr. Beauchamp has humbly and honestly recognized that these principles are broad, general, and subject to additions or adjustments. So, for me at least, this misunderstanding has been overcome. The question that remains is: Why were these four principles in particular chosen, and how are they specific to medicine?

Tom Beauchamp

First of the all, the point was made that they are not specific to medicine, and that is absolutely right. They are intentionally not specific to medicine. They are drawn from the common morality that we all share. There is no doubt that they could be applied in many different areas. They are going to get different applications within the different areas because of the context. As I said earlier, business ethics is not journalism ethics and also not medical ethics. However, as you begin to apply them in those areas, you will get something that becomes highly specific to them. To put it in another way, we draw from the common morality. The common morality is that which we all share before we try to take it into medicine or we try to take it anywhere else.

Also, with the way in which the question was cast, it is as if these issues are all about the doctor–patient relationship. Of course, that is not the way we see it at all. It is a much broader territory of medicine. For example, it covers the issues of public health. Public health is not about a doctor–patient relationship *per se*. It involves a lot of policy structures, for example, to protect the health of the public. We also have extensive discussions in the book on research ethics. Research ethics is not principally about a patient–physician relationship except in the context of treatment. Most research is not actually in a treatment context. So it has to be medicine broadly understood. The framework, the core principles, needs to be general enough so it can be used in all of those different areas. Another point made was that these principles apply to all areas of the moral life. Yes, of course that is right. That is one reason we picked them: they are general and apply very broadly in the moral life.

Finally, in terms of application in a medical context *per se*, I think what happens is something like this, put simply: you have a principle like respect for autonomy. It obviously applies all the way across the moral life. However, when it comes to medicine, how does respect for autonomy apply in the medical context? One way it applies, a major way, is with informed consent. Informed consent is a doctrine that really is unique to medicine and research. It has never been applied in any other context. We explain what the connection is between respect for autonomy and what the doctor owes the patient or a research subject, what informed consent is. That then leads to further problems, particularly in treatment contexts. It leads to problems of medical paternalism. So this is how it goes in making these general principles specific to the medical context. One discussion leads to another discussion, which leads to yet another discussion, and this is basically the way Childress and I constructed the book. Eventually you get this hopefully reasonably comprehensive book that is very well suited to medicine broadly understood.

Jasser Auda

I remember a movie called *Lost in Translation* about missing the meaning during interpretation. I listen to what you are saying and to the translation and, although the live interpreters' translation is excellent, some vocabulary needs examination and requires clarification. Perhaps we can discuss this further another time. It is an important issue because Sheikh Al-Qaradaghi, for instance, talked about *naf'*. This Arabic word has the meaning of utility (utilitarian) and benefit (beneficence) at the same time. The meaning of beneficence is totally different from utilitarianism. In Arabic, we would say utilitarianism is *al-naf'īyah al-māddīyah*, and we would say beneficence is *maṣlaḥah*. I believe when Dr. Beauchamp speaks of beneficence, he means it in the *maṣlaḥah* sense and not in the materialistic or utilitarian sense, which he himself rejects in his book.

Another example is when we talked about *taqwá*, which was translated as being God-fearing. However, if *taqwá* had been translated as conscientiousness, then it could have been understood in a neutral meaning that applies to all physicians, whether religious or not.

One speaker also talked about the "atheist" culture. In his translation, the translator did not mention atheism but instead used the term "secularism." I think it was a good and correct translation because the translator understood that the speaker meant secularism and not atheism. Yet, even the term "secularism" in English requires a compatible Arabic meaning because "secularism" in the English language does not necessarily mean the absence of religion; rather, it means the separation of church and state, which is another topic altogether. I think even if we are talking about secularism in a Western understanding, it is not void of religion. The American culture itself is full of religion, and it is only the state that is secular.

Finally, Dr. Beauchamp talked about the "basis." These values were translated as *mabādi'* ("principles"). However, this is not an accurate translation (even though it is a translation I took part in admittedly). Rather, the "basis" as described by Dr. Beauchamp means the fundamental [literally: "the mothers of"] values. Dr. Beauchamp was saying that these four are the "mothers of values," not all the values. Scholars of Islamic legal thought (*uṣūlīyūn*) would say they are the issues to which all other issues refer back. So Dr. Beauchamp was talking about the "mothers of values" and not "principles" in its exclusive meaning. He was talking about the large fundamentals in the subject of values, as I understand it.

Mohammed Ghaly

I also have some comments about translation issues. For example, I think Sheikh Al-Qaradaghi discussed the integration of achieving benefit (beneficence) and preventing harm (nonmaleficence). Beneficence was translated as *iḥsān* in Arabic, which is not entirely correct because *iḥsān* has a much more general meaning in Arabic, and Dr. Beauchamp is in fact not talking about *iḥsān* with all its implications. No doubt there are language technicalities that have impacted this discussion.

Mohammed Ali Al-Bar

I have seen the second, fifth, and seventh editions of Dr. Beauchamp's book. Being such a prominent figure, it is not surprising that Dr. Beauchamp received many remarks and points of criticism, and it is admirable how much he changed between one edition and the next. In earlier editions of the book, the principle of autonomy took the shape of Western liberal utilitarian philosophy and relied completely on that philosophy. It granted the human a great amount of personal freedom, though this may have conflicted with other philosophies such as Kant's philosophy, communitarian philosophies (i.e. Marxism or socialism), or different religions. In the last edition in particular and in the research paper that was disseminated to us, the tendency towards this philosophical direction seems to have been reduced, although it is still present as far as I can see.

Coming now to social justice, I have a comment regarding something I read in the fifth edition of Dr. Beauchamp's book. There, he mentions research done on a group of African-Americans who did not have health insurance. They were emergency room patients and were treated by having their blood pressure measured there and being prescribed medicine for high blood pressure. A study found that these patients were not benefiting from this treatment for high blood pressure because they were not being followed up by a doctor and in some cases were not able to purchase the necessary medication for themselves. The conclusion was that there was no need to concern themselves with this group of people. These were the medical opinions given, but Dr. Beauchamp did not seem to criticize them. Perhaps my English is not very strong, but this was my understanding of his book. It was clear to me that he did not criticize these opinions, although he argues that he does.

Mohammed Ghaly

Dr. Beauchamp has said that his criticism was clear in his text on social justice.

Mohammed Ali Al-Bar

Once again, I am referring specifically to the fifth edition in this regard. Dr. Beauchamp did not include criticism of the injustice and unfairness of the system except in the seventh edition of the book as well as in the paper we received from him. I am very pleased to see this change because Dr. Beauchamp is a very prominent figure in the world of bioethics whose ethical methodology impacts communities all around the world and thus requires constant revisiting and revision. I am pleased to see that he has started to review the sections on social justice and the distribution of medical services.

It is difficult to justify that in the United States, which has some of the finest doctors and the best hospitals and produces some of the best medical advancements, there are 50 million people without health insurance. The United States spends around $8,000 per person, whereas countries in Northern Europe (which spends $2,000–$3,000 per person) and others like Malaysia (which spends $680 per person) spend far less. Yet the infant mortality rate in Malaysia is lower than in the United States. This is appalling. Even Cuba, which is not considered a very advanced country by many standards, has a much better medical situation. In fact, many Americans go to Cuba in order to receive free treatment. It is imperative that the United States government provides medical insurance for its own citizens. The insurance companies are monsters. A large company gets cheap insurance if it has at least 10,000 employees, but small businesses with fewer employees are charged higher prices. I am appalled at this system and how the United States, with all its great minds, can accept such exploitation. Ethically speaking, as a human being, I must criticize this system as a failed system.

Everyone looks to the American system as the ultimate system to be followed. This is very far from the truth — and as a physician, I am talking specifically about the health sector. The system must be revisited. I am from Saudi Arabia. Our government in Saudi Arabia blindly follows the footsteps of the American system and consequently has huge expenses that are even larger than that of the United States. This is catastrophic. The United States should not be viewed as the role model in healthcare for the rest of the world. Perhaps Singapore, Sweden, Norway, Switzerland, Canada, or the United Kingdom could potentially be role models in this regard, but not the United States. The United States has the highest number of doctors, the best resources, the best brains, and the best hospitals, yet these excellent services do not reach all people; they are only accessible to a small group of people. There are a few millionaires in the United States who have access to everything, but there is a larger group of people who do not have access to proper medical services. This is an unjust system.

Mohammed Ghaly

Dr. Al-Bar's comments can be divided into two main points. The first point concerns the changes that occurred between editions of your book. Were these changes due to a change in ideas and perceptions? Are you and Dr. Childress busy now adding ethical values, principles, etc.? The second point concerns your ethical stand regarding what is happening in the health sector in the United States in terms of justice. I will give you a chance to comment on these two points, Dr. Beauchamp, but first Sheikh Abu Ghuddah would like to comment on the subject of social justice and the related Islamic point of view.

Abdul Sattar Abu Ghuddah

Earlier I discussed the concept of justice in the distribution of social services. Social services were distributed well, by means of the endowment system. Public hospitals were established by generous individuals through charity in the form of endowments. These hospitals used to be open to everyone for free. All medical services including residence, prescription, medication, treatment, good nutrition, and care for hygiene were free of charge. I also mentioned that one of the doctors, Dr. Ahmad Issa, wrote a 400-page book[1] describing hospitals during the Islamic civilization. These hospitals used to be called *bīmāristān*. *Bīmār* is a patient and *istān* is a place. In other words, the hospitals were called "the place of patients." This book highlighted that in every Islamic capital, or in every major city, there used to be a large *bīmāristān* like a medical city and included a school for new doctors, who were educated and assessed by the doctor-in-chief. This was all for free, made possible by the contributions of generous individuals, whether rulers or citizens.

This created environments of social justice that ensured the distribution of medical and health services for free without any discrimination between those who did and those who did not have medical insurance. Any human suffering from pain or illness could go to the *bīmāristān*, where he would be diagnosed and issued medication even if his case was a minor one. If there was a need for him to sleep in the hospital, he would be admitted for several days if necessary, until he recovered completely, God willing. These are examples from our Islamic civilization that are thoroughly documented. Basically, these huge hospitals could be found in every major Islamic city and were sustained through the endowment system.

Tom Beauchamp

First of all, a question has been raised about whether there are differences across the editions. The answer is yes. If you go back to the first edition and then look at the seventh edition, there have been vast changes. One thing to bear in mind is that when we started, there was nothing. That is to say, we had nothing to work from because there was no biomedical ethics. There were no principles of biomedical ethics, at least not in a moral secular context. So yes, there have been quite a few changes over the years as the field has advanced, and the book would try to take account of those advances.

[1] Editor's note: It seems the speaker is referring to: Ahmad 'Isa (1938). *The History of the Bimaristans in Islam* (*Tārīkh al-bīmāristānāt fī al-Islām*). Damascus: Jamiat al-Tamaddun al-Islami.

There was a point about liberalism in particular. I would say liberalism is no longer discussed much at all. It was discussed in our book more during a period in which communitarian theories were getting a great deal of attention. Communitarian theories are nowadays not receiving very much attention. Consequently, the discussion of liberalism and communitarianism has been reduced. At the same time, we have increased the discussion of rights, human rights in particular. There was a big change in the seventh edition about discussion of rights, and there has been some clarification of the theory of justice. I would say what has happened there is that the theoretical side has increased and the conceptual side (just analyzing the concept of justice) has been reduced somewhat. I do think that there is the same treatment of the problem presented by Weinstein and Stason, the hypertension problem. There is the very same treatment in our book, in the fifth edition and in the seventh edition. The important thing in this regard is you should read the chapter on justice, not just the chapter where we are dealing with Weinstein and Stason and hypertension. This is because in that chapter we deal with the utilitarian character of this theory. We are not trying to deal with our theory of justice at all, so you have to get those together.

Now there were a number of points about the United States system. The United States system is, in my opinion, a morally outrageous system. I think we are largely in agreement there. I would also agree that insurance companies in particular, but not so much federal insurance since federal insurance in the United States is actually quite good in many respects for those people that it covers. Insurance companies, however, which of course cover most people in the country, I would agree, are quite greedy. It is also out of hand because of certain political features in the American system, lobbying in particular because they have a lot of power through lobbies. I think a part of this is what you refer to as materialism. Materialism is not a term that we use much any longer. Many years ago, it was used a great deal in these discussions, but I think I understand what you mean by it.

It should be borne in mind that here in the United States we do have a new law that is just going into effect, the Affordable Care Act. The Affordable Care Act brings the laws of this country much more in line with European countries like Germany and Switzerland, for example.

They were studied very carefully in the construction of the new law here. We are yet to see if the coverage will be as complete in this country as it is in many other countries. Actually, one should be cautious in predicting that too because things might actually get worse. My own belief is that things are going to get worse in most countries. The very simple reason for this is money. The rising cost of the technology that is required to produce first-rate medicine for everyone increases dramatically every year. It is unclear how much the economic system in different countries can keep up with it. I am mildly pessimistic there, although I am mildly optimistic that the new system that we have in the United States will be an improvement. Also, it is very important to separate the medical system in the United States from the insurance system. They often are not separated, particularly by politicians in this country. That is a huge mistake in my view. Insurance is totally separate from medicine. What people should concentrate their criticisms on, I think, are the insurance scheme and how people get reimbursed for their costs. You might put it in the following way. We have a terrible insurance system in the United States for all the reasons that were mentioned about greed and so on. We have a very good medical system. What we have to do is get the two together so that we cover more people. I think that covers most of the points.

Mohammed Ghaly

Dr. Beauchamp, I would like to ask a question about an issue you mentioned in your paper and in your presentation. It concerns the problem of structuring, organizing, and prioritizing the four principles. There is a big emphasis on autonomy, and some say that you give it priority over the rest of the other principles. How do you prioritize and organize these principles, or does it depend on the context?

Tom Beauchamp

As a quick answer to that question, it all depends on the context. There is no prioritization given to any one of these principles. I do not see how it is even possible to contemplate doing that because you want to apply the principles or put them to work in a certain context, and some are simply going to be much more important than others. Take my example of informed consent, for instance. Respect for autonomy turns out to be remarkably important in most informed consent contexts. It does not follow, however, that beneficence or nonmaleficence in particular are not important in an informed consent context. I think they are very important. After all, protecting people against harm is part of the rationale of having an informed consent, but respect for autonomy is particularly important there. It is even more so when you have refusals of treatment — not an informed consent to a treatment but an informed refusal of a treatment.

In other contexts, for example, we have just been discussing healthcare systems and coverage for people, respect for autonomy is not very important in those contexts by comparison to justice. Justice really becomes all-important. I think that is true in the national system, and I think it is true internationally as well. So you have to look at each given context and what rises to the surface as the most important set of considerations and specify accordingly. So I think maybe the direct answer to your question is no *a priori* prioritization ever works. You have to look carefully at the context and what is needed in that context.

Annelien Bredenoord

I have one question. You started by saying that the principle of respect for autonomy has been deeply misunderstood, and I think it might be interesting for our discussion if you could further elaborate on that because I think it has not only been misunderstood by Western critics but particularly also by Asian or Islamic critics. I would be interested to hear from you what exactly has been the misunderstanding of autonomy. Also, do you see differences between different cultures on how they conceive this concept?

Mohammed Ghaly

Just to add to that, some intellectuals and scholars explain the principle of autonomy to mean that a patient has full freedom to do whatever he or she wants. Could you please elaborate on that too?

Tom Beauchamp

First about the principle of respect for autonomy and how it has been misunderstood and what the proper application is. Let us first deal with the question of why it has been misunderstood. I am honestly not sure about this, but the one thing I feel fairly strongly about is that it is not an East–West difference as you can tell from what I said in my talk. I do not believe in East–West differences. As best I can see, historically the first criticisms outside the United States of our theory of autonomy actually came from Europe and from a very surprising source. For example, one of the early critics was Professor Søren Holm, who himself is Scandinavian and is now teaching in the United Kingdom. He was unhappy with the idea that respect for autonomy was a basic principle of biomedical ethics. From his perspective, it was not, and he thought that it basically came out of the American culture. This is something that I have heard all over the world, so it has to be something that has bothered a number of people: that it is really not a universal principle and instead is this sort of individualism of the United States that is being brought in as if it were a universal principle. I think that is a huge mistake, but there is no doubt that a number of people have thought that. So one source then is the framing of the language of autonomy in terms of individualism or egoism or something like that.

Also, because of the rise of political philosophy and the importance in political philosophy of liberalism, autonomy has been thought to be necessarily attached to a political philosophy of liberalism, which I think is not true. Now it certainly is true that a liberal political philosophy might pay great attention to the principle of respect for autonomy, but the principle of respect for autonomy is independent of any particular political philosophy. Nonetheless, I think that has been a source of the problem.

The last-mentioned problem is the one of absolute freedom. If you look at the early criticisms that emerged from the medical literature — this was true not only in the United States but also internationally — that was a common interpretation of the idea of respect for autonomy. It made the patient have the upper hand rather than the doctor having the upper hand. The patient had absolute freedom to reject what the doctor is recommending, and so on. I think what I did was to "absolutize" the principle of autonomy in a way in which I have tried to make clear. We simply do not do it, as it does not have any kind of absolutist value of this sort. We are not at the moment trying to say what is correct and what is incorrect so much as, why did we get these many different misinterpretations? I think basically those are the reasons for these misinterpretations, although I am sure there are other reasons as well.

Hassan Chamsi-Pasha

Thank you for this exceptional contribution, Dr. Beauchamp. I have two comments. The first is about preventive medicine. As you know, in the West and particularly in the United States, most of the money is spent on treatment — like, as you said, on new gadgets like internal cardiac defibrillators or cardiac resynchronization therapy, etc. — while very little is spent on prevention. I will give a small example. An ICD or internal cardiac defibrillator reduces mortality by about 30 percent in those patients who have had a heart attack. This costs about $25,000 and according to American guidelines it is a Class One indication. The same applies to the flu vaccine for cardiac patients. It reduces mortality also by about 30 percent, and the vaccine only costs about $25. Not much attention is paid to the flu vaccine because not many people make money out of it — $25 is nothing — while companies push for the internal cardiac defibrillator. This is where most of the money goes. This is a very important issue, in my opinion: that we spend very little on preventive medicine, on reducing the risks of coronary artery disease, while we spend billions and billions of dollars on treating heart disease.

The second comment is about respect for autonomy. As a cardiologist, I can say that while we undoubtedly respect the importance of the informed consent of a patient, we do not take any patient for cardiac catheterization or cardiac surgery without informing one of his relatives at least. In this society, in the Eastern culture, the family is very supportive, and they ask to know and want to know about any procedure that will be undergone by their father, their mother, their sister, or their brother. So we do not take any patient for cardiac surgery without informing the family. This is completely different from what happens in the West. Once again, I will give a small example. Last week, I had a 24-year-old female who had five congenital anomalies. She was also anemic and hypoxic. I was asked to do a transesophageal echo for her, but I said I would not do it without informing the family first because this is a risky procedure. It is a semi-invasive transesophageal echocardiography, and I could expose her to danger. I would not put my transesophageal probe in her throat and expose her to the danger of going into cardiac arrest or at least becoming hypoxic and put on a ventilator without informing the family so that they are aware of what I am doing. I would also like to hear your comments about this please.

Tom Beauchamp

From my perspective those are very congenial questions. On the points about preventive medicine, I could not agree with you more. You gave us some interesting examples about lowering costs or how low the costs are, and what the product is. One of my favorite examples is preventing catheter infection in ICUs. I like this example because it is completely free. It does not cost anything to have a program in which you wash your hands and go through several other things that prevent catheter infections. It costs nothing, and it saves not just a few lives — it saves hundreds of thousands of lives that are lost from catheter infections. It is an injustice in the system that we do not lay greater emphasis on preventive medicine of just this sort that I think you and I would agree on.

Secondly, on the part about informing the family, this interests me a little bit because you seem to introduce again a difference between the East and the West. I have not found that to be the case. I think that internationally there is a great deal of interest in effectively all cultures on proper information for the family. There are some differences as to what proper information is and exactly how to do it, but I think internationally there is very little difference now. Informed consent is more or less required everywhere. We are still in the process, though, of people understanding this very well. I was recently at a conference in Japan, and a professor from Japan and I were both giving talks about informed consent. He said in his talk that it is now undoubtedly a worldwide phenomenon and that it has been very carefully studied and so on. His audience in Japan was in disbelief. They responded, "But we do not do that kind of informed consent in Japan." He said, "Yes we do, you just do not know about it." In other words, the rise of informed consent in the way in which it has been infused through systems around the world has been so rapid that a lot of people are simply behind the times about how much it is done. This is true in terms of both first party and what you were talking about, which is third party (the family). So I think I am in complete agreement with you. I just would not want to make the East–West distinction that you at one point suggested.

Tariq Ramadan

What is the translation of the word "beneficence" in Arabic? Is *iḥsān* not acceptable? Dr. Jasser spoke about *maṣlaḥah*. What Arabic translation for "autonomy"?

Mohammed Ghaly

Dr. Beauchamp, if you have comments to offer, please go ahead.

Tom Beauchamp

Beneficence divides down into different parts. I will read what I said earlier. Beneficence represents a group of principles requiring both lessening of and prevention of harm as well as provision of benefits to others. That is as good of a short definition as I can give you of beneficence.

Mohammed Ali Al-Bar

I think the word *iḥsān* [translated by the Arabic-to-English interpreter as "philanthropy"] is a good translation for beneficence because beneficence in medical terms, from the time of Hippocrates until today, means that one should be good to the patient in all possible ways. This does not only refer to providing him with drugs or treating him well but also trying to do your utmost to serve the patient. That is really what *iḥsān* is about. It is about striving to be perfect in your treatment of the patient. In other words, you should be nice and good to him, treat his illness, alleviate his pain, treat him psychologically and do everything you can to treat him. So I think *iḥsān* will make a good translation for beneficence. Autonomy is a lot more difficult to translate because it has to do with the individual, the person.

Tom Beauchamp

No doubt philanthropy is a word that is going to be used somewhat differently in different cultures, and there will be different understandings of it in English. Ordinarily in English, we would not use the terms beneficence and philanthropy as synonymous. However, philanthropy is one kind of beneficence, there is no doubt about that. What makes it more complicated in the context we are in is that I am thinking of beneficence as a principle of obligation. You are obligated to provide these benefits. Ordinarily, philanthropy is not considered something you are obligated to do but rather is a moral ideal in the moral life. It is something that you can do to provide goods or services for others, but it is not something that is obligatory on you to do. That is the way I would draw the distinctions here. They are close but not identical.

Mohammed Ghaly

Dr. Beauchamp has further complicated the matter but in a beneficial way. He stated that philanthropy is a type of beneficence but it is not mandatory or obligatory. He is right in that beneficence is obligatory and that [the Arabic word] *iḥsān* does in fact refer to something more than obligatory.

Mohammed Ali Al-Bar

In his book, Dr. Beauchamp discussed supererogatory acts and mandatory duties, and he did distinguish between them. Islamic law also includes this distinction. We have mandatory duties, and we have supererogatory philanthropic actions.

I differ with him in one example he mentioned concerning the story about the Samaritan in the Bible. Dr. Beauchamp says that Jesus gave an example to his companions through this Samaritan. While on a journey, the Samaritan found someone on the way who was injured, so he stopped. By the way, the Samaritans were a group looked down upon by the Jews. The Samaritan went to the injured man, tried to treat his injuries, and entrusted him to someone, promising to come back to take care of him and cover the costs of doing so. Indeed, the gentleman did get better. Dr. Beauchamp considered this act to be supererogatory, not mandatory.

From the words of Jesus, peace be upon him, in the Gospel, it was clear that Jesus was telling his companions and disciples that this is the least you can do for the sick person; in other words, it is obligatory. According to Dr. Beauchamp, this is not obligatory, and I have an issue with that. From my perspective, what Jesus, peace be upon him, said clarifies how much people should care about other people. The gentleman is on the street; he might die. It is an obligation to save his life. The position taken by Jesus, peace be upon him, was very noble. Of course, he is a prophet and is among the best of humankind, but nevertheless he was setting an example for his disciples and companions that this is the least of the mandatory. Dr. Beauchamp considered this to be supererogatory, not mandatory.

Jasser Auda

Dr. Beauchamp said the definition of beneficence was basically about bringing about good and preventing harm. The definition translates seamlessly to an Arabic phrase we ourselves use very often: *taḥqīq al-maṣlaḥah* (realizing benefit) and *dar' al-mafsadah* (repelling harm), respectively.

In regards to autonomy, it was translated as *istiqlālīyah*, which means independence and is different [from autonomy]. Autonomy was also translated as *dhātīyah*, which means individualism. Autonomy was also translated as *ḥurrīyah* (freedom), but I do not think autonomy is about freedom in its absolute sense. Rather, autonomy should be translated as *ḥurrīyat al-qarār* ("the freedom of action" [a person's freedom to act as he chooses]), which is the Islamic term. I think *ḥurrīyat al-qarār* is the translation closest to the meaning of autonomy. Autonomy is not about *istiqlālīyah* or *dhātīyah*, both of which are very different from autonomy.

Mohammed Ali Al-Bar

Autonomy is part and parcel of independence and individuality according to liberalist thought.

Jasser Auda

Dr. Beauchamp has clarified that he is against the liberalist approach. So we have to be aware of all definitions.

Mohammed Ghaly

My personal opinion — and God knows best — is that beneficence and nonmaleficence are *jalb al-maṣāliḥ* (bringing about benefits) and *dar' al-mafāsid* (repelling harms), respectively. That is how they should be translated in Islamic legal terminology. Alternatively, we can say *taḥqīq al-maṣlaḥah* (realizing benefit) and *daf' al-adhá* (repelling harm) if we want the general Arabic translation. However, using the term *iḥsān* is problematic because *iḥsān* is also about perfecting work, and it also means giving money to people in charity. Furthermore in the Islamic tradition, *iḥsān* is a very complex and rich concept and encompasses much more than what we are talking about. For this reason, Sheikh Al-Qaradaghi had a point when he said that since *iḥsān* encompasses both concepts of beneficence and nonmaleficence (and more), there is no need to include them as separate principles. Therefore, using *iḥsān* could be accurate if we combined the two concepts of beneficence and nonmaleficence. Dr. Beauchamp is opposed to this because beneficence is about doing and nonmaleficence is about not doing.

I think the bigger issue is autonomy. The closest we got was the comment made by Dr. Jasser that it is about freedom of action, and we might also add the phrase "with responsibility." Even in Dr. Beauchamp's paper, he says it is not only about liberty, but it also has to do with agency. So it is freedom plus action plus bearing the responsibility of that action. Dr. Beauchamp clarified that among the most commonly misunderstood principles is autonomy. He clarified that, for example, autonomy may occasionally involve limiting and constraining the freedom of the patient.

So it is not necessarily about allowing the patient to do whatever he wants. Therefore, I think that "freedom of action with responsibility" might be a good translation.

Jasser Auda

However, I think the concept of independence is indeed present in the meaning of autonomy.

Mohammed Ghaly

Yes, independence is there, but it is not absolute.

Jasser Auda

Yes, it is not absolute, but it is there. I think autonomy cannot be translated into *ḥurrīyah* (freedom) alone or *istiqlālīyah* (independence) alone. I think it requires the use of more than one term.

Mohammed Ghaly

Of course, one of the beautiful things about our meeting today is the issue of terminology. When different ideas meet, it is imperative to fix the definitions of the terms we use. Many of you know what Hunayn bin Ishaq, an Arab philosopher, had to go through when he translated Greek texts. He would constantly amend, review, and reamend his own translations. Sometimes he would recognize that certain concepts were simply too complex for him to translate concisely. No doubt the translation of philosophical concepts especially, as in our discussion today on bioethics, requires review several times over.

Tom Beauchamp

I have a comment on the Samaritan story. I think it is quite clear in the way in which we frame the language of a moral ideal versus that which is obligatory today. What the Samaritan did in the story is a matter of following a moral idea and not something that is morally obligatory. Of course, that does not mean that you could not have a religion in which it was made mandatory. Of course you could.

The full story of what the Samaritan did is really quite remarkable. It would be the equivalent today of us finding someone on the street who is very sick and ill and probably starving and injured, getting them in our car, taking them to a hospital, putting them in the hospital, paying for the cost of their hospitalization, taking care of them while they are in the hospital and when they are released from the hospital, taking them home and continuing to take care of them and so on. That surely has got to be supererogatory in the matter of our moral ideals. That is the reason why it is interpreted in that way.

I also have a comment on the meaning of autonomy. Originally, autonomy comes from the Greek word *autonomos* and originally had a political application, not a moral application. In the context of political states, it basically meant sovereignty. As it got translated into moral philosophy, the meaning basically became "self-rule" or giving oneself the law, which could be the moral law or could just be giving oneself a different kind of rule. As you rightly pointed out, in my way of interpreting it, the critical context is there is liberty — that is to say, there is no controlling influence that is operative — and there is agency on the part of the individual in giving oneself one's reason, one's rule, one's principle or whatever.

I do not think that in any respect Childress and I speak against liberalism in talking about autonomy, but we certainly do not speak in favor of it either, except insofar [the following is true]. If you believe that support of human rights theory is inherently a part of a liberal political philosophy, then we do place it in the liberal political context because we certainly believe strongly in human rights. However, in general, we try to stay away from that particular commitment — that is to say a liberal political philosophy.

Script of Oral Discussions (Day 2, Session 3)

After **Tom Beauchamp** presented his paper, the following discussion took place.

Mohammed Ghaly

Dr. Beauchamp said the four principles are universal on the one hand and localized and particular on the other. They are neither purely universal nor purely particular. He explained that the four principles are universal in principle, meaning everyone does agree that justice, beneficence, nonmaleficence, and autonomy are important. However, applying the principles to make them particular is a different issue altogether. The difference does not emerge only because of adherence to a certain religion or culture; rather, differences may emerge because of differences in various fields and disciplines. For example, when we apply justice in the field of economics, medicine, or politics, each application yields a different outcome. So despite the universality of the principle, its applications do differ even for individuals who adhere to the same religion. It is not about religions but rather about differences inherent in various disciplines and professions. Still, this does not mean that the four principles are not universal.

So Dr. Beauchamp maintains that part of it is universal and another part is particular to the local circumstances where it is applied.

Dr. Beauchamp also talked about cultural diversity. He realizes that a universal morality may seem threatening to cultural diversity. However, he thinks the opposite is actually true: the principles support and encourage cultural diversity. Cultural diversity does not necessarily mean pluralism, and Dr. Beauchamp thinks that if we accept pluralism, this will contribute to a "melting" [or softening] of ethics. Rather, if we all accept the same principles but differ in our implementation of those principles because of our different cultures, this is closer to living harmoniously with one another. Therefore, the presence of universal principles does not cancel out cultural diversity. The same goes for religious diversity.

Ali Al-Qaradaghi

Dr. Beauchamp addressed some of the questions raised yesterday about the fact that the four principles are not specific to medicine. He clarified that even though the principles are general, they can be applied specifically to medical issues. I share this opinion. I think the generality of the principles does not contradict the specificity of their application to medicine. Similarly, if we take the higher objectives of Sharia as a framework, they themselves will be ratified in the specification process.

However, I would like to make some clarifications. Islam is creed, law, ethics, and ritual acts of worship. Ritual acts of worship are about the religious behavior and conduct of the faithful. While they are not explicitly or manifestly about ethics, they do have ethical ramifications. God says, "…Indeed, prayer prohibits immorality and wrongdoing…" (Qur'an 29:45). Although the act of prayer itself is not about ethics, it still has ethical implications. This also applies to almsgiving (*zakāh*). God says, "Take, [O, Muhammad], from their wealth a charity by which you purify them and cause them increase" (Qur'an 9:103). There is a difference between the action and the effect, between the means and the end. Therefore, in my opinion, religious specificities do remain within the realm of ritual acts of worship, while general, unchanging ethics are part of what Imam Al-Shatibi called *al-dīn al-'ām* (general religion), and they are part of human nature (*fiṭrah*).

We mentioned previously the following section from a Qur'anic verse: "The innate disposition [*fiṭrah*] from God upon which He originated (or created) mankind" (Qur'an 30:30). The verse then continues, "That is the upright religion." In other words, God made the human with an innate disposition (*fiṭrah*) that is agreed upon and shared by all humanity and people of religion as part of the steadfast, unchangeable religion. Again, we are talking about things that are agreed upon, such as prohibiting immorality or wrongdoing — even if we may differ as to what exactly is immoral or wrong. In other words, these general ethics are part and parcel of the human's innate disposition (*fiṭrah*), and before, simultaneously, or after, they became part of religion. Each religion contributed certain specifics or specifications to these ethics, but the foundations of ethics do not at all differ between religions.

So I just wanted to clarify to Dr. Beauchamp the distinction between ritual acts of worship — which are not ethics but have certain ethical implications — like prayer and between general ethics that can be applied to all humanity. In other words, if we examine the Islamic system as a whole, including the ethical values it calls for, I think it would be accepted by all rational thinking people across the world.

One more thing: differences between cultures and peoples should be taken into consideration, but only after a firm acceptance of the core principles. It is for this reason that Sharia contains absolute texts that are immutable, unchanging across time and place, and whose meanings are clear-cut. Only their applications may change according to circumstances of time and place.

Mohammed Ali Al-Bar

I have a comment related to the ethics of medical research or biological research more generally. There are a number of examples of harms that resulted from human experimentation, starting from the beginning of the 20th century up until the beginning of the 21st century. The first event that drew attention to and laid the foundations for these issues was the trials of Nuremberg in which the Nazis had conducted experiments on the Jews. This led to a lot of controversy, and the doctors participating in the inhumane human experiments were executed. It was later revealed that the same Nuremberg experiments carried out by the Nazis were replicated in America and Europe in an even more disgraceful manner. This is recorded in medical research history. I referred to this in my own research and highlighted the mass killings that occurred due to these events. Arising from this, foundations and regulations for medical research were established. One example is the Belmont Report. They are very good foundations and regulations, but they can be manipulated and circumvented, even in the United States.

As for nations of the Third World, these regulations did not exist in the first place, so it was easy to get away with unethical medical research. I will give you a case in point. In 1996, the company Pfizer conducted experiments on Nigerian children. It was testing a new medication for *meningitis*. They claimed this medication was ready and licensed and that they were donating it to the poor. Nigeria was initially very pleased with this, but it ended up killing a number of children and injured many others. Once this was exposed, the Nigerian government sued the company and received $75 million in compensation after the company confessed and acknowledged its actions. In 2009, Pfizer was also penalized by the American F.D.A. with a $2.3 billion fine for the simple reason that the company had conducted experiments on four of their medications at a time when they were "off label." They were without a license and yet were distributed to doctors who used them without official recognition by the F.D.A. This was considered unlawful, and the F.D.A. fined the company with $2.3 billion, although no one was harmed. Compare this with the Nigerian case in which children were killed and many others were harmed and yet the compensation was only about $75 million, which of course did not trickle down to the victims.

In 2012, the British drug maker GlaxoSmithKline was fined approximately $3 billion for the biggest fraud in American healthcare. Keep in mind that this took place in 2012, which is only a few months ago. This company was fined for distributing 10 drugs, including Avandia antidiabetic, marketed globally as an efficacious drug for diabetes but later as causing heart disease. The company was well aware of the side effect but concealed it. Experts in the field stated that $3 billion is a trivial amount for the company, given the approximately $30 billion it had reaped from those 10 drugs. This was in the United States. How much did they pay the Third World nations where these 10 drugs were distributed? Nothing at all.

I also have a personal experience that took place in Saudi Arabia. There are new drugs that are used to treat cancer patients and other serious diseases. I was a member of some ethical committees responsible for permitting or restricting the experimenting of drugs on people. I was pleasantly surprised that Pfizer and other leading companies like Glaxo would state that a certain drug might cause blindness, heart disease, or other harm, etc. This was good transparent practice. However, included in the same report was a section stating that if you incur one of these diseases or pass away, the company would not be responsible for any compensation, and treatment is based on your own health insurance. I was completely opposed to the company's refusal to treat or compensate the patient who incurred a disease due to this drug, especially because the company admits that the drug may cause certain diseases. I resigned from one of the committees because the chair of the committee used to receive money from the company itself and he wanted us to sign the report, and of course I was against that. If this is what happens in a rich country like Saudi Arabia, where its residents are not much in need of money, imagine what happens in poor countries.

As made evident by these examples, there is outrageous exploitation taking place by Western leading companies in the Third World. These companies are allowed to conduct research through bribing researchers and high profile personalities in order to facilitate the circulation and usage of the experimental drug. They do not provide any sort of compensation for the poor people who suffer illnesses due to these drugs, even though companies have started admitting that many suffer due to their experimental drugs. Acknowledgement is a good first step, but there is a necessary second step. When I refused these actions on many occasions, I found that my opposition led to the company being forced to acknowledge the need for it to compensate — or at least medically treat — those affected by the drug. This is a positive thing; it suggests that if doctors stand up for ethical issues, the companies might meet ethical demands, although admittedly in most cases the companies do not end up meeting them, especially in Third World companies. I am confident that ethical demands are met in the United States but only after the company is exposed to the public. The point I am trying to make is that manipulation and fraud continues to take place even in the United States. In the Third World, fraud occurs even more so and on a larger scale, as people can be bribed with small amounts of money.

Mohammed Ghaly

Dr. Al-Bar has provided many examples over the past two days regarding breaches and violations that happen despite the existence of principles of medical ethics and despite there being agreements and contracts involving those ethics. In personal exchanges between Dr. Al-Bar and myself, I communicated to him an idea that is my own personal opinion and may not be completely correct. It is that one of the main reasons these violations were exposed was the existence of the field of medical ethics. If we did not agree upon certain principles, we could not have called them violations. It follows that these principles are exposing, and without them many things would have gone unnoticed. Of course, it is not enough to have principles or rules; another important matter is the mechanisms by which to apply the principles. This could be one question for our final day's discussions.

Hassan Chamsi-Pasha

My question is about the recent concept of defensive medicine that has become widespread. Doctors sometimes conduct X-ray examinations or medical interventions in order to protect themselves from blame or legal action that may arise due to them not carrying out a certain test or medical procedure. Despite this, the cost of medical insurance for doctors has greatly increased especially in the United States and Europe and particularly for gynecologists and obstetricians. I believe Dr. Beauchamp knows that the insurance rate or insurance fees on these doctors have increased significantly.

My question is: To what extent can we apply the four principles to limit the spread of the concept of defensive medicine? It may cause the patient unnecessary complications and yet many doctors do it to protect themselves or out of fear of accusations from their patients. I will also ask why this phenomenon has been spreading although the four principles have also been spreading widely over the last 30 or 40 years in the United States and Europe?

Mohammed Ghaly

Another question to note is how the principles of biomedical ethics or biomedical ethics as a field in general can be more effective and how satisfied are we with the *status quo* of medicine and medical ethics in general?

Abdullah Bin Bayyah

Edgar Morin's book, written in French, *La Voie*: *Pour l'Avenir de l'humanité* (*The Way*: *For the Future of Humanity*) covers many of the issues being spoken about here because they are of interest to the future of humanity. According to Edgar Morin, scientific research makes *promises et menaces* (promises and threats). It promises benefits, but it also warns of evils or harms. As I thought about this I came to the conclusion that this is part of an important principle in Islam jurisprudence: removing the means to error (*sadd al-dharā'i'*). Muslim scholars agree on the necessity of avoiding harm if it is certain, but if the harm is not certain their opinions start to differ.

The matter has to do with verifying the underlying character of certain issues (*taḥqīq al-manāṭ*), which is a topic we have been studying and will be tackling in an upcoming conference in Kuwait. We are interested in *taḥqīq al-manāṭ* in both the current reality (*wāqi'*) and predictable incidents of the future (*tawaqqu'*). We have been studying this topic for a year or so, and we find that the entirety of Islamic jurisprudence (*fiqh*) must be reviewed in light of both current reality and future expectations because the reality of the modern world in the fields of economics, society, politics, scientific discoveries, and international relations is unprecedented in human history. Therefore, we need to review the entirety of Islamic law. So far, we have categorized it into disciplines and domains. The current challenge is how to generate a clear description of the reality. According to the system of an early Muslim scholar, Abu Hamid Al-Ghazali, there are five scales for qualifying reality in order to better understand it: the scale of the senses, the scale of language, the scale of customs, the scale of the intellect, and the scale of nature. He mentioned this in one book, and I do not know of any other Muslim scholars who dealt with this in the issue of *taḥqīq al-manāṭ*. I see this as an incredibly important issue pertinent not only to Muslims, but to humanity at large.

Hence, in my opinion, there are two main issues that we need to address. The first is *ta'ṣīl*, to develop a framework rooted in the Islamic tradition. The second is *tawṣīl*, to communicate this framework to the public. There is a problem that Dr. Al-Bar pointed out: although these ethics and morals exist, people do not act according to them. This is because the ethics and morals have failed to reach their consumers; they may have only reached physicians and companies. The responsibility of industrial capitalism is huge in this regard because industrial capitalism often runs away from ethical responsibility, not only in the field of scientific discoveries but also in the domains of labor, production, distribution, and so on. We must say that this ruthless industrial capitalism must review and re-evaluate itself.

Regarding other ethical values, whether they are religious, based on tradition, or stemming from a social ethical system, it should help find an end to the great greed that does not ask about why but rather about how: How to acquire wealth? How to make a scientific discovery? However, the question, "Why?" which is a philosophical question, necessarily must precede the question, "How?" In *taḥqīq al-manāṭ*, we established three questions. The first question is, "What?" as in, "What did your Lord say?" The second question is, "Why?" and this is the domain of *ta'līl* (justification). The third is, "How?" and this is the domain of *tanzīl* (application).

We are speaking about the third, *tanzīl*. Here, *ta'ṣīl* is important and *tawṣīl* is important too. Communicating this knowledge and educating societies about it is critical so that they may claim their own rights. There have been discussions about harmful drugs administered to patients who are unaware that the drugs they take are indeed harmful. I think often the consumer is not aware of what is happening, so communication is imperative in this regard. As we said, the promotion and spread of knowledge is key. Biological research studies must focus on preventing harm before seeking what we call "the fake interests" because the prevention of harm is prioritized over the bringing about of interests.

Abdul Sattar Abu Ghuddah

My question is about whether all the principles should be taken together or whether there is some prioritization or ordering among them. Also, Sheikh Al-Qaradaghi mentioned that the number of the higher objectives of Sharia could reach nine, the ninth one being preservation of the environment. I would like to ask about the ordering of these objectives. We believe the objectives must all be accepted, but do they follow a particular order? Sheikh Raissouni mentioned that while the actual ordering is not agreed upon, the concept of ordering is established.

Abdullah Bin Bayyah

In *Chapters of the Higher Objectives* (*Mashāhid min al-maqāṣid*), I discussed the issue of ordering and I found that each higher objective or principle has within itself levels. For example, some scholars say that business or selling is counted among the group of needs (*ḥājīyāt*) while Imam Al-Haramayn says it is among the group of necessities (*ḍarūrīyāt*). In fact, selling is of different types.

The early Muslim scholars did not reach a consensus on one ordering for the necessities, although they did agree on the necessities being comprised of five benefits [to be preserved]: religion, life, offspring, the intellect, and wealth. Some of them prioritized religion over life — and this was the majority opinion — while others prioritized life over religion, and so they differed on the rest of the necessities.

Back to my earlier point, selling is sometimes considered a necessity and at other times is considered a need. Selling food is among the necessities, based on the texts of Sharia, because of the necessity of food. Selling luxury items is neither among the necessities nor is it among the needs; it is counted among the luxuries (*taḥsīnīyāt*).

Early Muslim scholars dealt with a number of detailed issues in the medical field such as mercy killing. They said that mercy killing is prohibited in Islam. I point here to the words of the Maliki jurist al-Zurqani, who said that expediting death is prohibited and that there came a time in Egypt when physicians would hasten the death of patients whom they deemed terminally ill. So these issues were relevant even then.

The early Muslim scholars also dealt with the question of the liability (*taḍmīn*) of the physician. They made a distinction between being liable and being sinful. The scholars said that if a patient asks the physician to amputate his or her hand — while the patient is healthy and completely sane — the physician is not liable for complying with the patient's request [and thus would not pay a *diyah*], but the physician is considered to have committed a sin.

Mohammed Ghaly

Dr. Beauchamp, I would like to reiterate the two main questions to you. The first is the one I mentioned about how to make these general principles effective and what is your opinion on the current situation — is it getting better or is it getting worse? The second question, which came from Sheikh Abu Ghuddah, was about the four principles. Are they complementary? Are they one indivisible set that should be considered all together, or can we take one principle and leave another? Also, is there a hierarchy for the four principles? Can they be ranked from one to four or not? If you have any further comments on what you have heard, also please go ahead.

Tom Beauchamp

Let us talk a little bit about making them effective and how we can get to a better situation and avoid the worse situations. As you know, I think there is a methodology that underlies the so-called "principlist" approach, and it has to do with the business of specification. Specification is not something that one just wakes up one morning and says, "Well, I am going to specify a principle in such a way." At least it cannot be done responsibly that way. It takes a lot of arguments and dealing extensively with cases.

For example, let us take the discussion that just occurred about the cases presented by Dr. Al-Bar regarding Pfizer and GlaxoSmithKline. This is an area I know a fair amount about. It is a very difficult territory; there have been a lot of abuses in that area. There are also, however, some fairly exemplary pharmaceutical companies that have bioethics committees, not only for human research but also in some cases for animal research. So, it is something that can be controlled. It can be brought under control, monitored, it can be supported from the position of the CEO down to all employees. Unfortunately, though, most pharmaceutical companies do not have a structure like that in place. Also, at least in the United States, they are not very carefully monitored by the government because they are private corporations and also because we do not have a very good system, frankly, in the United States for monitoring these fundamentally ethical problems, the problems of Pfizer and GlaxoSmithKline that Dr. Al-Bar was mentioning. I think the best solution is to have both internal committees that debate these issues and formulate policies that are then reviewed at a higher level as well as have external people as well.

There is really no way to shortcut this. It is similar to writing a book. You do not get up one morning and write a book. It takes a lot of extensive research and arguments and so on. The same applies to ethics. It takes embedding the stuff in material and sometimes the material is highly unfamiliar to people so they have to come to grips with it. Earlier I mentioned the discussion I had at a seminar in Japan where people simply did not understand what informed consent was and how important it had become, even in their own country. They had to be updated on what the situation was and then they had to formulate the policies of informed consent and informed refusal and so on in very difficult circumstances. So that is just a way of saying there really is no shortcut. It takes extensive debate and argument considering the examples and counter-examples, looking into problems and how those problems can be rectified. It has to be done both internally within organizations as well as by external observers and critics of those organizations. That would be my basic answer to the first question.

The second question asked whether the four principles are complementary and do all the four go together as a set. Yes, I think they all four go together as a set. That is the whole idea. As to whether they are complementary, I suppose it depends a little bit on what is meant by complementary. I would rather use a term such as *comprehensive*. I think they are reasonably comprehensive, and of course by specification they can be made even more comprehensive.

The one thing that is important here that we have discussed a good bit is the possibility of conflict. These principles can certainly constantly encounter situations of conflict. The chief example I used in my talk yesterday was the problem of paternalism, where respect for autonomy comes in conflict with beneficence or, since we are dealing with medicine, medical beneficence. There is a constant potential for conflict between respect for autonomy and beneficence. I would say the same thing here that I was just saying in general: there really is no shortcut for this. I think it is a huge mistake for people to say, well I am a paternalist or I am an anti-paternalist. You have to argue each issue out as it comes along. Paternalism can arise almost anywhere, not only in clinical medicine, which is where people often think about it. It could also arise in, for example, public policy. Earlier someone mentioned the F.D.A. in the United States. The F.D.A. is a paternalist organization. That is what it is in the business to do. It is in the business of protecting you against yourself by not allowing you to purchase certain kinds of medicine before they are ready to be purchased in addition to requiring prescriptions. That is basically a paternalist organization. Is that good or is it bad? Well, maybe some features of it are good and some features of it are bad. However, one cannot just decide that *a priori*. It must be argued out at some length. That is what I would say about them being complementary.

The third part is whether the principles can be prioritized. As I think I said with some firmness yesterday, there is not. I do not believe in the idea of prioritizing principles. I have never seen a system in which there was an attempt at prioritizing that was successful. Professor John Rawls wrote probably the best-known book of philosophy in the 20th century, *A Theory of Justice*. He attempted to do this just with the principles of justice in his case. I think that by almost all accounts it was a complete failure. So even in the very best academic works or public policies where prioritizing has been attempted, it simply does not work. The reason is quite simple. In a policy or formulation of abstract principles, you cannot anticipate all of the cases that will ultimately fall under those principles.

Therefore, you cannot know how important one principle will be by contrast to the other. To go back to the paternalism example, in some cases it is extremely important to get a medicine started on a patient or to perform a medical intervention because otherwise they will die. Let us say you have a severe threat that is operative. In other cases, there is not much of a threat at all. It is a very small operation. Each situation presents a different context with a different set of considerations that need to be balanced. So I am not a prioritizer; I am a balancer and a specification person as you can see.

Tariq Ramadan

Earlier, Sheikh Raissouni asked a very important question: What is medicine? Dr. Beauchamp, you said you developed these principles in the 1970s because at that time bioethics did not exist. In other words, bioethics is something specific, and medicine in earlier days is not the same as the medicine we are talking about today. So while the papers presented during this seminar argue that there were similar issues [in medicine] before and there are answers to these issues from the past, you are saying there is a difference in the nature of medicine before and now. I believe this is an important point worthy of discussion. So what exactly is the difference, and what exactly do you mean when you say nothing was there before?

Tom Beauchamp

I certainly do not say that nothing was there before. Both medicine and medical ethics have a history of several thousand years. Much of it is interesting, but the important realization that occurred, I believe, was closer to the 1960s. The realization began to seep in that most of it is quite irrelevant to modern problems. That was the tipping point. Let me give you a particular event that happened in my own life that had to do with when I was recruited into bioethics by a man in medicine. He was an obstetrician and gynecologist (OB/GYN) named André Hellegers. He was the director of our institute at Georgetown University. When I got to know André, he had the view, and I think it was fundamentally a right view, that medicine had completely lost its way because of developments in modern medicine. It [medicine] thought that something like the Hippocratic tradition was going to be a sufficient medical ethics because it had thought in that way for centuries. In his view, and again I think he was correct, it is utterly inadequate to resolve most of the problems that have come into medicine.

Take one example that was occurring at that time regarding what to do in the way of distributing dialysis machines. We suddenly had, in the United States, legislation — a national law — that said everybody gets a dialysis. Is that a right law? Do we do that with all of medicine? We never had dialysis machines before, and generalizing from dialysis machines, we never had anything like the kind of power in medicine, scientific power, to actually cure people. Medicine for centuries and centuries had been largely a matter of giving people hope with very little science behind it. What happened in the early part of the 20th century was interesting. The most notable country here was Germany because Germany was the most advanced scientific country early on and began to refashion the way in which medicine was taught along scientific lines. The United States began to learn from the German example around the 1920s or so and began to redesign all of its medical schools and its entire system.

So what was happening is the science was getting ahead of the ethics. The ethics was not changing and yet the science advanced rapidly. Suddenly there was this enormous amount of scientific research being done and brought into medicine, and new technology developed and we simply did not know what to do with it. Furthermore, the Hippocratic tradition was not helping us at all. So when I talk about fundamental change, that is the kind of fundamental change that I mean. You needed a new biomedical ethics to come to grips with a period in which hundreds of new problems that had no precedence at all in the Hippocratic tradition were coming along.

I will give one example. In the Hippocratic tradition and all these medical ethics traditions from thousands of years ago that I mentioned, there is no research ethics whatsoever. Suddenly we found the major problems that we had had to do with, for example, cases like the Nuremberg trials that someone mentioned earlier. That is very interesting because the trial took place in Germany, the most scientifically advanced country in the world. One of the problems is that ethics had not kept up with reality there. Of course you also had a crazy political regime in Germany, but there was a parallel problem about the ethics.

Let us come back now to the question that was set in the 1970s, and let us take research ethics as an example because it is the simplest one. The discussion of research ethics really only began in the 1970s. Something like the four principles or the idea of having principles that can be embedded in discussions of medical research was all new. It had to be completely created because there was no precedence for it whatsoever. Hence, when I make these sharp breaks and put it in that way, that is the kind of thing I am talking about.

Tariq Ramadan

Just to follow up, would you say that with all the technology we have now you would give a new definition to medicine, or is it the same?

Tom Beauchamp

That is a very good question. It is fundamentally a definitional or a conceptual question, and the territory has to be much broader. In other words, if you are going to recast the definition, which it probably should be, the territory will have to be a lot broader than it covers, and the ethics is going to have to track the changes in that territory. Again, perhaps an example would help a lot. In my career, I spent a great deal of time arguing — gently, but arguing — with a colleague of mine named Edmund Pellegrino. Pellegrino believes that the fundamental ethics in a clinical context, in clinical medicine, has to do with the patient–physician relationship. He views it as a one-on-one relationship, the doctor and the patient. That is fundamentally what medicine is about, and it is fundamentally what medical ethics is about. I think that is far too narrow. Medicine is far, far more than that. It infuses into territories like biomedical research, public health, and so on in ways in which it has not in the past. The encounter between physicians and patients is nothing like one-on-one anymore. So those are just a couple of the many issues we have to think about in order to address your question intelligently and comprehensively. Do I think there has been a fundamental change in the healthcare system? Absolutely I do, so in terms of definitions, we have to catch up with what those changes are. This will perhaps help us restructure and rethink the nature of the system as we continue to create it.

Mohammed Ghaly

The change that has been occurring in medicine — and it is a fundamental change as Dr. Beauchamp says — requires a fundamental change in the ethics of medicine. I think it is not enough to point out that something that occurred was ethically wrong. It is also necessary to figure out how to proceed.

Tariq Ramadan

Given what Professor Beauchamp just mentioned about the fundamental changes in medicine and the changing realities, I do not think it is possible to order or prioritize the higher objectives of Sharia in any particular way. Dr. Beauchamp says that there is no way to order the four principles in any particular way; they form a set together. Given what I hear now about the change in medicine and the new questions that arise, ordering does not seem feasible. Is it possible now to maintain the order and prioritization of the higher objectives of Sharia as they have been before?

Abdullah Bin Bayyah

It is possible to say that the higher objectives of Sharia are the products of the human intellect, of human rationality, meaning what are the needs and necessities of man on earth? For the religious person, Muslim and non-Muslim alike, the central point is the person's relationship with God. That is why they say religion. In this sense we mean religion in general, in the sense stated in the verse, "He [God] has ordained for you of religion what He enjoined upon Noah and that which We have revealed to you, [O Muhammad], and what We enjoined upon Abraham and Moses and Jesus — to establish the religion and not be divided therein…" (Qur'an 42:13). So we mean religion in the general sense of the word.

Wealth is also one of the higher objectives of Sharia. Most scholars of Islamic legal theory (*uṣūlīyūn*) put the higher objectives of Sharia in the following order: religion, life, wealth, intellect, and offspring or honor (or whichever wording they used). If man exists in order to maintain his life, he needs to own property. As God states, "And the earth He [God] laid [out] for the creatures. Therein are fruit and palm trees having sheaths [of dates] and grain having husks and scented plants" (Qur'an 55:10–12). God created earth with abundant benefits for man, and the first notion of ownership was ownership of the land that a person revives with his own hands. Therefore, it is natural that the higher objective of wealth would come after the higher objective of life in terms of order and priority.

Similarly, it is natural to care about the higher objective of the intellect of the human because intellect is what distinguishes humans from animals. Of course, the discrepancy here is in the means and not in the fundamentals themselves. I believe all religions agree on the need to protect and preserve the intellect. Our Islamic literature tells us this is a point agreed upon by all sects and religions.

The preservation of offspring or lineage is also important. A person's lineage requires certain conditions such as having parents: a father and a mother. The new ethics — or allow me to say the new "nonethics" — wants to cancel the concept of motherhood and fatherhood, which is part of a human's natural disposition (*fiṭrah*). In my opinion, I do not see anything new. I see that the novelty happens in the details and not in the tenets or the foundations (*uṣūl*). This is true even in medicine. The etymology of the Arabic word for medicine, *ṭibb*, means that which treats man. Getting to know the context through the language points us to the general concept that everything that treats man is considered medicine.

Regarding the ordering of the higher objectives of Sharia set by the early scholars, it is important to view this issue as one of *kullī mushakkik*, which is defined as a concept that exists in its instances in varying degrees.[1] Such a concept requires verifying the underlying character (*taḥqīq al-manāṭ*) at every one of those varying degrees. Independent

[1] Editor's note: As an example, the color green is *kullī mushakkik* because different objects exhibit various shades of green. *Kullī mushakkik* stands in contrast to *kullī mutawāṭi'*, which refers to a concept that exists in its instances univocally. For example, humanity is *kullī matawāṭi'*: all humans are equal in their humanity.

legal reasoning (*ijtihād*) requires *taḥqīq al-manāṭ*, which means the application of agreed-upon rules on a foreign reality. In other words, the rules and values are well established, but the question is: what is the relationship of these rules and values to reality? This is a key challenge facing us today. Industrial capitalism has occluded the prospect of practicing *taḥqīq al-manāṭ*. Modern man's greed, his rush to gain money even at the detriment of others, and his lack of care and devotion to serving others sometimes means that he is indifferent to and careless about morality. This triggers the set of problems raised by Dr. Al-Bar earlier.

I am fond of *taḥqīq al-manāṭ* because it is my specialty and it is an area I am currently working on. If I may, please allow me a bit of digression. Here is a question: Is the president of a country considered a caliph? Or is he the guardian of a constitutional document, while a caliph was considered the guardian of both worldly life and of religion. I believe the latter is true, so questions arise about how to apply religious legislations to the realities of our modern life. What benefits and harms result from answering these questions in one way versus another? In the case of Egypt today, should priority go to society's safety and security or to the implementation of some religious rulings? I would say that the safety and security of society is the first higher objective of Sharia. Likewise, do we still have the same understanding of men being the protectors and maintainers of women? Is the working woman expected to singlehandedly provide care to her child, or does the man now have a large part in childcare? These questions need answers because of the new realities of our time. Similarly, is the idea of the abode of Islam (*dār al-Islām*) and the abode of non-Islam (*dār al-kufr*) still applicable today? Today, it is all considered one land. International relations have changed, international treaties and agreements are different, and the nature of war has changed. All of these issues present confusion, and we need to become like the *mujtahid* who exerts his or her utmost effort to arrive at a certain truth or what is close to it.

Mohammed Ghaly

So is the ordering [of the higher objectives of Sharia] based on independent legal reasoning (*ijtihād*), or is it fixed and unchanging?

Abdullah Bin Bayyah

The order of principles is based on independent legal reasoning (*ijtihād*), and it depends on a group of the governing texts and the comprehensive juristic rules *(al-qawā'id al-kullīyah)*. This means if you want to develop a higher objective, you have to look at the Sharia rulings that affirm it. As stated in a verse, "...And whoever denies the faith — his work has become worthless..." (Qur'an 5:5). So you must search for relevant texts that are certain and governing in order to decide on the higher objective. In other words, it is open for independent legal reasoning but this does not mean it can be arbitrarily decided; there is a system.

Ahmed Raissouni

We are now talking about the ordering of the five necessary higher objectives (*ḍarūrīyāt*) specifically and not about the ordering of all of the higher objectives of Sharia. The order of the five necessary objectives is of course an intellectual and rational endeavor, an example of independent legal reasoning. In fact, the specification of the five necessary objectives and their naming are based on human thought and reasoning formulated over a period of three or four centuries, and the efforts continue. The role of independent legal reasoning is clear, but independent legal reasoning is of course done using proof. So if scholars provide the textual evidence and valid reasoning, then this independent legal reasoning is binding just like it is in any other case, unless and until it is refuted by evidence — and nothing refutes this ordering.

However, the most important thing is the idea of ordering in the first place. Then comes the ordering that I mentioned, at least the three levels that are agreed upon by all who have addressed the issue of ordering. This is one aspect. A second aspect is that there is another ordering that has an effect on this issue. This other ordering has to do with the division of benefits (*maṣāliḥ*) respectively into necessities (*ḍarūrīyāt*), needs (*ḥājīyāt*), and luxuries (*taḥsīnīyāt*). It is interesting to note that we find certain behaviors, actions, and rulings that can sometimes be classified as necessities and other times as needs. Even food itself is an example. The default category food belongs to is that of necessities. However, in some instances food can be considered among needs and in other instances it can be considered among luxuries depending on one's context, for example.

The order here is agreed upon, that the necessities (*ḍarūrīyāt*) are above the needs (*ḥājīyāt*), which are above the luxuries (*taḥsīnīyāt*). This is in the form of a theoretical organizing table, but when we engage with reality, the process of application — or *taḥqīq al-manāṭ* as Sheikh Bin Bayyah calls it — requires precise considerations in every single case. As Sayf Al-Din Al-Amidi says, we might find what appears to be the preferring of the preservation of wealth over the preservation of religion. In other words, we may find a case where we prefer what is usually ordered lower over what is usually ordered higher. However, these are specific applications. A person, for the sake of his wealth, is exempted from performing *hajj*, which is a pillar of Islam. He is exempted from congregational prayer if he fears for his wealth. He is exempted from fasting if he fears for his health. These are specific applications that require going back to the categories of necessities, needs, and luxuries. In all cases, a need has never been given preference over a necessity, and a luxury has never been given preference over a need or necessity. This is what I would say generally on the topic of ordering.

I would also like to comment on Dr. Beauchamp's point about applying the four principles together, as a set. I would agree and I would say the same about both the set of four principles and the set of five necessary objectives: within each set, the elements are all equally important. This is because the necessary objectives of Sharia, as a whole group, are that without which life is unsustainable. By definition, if one necessity ceases, life itself ceases. If religion ceases, people become barbaric and harm each other. Even wealth, which is usually given a low priority in the ordering, is important because without it, crops would perish and people would die.

There was a discussion about the events currently taking place in Mali. Some of my colleagues said that self-determination is the solution for Northern Mali, while others said that we should not accept the division of Muslims. The answer was that the division of Muslims was happening anyway, so the priority should be to stop the bloodshed. Any kind of unity between the North and South would entail either fighting or self-determination. My point is that verifying the underlying character of certain issues (*taḥqīq al-manāṭ*) has its own calculations and its own vision as to how to fulfill a need.

Also, I will make a brief comment regarding the definition of medicine and changes in medicine, and I would like to hear others' opinions on this, especially Dr. Beauchamp. I believe the reality of medicine today has expanded beyond its previously known limits. Does this expansion mean that there is a new understanding of medicine, from the perspective of the World Health Organization, for example, or from the perspective of any other party? Has a new understanding emerged that includes mercy killing, abortion, and the torture of prisoners? Yes, military doctors now participate in the torture of prisoners, whether military or civilian. These are all new unethical and criminal roles practiced by doctors. Does the definition of medicine encompass this, or is this something else forcibly attributed to medicine? Is there a new definition of medicine other than the one mentioned by Dr. Al-Bar, which is preserving health and warding off harm? That, or something similar, has been the definition for a long time. However, nowadays there are widespread medical practices that are not encompassed by that definition whatsoever. An example is plastic surgery. We heard about the scandal that happened a few months ago in France regarding the artificial body parts that led to cancer. Plastic surgery has started to contribute to deformations, lesions, and impairments while this is not from the core of the medical field. It is not one of the roles of the doctor to beautify a man or a woman; instead, a doctor is responsible for treating illness and preserving health. Do we have a new understanding of medicine that goes beyond our traditional understanding?

Tom Beauchamp

I think we are in a period in which we are attempting to rethink the doctor–patient relationship and all the functions of the physician. Just think about the people being produced by medical schools and then what people can do when they come out of medical schools. They can be involved in public health, they can be involved in the medical humanities, or they can be involved in the basic sciences among other things. They may have no contact with patients whatsoever, or they might have 100 percent contact with patients. Doctors can do a lot of things, and [their role] is going to change even more dramatically. People who are trained to be physicians are going to be able to do a great deal more in terms of diversity than they were in the past and will continue to adjust the system to their being able to do that. Probably some of these things will be good, and probably some of them will be bad.

That is part of where ethics comes into the situation. For example, we now have many more conflicts of interest than we have ever historically had in medicine. The biggest one historically was of course fee-for-service that led to certain kinds of problems. How are we going to handle these problems arising from conflict of interest? It is the same point I made earlier: as we expand the number of things that physicians and people involved in the healthcare system can do for people and the things that can go wrong ethically, we will need new ways of regulating that and controlling it and so on.

Tariq Ramadan

I have a question for Sheikh Bin Bayyah. You said that the foundations of religion (*uṣūl*) do not change and rather the issue is about verifying the underlying ground (*taḥqīq al-manāṭ*) and applying those foundations in the context (*tanzīl*). Dr. Beauchamp said something else. He said that the changes in medicine now spurred them to come up with four principles that are derived from reality, from the changes in medicine and from changes in the doctor–patient relationship. This brings me to the issue raised by Sheikh Al-Qaradaghi regarding the preservation of society. The security of society is a new concept and is very important. So there is a change here in the foundation, and it is possible sometimes that the ordering would change. So is this possible? Or do we have to go back to the tradition of what the earlier Muslim scholars, and would that be enough as a response? We have to realize that it is no longer only about the doctor–patient relationship. Rather, it is about the preservation of the safety of society.

Jasser Auda

I would like to add to this last question regarding the fact that objectives have to do with the individual. I mean they are intended to preserve the life of the individual, the mind of the individual, the honor of the individual, etc. Dr. Ramadan, on the other hand, spoke about society and that the old ethics relevant to individuals can no longer cater for the needs of society. So if, in the science of the higher objectives of Sharia, we were discussing the life of the individual and the honor of the individual, etc., now at the societal level things become more complicated when we discuss the "life" of the society or the "honor" of the society. My question is about the social or societal dimension of the higher objectives of Sharia: Does it affect or put pressure on the theory [of higher objectives]? Is there a need to change the theory to become a theory for the society instead of a theory for the individual, which is what it has historically been?

Ali Al-Qaradaghi

As I explained earlier, the safety of society and the safety of the state have been given two criteria [individual and communal] in Islamic law (Sharia). These two criteria are not entirely encompassed by concept of the higher objectives of Sharia because the Islamic legal jurists (*fuqahā'*), may God reward them greatly, focused on the individual because the individual is the basic unit [of society]. However, reality dictates that safety is the safety of society, and it includes political, economic, societal, and environmental security. I will not elaborate on these issues now but rather will talk about what the scholars of legal theory (*uṣūl*) have contributed on the matter.

As Sheikh Raissouni said, the higher objectives of Sharia are a topic that has been discussed for several centuries, starting with Imam Al-Haramayn and continuing into the present day. We are all trying to understand it. For example, in my opinion, the order of the higher objectives is based on independent legal reasoning (*ijtihād*) which is not conclusive in nature. In other words, the order is based on independent legal reasoning that is open to discussion and revision, but it remains a sort of a general principle. For example, we all say that religion is prioritized above life. If we specify "religion" to mean the religion of the individual, when an individual's religion threatens his life, then in that situation, it is accepted that life is prioritized over religion, as long as he is in his heart still steadfast on the truth. However, if we specify "religion" to mean the religion of the society, when religion in total is jeopardized, this is where we would say that religion is indeed prioritized over life. In this case there would be *jihād* within its proper limits or norms, and *jihād* is not defined as the killing of the soul for just any reason. Therefore, it is incredibly important that we look at the issue at the individual level and the societal level.

Here are some more examples: whoever is killed defending his wealth is considered a martyr; whoever is killed defending his honor (*'irḍ*) is considered a martyr; and whoever is killed defending his soul is considered a martyr. These cases indicate that the prioritization can change depending on the situation. In my opinion, we need to work more on this issue. The matter requires the establishment of groundwork and standards because so far we can only talk about generalities: in general, religion is prioritized over life, for example.

What I mean by "religion" here is not Islam in its entirety because the preservation of life, honor, and wealth are all a part of Islam. By religion I mean specifically the aspects of Islam relating to ritual worship and the like. The higher objectives of Sharia are not evidence by themselves, standing alone. I cannot come to a conclusion where my only evidence is the higher objectives. The higher objectives of Sharia serve as standards and criteria (*mi'yārīyah*): they are only a scale by which to weigh evidences against each other. They are part of Islam and cannot function as independent evidence by themselves.

Abdullah Bin Bayyah

To be honest, I am afraid that we will end up in what is called a Byzantine discussion. Reality is not always what we see. "And you see the mountains, thinking them rigid, while they will pass as the passing of clouds. [It is] the work of God, who perfected all things…" (Qur'an 27:88). What we see could be misleading. Since the beginning of humanity's existence, humans have had needs like wealth. I do not agree that the legal jurists focused exclusively on individual issues [when it comes to the higher purposes of Sharia]. Rather, when we say preservation of "individual" life, we also mean the preservation of the society and its safety. Indeed, if the need is a public one, then it is emphasized as such. It is as Al-Ghazali said and also as stated in *Al-ḥāshīyāt*: a certain need is either a public one or an individual one. So I urge us to not jump to conclusions about what the early scholars said.

If we say that religion came to preserve for people both their worldly benefit and their benefit in the Hereafter, this demonstrates the centrality of religion as a higher objective since the loss of the Hereafter is a great loss, at least in the eyes of the believer. In my opinion, the changes happening around us are immense, but the basic needs of humans will stay for as long as humans walk the Earth. No doubt man needs to eat, to be clothed, to live, to die, etc. These needs do not change. If they change, all rulings change. If these basic human needs do not change, then the higher objectives of Sharia [still apply].

The higher objectives of Sharia provide a broad framework, and they are indeed "high" and thus do not produce rulings directly. Under them is a set of other objectives that come second to the higher ones but not necessarily secondary to them, and so on. For example, justice is considered a *kullī mushakkik* (a comprehensive concept comprising instances of varying degrees). Al-Shatibi said there are 70 degrees of justice, ranging from obligatory on one end to recommended to permissible on the other end. Similarly, the objectives of Sharia exist in levels or degrees. Nevertheless, one thing is clear. There do exist high objectives that apply to society in general and not only to individuals. Take the verse, "And there is for you in legal retribution [saving of] life, O you [people] of understanding, that you may become righteous" (Qur'an 2:179). Life for whom? The murderer's victim has died. Life here refers to the life of the society.

Muhammad Ali Al-Bar

Dr. Beauchamp said that before the 1970s, there was a different reality and thus they were obliged to come up with the four principles. In 1964, there was the Declaration of Helsinki and before that as well there were a number of similar efforts. The Declaration of Helsinki talked about a host of ethical principles including those associated with defining risks, how to protect the rights of participants of scientific experiments, the responsibilities of the doctor in preserving the life of patients, the importance of upholding scientific research standards, respecting the environment, and proper treatment of animals. It also discussed the need to provide a protocol to the Institutional Review Board; the importance of being transparent about the ethical issues involved in a scientific research project; disclosing all associated risks; conducting research only on individuals who are suited for such research; taking the voluntary permission of research participants after disclosing all relevant information; the need to get patient consent detailing the different types of consents, withdrawals, refusals, or participations; and more. The detailing of all these points did not start in the 1970s; rather, it was declared on an international scale with the Declaration of Helsinki in the year 1964, and other similar things did also exist.

Tom Beauchamp

I will comment briefly and then we can discuss. First of all I did not say the 1970s. I specifically said the 1960s was when I think the big change was made, and I mentioned the dialysis case. The dialysis case appeared 1 or 2 years before the Declaration of Helsinki. This was clearly a very instrumental period in the change. What is important to understand, and what I was emphasizing before, is why we had to have this change. Why it is a radical change to have something like the Declaration of Helsinki, which really is not a very good document. It was an early, rather poorly constructed document. It is very different today, but it was quite poorly constructed in the 1960s. The main point here is why we needed it. We needed it because we had nothing. We had nothing to cover that area whatsoever. That is the really important point.

Now let us step back a minute because someone earlier mentioned the Nuremberg trials. The Nuremberg trials are a fabulous example of how we missed the boat because we did not understand the need for change that we had. The Nuremberg trials were an American military tribunal. It was originally set up to be four different countries that would try the tribunals, but ultimately it became an American military tribunal. In the end, in my view, it was an absolute disaster. The trials did bring forward a lot of evidence, and the evidence was in many respects very carefully monitored. Some of the judges exhibited some good reasoning, but the truth of the matter is that it was a kind of mockery. Why? Because the American military at the time found guilty German physicians who were doing exactly what the American military was doing at the time. Now, what did we learn from German experimentation about what was lacking in our system? The answer is nothing.

It is often said that the Nuremberg trials were a great precedent and the Nuremberg Code is a great precedent. Historically, that is just very false. What happened in Germany in 1946 and 1947 was a finding of guilt — or innocence in some cases — of a group of German physicians, and then we walked away from it. I want to emphasize that we walked away from it. I want to emphasize it was not just the Americans who walked away from it. In my view, disgracefully, it was the whole world who walked away from it. No one took Nuremberg seriously. The Germans, at that time it was East Germany and West Germany, both rejected it wholly and completely. They took nothing away from it. The Americans, who had conducted the trials and had come up with the so-called Nuremberg Code, did not institute one single principle of that code anywhere in the culture or the government or anywhere else; nor did any other country. It was a huge lost opportunity. It was difficult to come to grips with the fact that we had no system to control science of the sort that had gotten out of control and, actually, was out of control in the United States at the same time.

I say you not only were having changes, you needed these changes, and we missed the boat. I think we bear — maybe the American military more than anybody else — we certainly bear as a culture in the United States and I think the world bears some guilt here for failing to understand because we went on with this kind of experimentation well beyond the Declaration of Helsinki. It went on and on for another 30 or 40 years during which a great many experimental subjects were being abused because we did not have anything put in place to control it. To be precise about this, in the case of the United States, it was not until roughly 1968 that we had any controls whatsoever put in place, and those were for entirely different reasons. They had nothing to do with the Declaration of Helsinki and nothing to do with the Nuremberg trials. They had to do with certain legal problems in the American system where we were concerned about the liability of the national institutes of health. So when I say there were dramatic changes in the 1960s and then again on the biomedical ethics side of it in the 1970s, I believe that that is entirely accurate and true.

People continue to praise the Nuremberg Code and its impact. There was nothing to be praised in the Nuremberg Code and its impact because there basically was no impact. I could go on and on about that and about the Declaration of Helsinki. The Declaration of Helsinki is nowadays being rejected more than it is being accepted, but that is a different story.

Annelien Bredenoord

I would like to ask you a question about what you call specification. In the end, the principles are abstract moral norms. In order for them to be an action guide or to be used for what we call applied ethics, they need to be specified to concrete cases. In the end, it could be very well possible that with different concrete specifications, there is pluralism at the level of specification. In other words, there could be several existing specifications that conflict with each other and that collide with each other. So when can you say that one specific specification is more justified than another specification?

You also say that a specification is justified if it is consistent and coherent: consistent with common morality and coherent within its own system. I think you can check whether it is coherent with its own system, but how can you check whether a specification is consistent with the norms of common morality because then you have to be quite lucid about what entails common morality. Perhaps you can elaborate on that.

Tom Beauchamp

There are lots of problems here. One is that we do not have as good an understanding of the common morality as a whole as we would like to have. I understand your question to be not about medical or biomedical ethics in particular but rather about the general problem of how to hold the whole thing together and know that one set of specifications is better than another.

There is a basic rule that I operate with, and Childress and I tried to spell it out to some length, although probably not a satisfactory length, but the idea is quite simple. Any set of specifications that is coherent with the general principles of the common morality — whatever those principles exactly turn out to be — if it is coherent both internally with itself and also coherent with the principles of the common morality, then it is acceptable. That can lead to many different, to take my example earlier, professional guidelines. There are many different professional guidelines, and each professional association may have a somewhat different one. To answer your question, yes, they can conflict with one another — there is no doubt about it. I think it is just a matter of fact that that is the case, and they justifiably conflict. The way I want to take that up is: everything is justified if it is coherent with common morality until the point at which it violates a principle of the common morality, in which case it is obviously no longer coherent. That is where I think problems begin.

So if you go back to what we were discussing a minute ago, the German experimentation and American experimentation in the 1930s or principally in the 1940s, they stepped over the line. They clearly stepped over the line and were violating those principles. So if you had tried to specify a moral system to govern what was being done (there actually were some attempts at the time to do that by the Department of Defense in the United States), they would have been over the line. In other words, they would not have what I would call a system of biomedical ethics that is coherent with the common morality. That is the basic answer to your question.

It is terribly complicated in part because we also do not have an adequate theory of coherence, a philosophical coherence theory. We have lots of them, but we still do not have an adequate account that engages in this area that we are talking about, which is applied ethics. That is, so to speak, still to be written.

Tariq Ramadan

Professor Beauchamp, I have one clarification about the terminology that we are using. We talked about medicine, we talked about bioethics, and while I was listening to you right now you used the term biomedical ethics. What is the difference between medicine and biomedicine?

Tom Beauchamp

I have never liked the word *bioethics*, and that is just a personal preference. It does not mean very much to me to abbreviate it. The word was adopted in the very late 1960s probably by two separate people, but I will not go into that history. It was a very shorthand way of attempting to get not only what we think of as *biomedical ethics* but also *bioethics* more broadly as when we speak today about something like *biodiversity*, so it incorporated an environmental ethics. I have always thought that the term *bioethics* was too unclear. Childress and I did not want to use it and so we put *biomedical ethics* in the title of our book. However, having said that, that is more a personal preference on my part than the way usage is actually developed. Usage today is such that, universally, the word *bioethics* is used far more than *biomedical* and it has become the standard word. To make this really simple, they are synonymous. I think nowadays they have become synonymous so *biomedical ethics* is *bioethics*, and there is no difference between them even though someone like me would like to draw a difference between them.

Mohammed Ghaly

I have one final question about the beginning of the story of writing your book in the 1970s. When you were sitting in your office together with Dr. Childress, how many ethical principles did you and Professor Childress have on the table before you arrived at the four principles? In other words, I am sure you had a list of possible principles and you had to choose some. How many did you originally have?

Tom Beauchamp

That is a historically interesting question and a little bit hard to unravel. You are asking a historical question about what happened. Two things were taking place. Childress and I were lecturing in a course for health professionals, and we were not using the language of principles — or rather, the language of principles was, so to speak, secondary. We were principally lecturing on ethical theories, and so then we would talk about the principles that can be justified in light of the ethical theories. At the same time as I was doing this, I went on the staff of the National Commission for the Protection of Human Subjects of Biomedical and Behavioral Research, where I wrote the Belmont Report for that National Commission.

So I was writing the Belmont Report at the same time Childress and I were lecturing in this course. After each lecture, Childress and I would sit down and try to figure out what we were learning from one another through our lectures as well as what I was learning at the National Commission. The National Commission, as you probably know, in the Belmont Report uses three categories: respect for persons, beneficence, and justice. I was not happy with the way in which they were using the language of respect for persons, and I was not happy with the way they were using the language of beneficence.

The biggest part of the early discussions that Childress and I had, although we already had those principles on the table, was exactly how we wanted to fashion the principles. So we decided to throw out the principle of respect for persons. There were a number of reasons for that. One, we simply thought it was far too confusing in the literature of what a person is. By the way, I believe that continues to be the case today. We did not think it is a manageable principle to develop along those lines. We also thought that when you are talking about first priorities, it was basically respect for autonomy, so that became the principle. Beneficence we thought was highly confused by the National Commission because it threw beneficence and nonmaleficence together into one principle. We decided that you had to break that out, and so we broke it out. Justice we thought was far too narrow as it was conceived by the National Commission because it basically had to do with the selection of subjects for research. We thought justice had to be considerably generalized, so we began to think about the scope of that principle.

It was in a context in which those were the principal things that were on the table that we eventually ended up with the basic understanding. It is the four folds concept when you think about it, so you have concepts like the concept of nonmaleficence and the concept of autonomy. You then fashion the principle around the concept, then you refine the principle to try to get it just right. That is the process we used.

Now you might have been asking if there were other principles on the table. We certainly looked at a lot, but we were never very attracted to any. I will give you a couple of examples. There were virtually no books at the time we started that discussed principles of medical ethics or biomedical ethics or whatever. The most plausible books or articles for that matter were old. I mean by this several years old treaties on principles in the Roman Catholic tradition. The Roman Catholic tradition has always been keen on developing principles. However, those were far too narrow and specific to the Roman Catholic religion, especially for what we wanted to do, which was basically a secular bioethics, as you know, that cut across all traditions. So we found that nothing in that tradition in the way of principles was going to help us. Another thing that of course was very much discussed at the time was the principle of utility. We decided that the principle of utility was simply unacceptable as a general principle and had to be folded under the principle of beneficence. So we went through a process of thinking like that, and that is how we ended up with what we have now.

Part III

Islamic Perspectives on the Principles of Biomedical Ethics

Ethics in Medicine: A Principle-Based Approach in Light of the Higher Objectives (*Maqāṣid*) of Sharia

Ahmed Raissouni

Abstract: The main premise of this chapter is that ethics is an indivisible whole and thus cannot be divided into various segments, each of which may fit within a specific aspect of life such as medicine, politics, finance, or social relations. However, specific principles and values can be more highlighted in particular fields because they will work more efficiently and be more productive than other clusters of values and principles. This chapter is divided into two main sections. The first section elaborates on the position of ethics in Sharia and its higher objectives arguing that life in its totality must be based on ethics. The second section focuses on ethics in the field of medicine arguing that the medical field in particular cannot survive unless it is based on ethics. Two main virtues are highlighted in this chapter because of their relevance to the field of medicine, both of which constitute two major principles of Islamic ethics as well, to wit, God-consciousness (*taqwá*) and mercy (*raḥmah*). The chapter also touches upon the overlap between the higher objectives of Sharia and those of medicine. The main objectives of Sharia are protecting (*ḥifẓ*) the so-called five necessities, namely religion, life, offspring, intellect, and wealth. Three of these five represent the main objectives of medicine, *viz*., protecting life, offspring, and intellect.

1. The Status of Ethics in Light of Sharia and its Higher Objectives

The high status conferred upon ethics in Islamic Sharia is evidenced through the following aspects:

1.1. *Ethics (akhlāq) and Creed ('aqīdah) Form the Basis of Sharia*

This first aspect is particularly discernible for those who reflect on the Qur'anic verses revealed in Mecca. The majority of these verses, as is well known, establish creed and morality as the foundations of the message brought forth by the Prophet Muhammad (PBUH) and of Islamic Sharia. These foundations were named "all-inclusive rules" (*al-qawā'id al-kullīyah*) by Imam Al-Shatibi. This category of rules encompasses Islamic creed and Islamic ethics. Al-Shatibi, may God have mercy upon him, states,

> Know that the "all-inclusive rules" were the first decrees … and the foremost of these decrees was belief in God, His Messenger, and the Last Day. These were followed by general principles such as ritual prayer, charity, etc.[1] Subsequently came the forbiddance of disbelief and any practices associated with it, such as engaging in animal slaughter in favor of falsely claimed deities or any parties other than God or enjoining upon themselves unfounded prohibitions and permissions, all of which contradict the principle of worshipping God alone. In addition, all good morals were enjoined, including justice, beneficence,

[1] These commands were mentioned in the portions of the Qur'an revealed in Mecca in a general form, without details about application. For this reason, Al-Shatibi considered them to be among the comprehensive principles (*kullīyāt*) and basic fundamentals (*uṣūl asāsīyah*).

> keeping promises, forgiveness, avoiding ignorance, repaying evil with benevolence, fearing only God, patience, gratitude, and others. Concurrently, immoral behavior was prohibited, including vice, maleficence, oppression, speaking without knowledge, engaging in fraud and duplicity, corruption, adultery, murder, infanticide, and several other transgressions that were common prior to the advent of Islam...[2]

In his exegesis of the verse revealed in Mecca, "He has ordained for you of religion what He enjoined upon Noah and that which We have revealed to you, [O Muhammad], and what We enjoined upon Abraham and Moses and Jesus — to establish the religion and not be divided therein..." (Qur'an 42:13), the judge Abu Bakr bin Al-'Arabi explained,

> It means that God ordained the same religion to both Muhammad and Noah, namely in the principles that both religions advocate: the belief in God as the only God, ritual prayer, almsgiving (*zakāt*), fasting, pilgrimage (*ḥajj*), getting closer to God by observing righteous deeds, seeking closeness to Him by what gets the heart and body organs focused on Him, truthfulness, fulfilling promises, restoring trusts to their owners, maintaining kinship relations, and forbidding: disbelief, murder, harming people, attacking animals in any way, committing obscenities, and engaging in violations of honor.[3]

It is worth noting that if we were to restrict ourselves only to the moral commandments and prohibitions conveyed through the early Qur'anic verses during the founding stages of the message of Islam, as highlighted by Al-Shatibi and Ibn Al-'Arabi, this would encompass the following:

Commandments: justice, beneficence, maintaining ties of kinship, keeping promises, honoring trusts, forgiveness, avoiding ignorance, repaying evil with benevolence, fearing only God, patience, gratitude, honesty, and seeking closeness to God through all good deeds.

Prohibitions: vice, maleficence, oppression, speaking without knowledge, engaging in fraud and duplicity, corruption, adultery, murder,

---

[2]Al-Shatibi (1997). *Al-muwāfaqāt fī uṣūl al-sharī'ah*, Cairo: Dar Ibn 'Affan: vol. 3, 335.
[3]Al-Qadi Abu Bakr bin Al-'Arabi (2003). *Rulings of the Qur'an* (*Aḥkām al-Qur'ān*), Beirut: Dar al-Kutub al-'Ilmiyah: vol. 4, 89–90.

infanticide, harming others, assaulting animals, committing obscenities, and violating honor.

1.2. *Abundant Texts and Expansive Ethical Discussions*

Ethical concepts and directives were not exclusive to the initial Qur'anic verses revealed in Mecca. Rather, they were expanded upon and reiterated across diverse Sharia texts and at all levels. An exploration of thematic classifications within the contents of the Qur'anic verses and Prophetic traditions clearly highlights the abundance, if not being the most abundant, of those themes and directives of a moral nature.

Perhaps the strongest evidence of the expansive space afforded to ethics in Islam is represented through the creation of a multivolume encyclopedia on ethics and morals under the supervision of Dr. Saleh bin Humayd and Mr. Abdul-Rahman bin Mulawwih. This encyclopedia was published in 11 volumes and was titled *Mawsu'at naḍrat al-na'īm fī makārim akhlāq al-raṣūl al-karīm*. It addressed 342 of the ethical and moral qualities included in the Qur'an and Prophetic Tradition (Sunna), encompassing internal and external (intrapersonal and interpersonal) ethics across all areas of public and private life. A thorough examination of the encyclopedia's index of topics explicitly reveals the high status of ethics in Islam, in addition to the pervasiveness and frequent occurrence of ethical directives across Qur'anic verses and Prophetic narrations.

1.3. *The Harmony between Ethics and Religion*

In a verse in which He is addressing the Prophet Muhammad — peace and blessings of God be upon him (PBUH) — God the Almighty says, "And indeed, you are of a great moral character" (Qur'an 68:4). The majority of Qur'an interpreters consider the great moral character of the Prophet (PBUH) to be the comprehensive representation of Islam and all Qur'anic teachings. In other words, the summation of Islam and the Qur'an in their entirety is represented through great moral character. The Prophet's wife 'A'ishah, may God be pleased with her, elaborated on this concept to those Companions who had asked her about the Prophet's character in reference to the above-mentioned verse; she replied, "His character was an embodiment of the Qur'an."[4]

Imam Al-Tabari says,

> The interpretation of God the Almighty's saying, "And indeed, you are of a great moral character" (Qur'an 68:4) is that God the Almighty says to His Prophet Muhammad, may the peace and blessings of God be upon him, that indeed, O Muhammad, you are of great manners, manners which constitute the manners of the Qur'an which God has inculcated into you and which are Islam and its legislations. The Qur'an interpreters said something similar to this explanation.[5]

Ibn 'Ashur said, "We have learned for sure that Islam is perfecting good morals and that the entire set of good morals boils down to God-consciousness (*taqwá*)."[6]

Accordingly, several scholars stated that, "Morality pervades religion; therefore, whoever exhibits better manners than you is superior to you in religious commitment."[7] Hence, the standard by which one's religiosity is measured is exemplary moral behavior, meaning that a person who practices good manners is considered righteous and vice versa.

Al-Bayhaqi reported through his chain of narrators on the authority of Ka'b bin Malik, may God be pleased with him, that a man from Banu Salamah relayed to him that he had asked the Messenger of God (PBUH) about Islam. The Messenger of God (PBUH) replied, "It is good manners." The man repeated the question, and the Messenger of God (PBUH) once again responded, "It is good manners," until he had repeated it five times.[8]

[4]Narrated by Ahmad in *Al-Musnad*, No. 24601 on the authority of 'A'ishah. It was also narrated by Muslim in *Ṣalāt al-musāfirīn wa-qaṣrihā*, No. 746 in the following words: "Indeed, the character of the Prophet of Allah (PBUH) was the Qur'an." It was also narrated by Abu Dawud in *Qiyām al-layl*, no. 1342 and Al-Nasa'i in *Al-Ṣalāh*, No. 424.

[5]Al-Tabari (2000). *Jāmi'al-bayān*, Beirut: Mu'assasat al-Risala, vol. 23, 528.

[6]Ibn 'Ashur (2001). *Uṣūl al-niẓām al-ijtimā'ī fī al-Islām*. Jordan: Dar Al-Nafa'is: 207.

[7]Al-Firuzabadi (1996). *Baṣā'ir dhawī al-tamyīz*, Cairo: Al-Majlis Al-A'la li al-Shu'un al-Islamiyah: vol. 2, 568.

[8]Narrated by Al-Bayhaqi in *Shu'ab al-īmān*, vol. 6, 242.

The Prophet (PBUH) clarified that the overarching purpose of his mission was to perfect noble character, as indicated by his statement, "I was only sent to perfect noble character (*makārim al-akhlāq*)."[9]

1.4. *Comprehensive Moral Principles in Islam*

Perhaps the most overarching purpose behind the cultivation of ethics across all divine messages is purification of the soul (*tazkiyah*). Purification of the soul involves purging the individual of any internal or external immorality and the fostering of internal and external virtues. In fact, this purification is seen as the common ground bringing together all divine messages. There are numerous Qur'anic verses that clearly refer to purification and edification as important aspirations. For example:

(1) "It is He who has sent among the unlettered a Messenger from themselves reciting to them His verses and purifying them and teaching them the Book and wisdom..." (Qur'an 62:2).
(2) "Our Lord, and send among them a messenger from themselves who will recite to them Your verses and teach them the Book and wisdom and purify them..." (Qur'an 2:129).
(3) "Just as We have sent among you a messenger from yourselves reciting to you Our verses and purifying you and teaching you the Book and wisdom..." (Qur'an 2:151).
(4) "Certainly did God confer [great] favor upon the believers when He sent among them a Messenger from themselves, reciting to them His verses and purifying them and teaching them the Book and wisdom..." (Qur'an 3:164).

In reference to the Qur'anic verses above, the eminent scholar Abu Al-Hasan Al-Nadwi, may God have mercy with him, said, "God the

[9]Narrated by Al-Bazzar in his *Musnad*, vol. 15, 364 and by Al-Bayhaqi in *Al-Kubrá*, vol. 10, 191, No. 21301 in this wording. It was also narrated by Ahmad in *Al-Musnad*, No. 8595; Al-Hakim in *Al-Mustadrak*, vol. 2, 670; and Al-Bayhaqi in *Shu'ab al-īmān*, vol. 10, 352, all three in the words "righteous manners." It was also narrated by Malik in *Al-muwaṭṭa'*, No. 3347 in the words "goodness of manners."

Almighty stated the main purposes and benefits of Prophet Muhammad's mission in several verses of the Qur'an," meaning the aforementioned verses. He then said: "The task of moral discipline and purification of the soul is highly valued in the Prophet's calling to Islam (*da'wah*) as asserted by the purposes of his mission."[10]

There are multitudes, perhaps hundreds, of psychological and behavioral qualities that constitute the elements of moral purification. Due to the diversity and interconnectedness of these elements, philosophers and ethicists attempted to trace them back to a central, governing framework of comprehensive principles. Thus, they defined four principles of virtue (which they considered to be the essence of all virtues) and determined their opposites to be the essence of all immorality. According to Ibn Miskawayh, "Philosophers unanimously hold that the four categories of virtue are: wisdom, abstinence (*'iffah*), courage, and justice."[11] He then said, "The opposites of these four are: ignorance, greed, cowardice, and injustice."[12] Following this, he outlined the various branches of virtues and vices based on these eight main categories.

Al-Ghazali said, "Although there are multiple virtues, they can be reduced to four all-inclusive categories: wisdom, courage, abstinence, and justice. In reasoning, wisdom is the virtue; in anger, courage is the virtue; in desire, abstinence is the virtue; and justice is the way in which these elements fall in the appropriate order. Through justice, perfection is attained in all matters. Hence, it is said that, "The heavens and the earth are founded on justice."[13]

Al-Ghazali went on to elaborate on these four principle virtues explaining that, "Psychological virtues ... include four types: intellect, which is perfected through knowledge; abstinence, which is perfected through piety (*wara'*); courage, which is perfected through perseverance; justice, which is perfected through equity. These are verifiably the fundamentals of religion."[14]

---

[10] Abu Al-Hasan Al-Nadwi, *Al-'aqīdah wal-'ibādah wal-sulūk*, 134.

[11] Ibn Miskawayh, *Tahdhīb al-akhlāq*, 19.

[12] *Ibid.*, 20.

[13] Al-Ghazali, *Mīzān al-'amal*, 27.

[14] *Ibid.*, 25.

According to the eminent scholar Shah Wali Allah Al-Dahlawi, happiness can be attained through four channels. Although these channels may differ in the labels and terminology used by philosophers and ethicists, they nonetheless share similar content and outcomes, particularly the second, third, and fourth channels. The four channels as identified by Al-Dahlawi are:

- Purification;
- Devoutness to God;
- Tolerance;
- Justice.

In his opinion, all Prophets were commissioned by God to preach these four virtues, and all divine ordinances emerge from these qualities and serve to delineate them.[15]

Muhammad Abdullah Draz, author of *Moral Code in the Qur'an* (*Dustūr al-akhlāq fī al-Qur'ān*), argues that, unlike other virtues, God-consciousness (*taqwá*) is pervasive across all ethical domains. Hence, it is the central and foundational virtue in Islamic Sharia whereas all other virtues and values are single-sided in both content and domain. He asserts,

> Traditionally, ethical laws were designated according to their dominant quality, i.e. individual or collective, spiritual or corporeal, Sharia of justice or Sharia of mercy and so on. However, in my opinion, this one-dimensional designation is incompatible within this context. This is because Islamic Sharia recommends observing justice and mercy together and emphasizes the complementary harmony between the individual and the collective and the divine and the human. Therefore, if we were to consider a central virtue in this framework, one foundational principle that embraces all commandments, the concept of God-consciousness would suffice. In other words, how else could God-consciousness be expressed other than through a deeply profound respect for Sharia?[16]

---

[15] Al-Dahlawi (1999). *Ḥujjat Allah al-bālighah.* 1st edn. vol. 1: Riyadh: Dar Al-Kawthar: 191–194.

[16] Muhammad Abdullah Draz, *Dustūr al-akhlāq fī al-Qur'ān*: 681.

This meaning was also emphasized by Ibn 'Ashur who said, "The entire set of good morals boils down to God-consciousness."[17]

Among the contemporary scholars interested in this topic was Sheikh Abdurrahman Habannakah Al-Maydani, who wrote a book entitled *Islamic Ethics and Its Foundations* (*Al-akhlāq al-Islāmīyah wa-ususuhā*). He explored the commendable and prescribed ethical qualities, tracing them back to their overarching principles. He then examined the different moral subdivisions under each principle including their immoral opposites. In his description of the nature and outcomes of his work, he explains, "As I investigated the types of morals utilizing a survey, which I do not claim to be perfect, and then classified them, I arrived at the following comprehensive principles:

First principle: Loving and Prioritizing Truth
Second principle: Mercy
Third principle: Love
Fourth principle: Social Incentive
Fifth principle: Willpower
Sixth principle: Patience
Seventh principle: Generosity
Eighth principle: High Resolve
Ninth principle: Benevolence

These principles that constitute the fundamentals of moral behavior have opposites that constitute the fundamentals of vice and immorality."[18]

After expending nine chapters in discussing each of these nine principles, the author included a 10th chapter addressing two additional virtues which he classified as subdivisions under more than one ethical principle; these virtues are abstinence (as well as its opposite), and courage (and its opposite).[19] It is well known that ethicists consider these two virtues to be among the four main principles.

---

[17] Ibn 'Ashur, *Uṣūl al-niẓām al-ijtimā'ī*, 207.
[18] Abdulrahman Habannakah Al-Maydani, *Al-akhlāq al-Islāmīyah wa-ususuhā*, vol. 1, 517.
[19] *Ibid.*, vol. 2, 581.

2. Ethics and Medicine

All fields and spheres of life require ethics, particularly as they grow and advance. The field of medicine is no exception, rather, ethics lie at the core of the medical profession and they are a necessity for its ongoing sustainability. Given that Sharia scholars maintain that "morality pervades religion; therefore, whoever exhibits better manners than you is superior to you in religious commitment," it becomes incumbent upon scholars of medicine to similarly advise one another that "morality pervades medicine; therefore, whoever exhibits better manners than you is superior to you in medical practice." Moreover, while the status of a physician may be determined based on his knowledge, expertise, and skill, his genuine success is contingent upon his overall moral behavior, including his conscientiousness, mercy, gentleness, compassion, leniency, patience, forbearance, and humility.

2.1. *Objectives of Sharia and Objectives of Medicine*

It is well known that the five objectives of Sharia (*maqāṣid al-sharīʻah*) are to protect[20] the five necessities: preserving religion (*dīn*), life (*nafs*), offspring (*nasl*), intellect (*ʻaql*), and wealth (*māl*).

The objectives of medicine, on the other hand, can be summarized as the protection of life, offspring, and intellect and thus share three of the objectives of Sharia. However, it must be noted that the protection of these three shared objectives also serve in the protection of religion and wealth. Hence, the objectives of medicine are included in and closely associated with the objectives of Sharia. It goes without saying that the protection of life, whether in Sharia or in medicine, is not limited to physical protection. Rather, protection of life also includes maintaining a safe, healthy, and balanced psychological state. Sharia then takes this a step further and,

[20] Preserving the necessities and other benefits is not limited, as some believe, to maintaining and protecting what already exists of those necessities and benefits, which the scholars call "preserving the nonexistent" (*al-ḥifẓ al-ʻadamī*). Instead, preserving the necessities first entails seeking to establish the necessities, foster them, and provide all the means leading to their establishment, which the scholars call "preserving the existent" (*al-ḥifẓ al-wujūdī*). Any type of preservation has two aspects relating first to what is existent and second to what is non-existent.

almost exclusively, advocates the preservation of spiritual well-being. This is perhaps the reason behind many Muslim scholars asserting that "Sharia is the greatest phyisician."[21]

What remains paramount is that the "human being" is the focal point for both the objectives of Sharia and those of medicine with the purpose of both being the preservation of people's physical, psychological, and mental well-being in their pursuit of happiness. The mission of medicine is to heal and spread mercy, while religion's mission is a more comprehensive healing and more expansive mercy. In the Qur'an, God proclaims, "And We send down of the Qur'an that which is healing and mercy for the believers…" (Qur'an 17:82). Thus, healing and mercy are the two objectives at which the missions of medicine and Sharia intersect, despite the differing scopes covered by each.

Sharia scholars summarize the objectives and necessities of Sharia with two concise expressions, namely preserving religion and preserving life. In other words, safeguarding the interests of people is contingent upon the preservation of their religion and their lives. Similarly, happiness in this world and in the afterlife is founded on the preservation of people's religion and lives, and the preservation of both these aspects is considered to be the pillars of cultures and civilizations. In fact, the basis of any form of development and progress is the preservation of life and religion.

Interpreters of the Qur'an frequently highlight the significance of the Qur'anic verse, "It is He who shows you His signs and sends down to you from the sky, provision. But none will remember except he who turns back [in repentance]" (Qur'an 40:13). This verse establishes a connection between the revelation of signs and miracles alluding to God and His messengers on the one hand and gratitude for the divine blessing of His provision of sustenance from the sky on the other hand. Scholars explain that the implication behind this connection is that these two elements form the overarching objectives of Sharia, where one refers to preserving religion (revealing signs and miracles) and the other refers to preserving life (providing sustenance).

Al-Fakhr Al-Razi stated, "Know that the most significant of duties is protecting the interests of religion and the interests of life. God the

[21] Al-Shatibi, *Al-muwāfaqāt*, vol. 3, 181.

Almighty protects the interests of religion through the revelation of signs and scriptures, and protects life through providing sustenance from the sky. As such, signs are to religion what sustenance is for life: signs enliven religion while sustenance enlivens life. Endowing mankind with both is a perfect blessing."[22]

Commenting on the Qur'anic verse above, Al-Qurtubi says, "The signs revealed by God indicating His oneness and power are combined with His provision of sustenance because signs are essential for the continuity of religion and sustenance is essential for the continuity of life."[23]

It has been established within religious culture, Islamic, and others, that all sciences revolve around preserving religion and life, keeping in mind that a substantial portion of religion is devoted to preserving life.

It is narrated that Harun Al-Rashid, the Abbasid caliph, had employed a skillful Christian physician. In a conversation with 'Ali bin Al-Husayn, the physician said, "Your Book (i.e. Qur'an) lacks any information about medicine despite the two main branches of knowledge being knowledge of religion and knowledge of the human body." 'Ali, in turn, replied, "God summed up the entire field of medicine with half a verse in our Book." The physician asked him what this verse was, and he answered, "God Almighty says, '...and eat and drink, but be not excessive...' [Qur'an 7:31]." The Christian then said, "There is also no reference to the field of medicine in any of your Prophet's narrations." Once again, 'Ali replied, "The Messenger of God, may the peace and blessings of God be upon him, summarized the field of medicine using a few words." The physician asked what they were, and 'Ali answered, "The stomach is the abode of diseases, diet is at the forefront of all cures, and each body must be treated in the way to which it has been accustomed." At this, the Christian said, "Your Book and your Prophet have left nothing in the field of medicine for Galen."[24]

---

[22] Al-Fakhr Al-Razi (2000). *Mafātīḥ al-ghayb*, 1st edn. Beirut: Dar Al-Kutub Al-'Ilmiyah, vol. 27, 38.
[23] Al-Qurtubi (2003). *Tafsīr Al-Qurṭubī*, ed. Hisham Samir Al-Bukhari. Riyadh: Dar 'Alam Al-Kutub, vol. 15, 299.
[24] Al-Qurtubi. *Tafsīr Al-Qurṭubī*, vol. 7, 192.

One of the rules underpinning Islamic jurisprudence and the objectives of Sharia outlines that "general interests have precedence over private interests." In the application of this rule, we find a close connection between observing the objectives of medicine and observing the objectives of Sharia, as well as between preserving life and preserving religion. In adherence to this rule, jurists have declared that it is an obligation to prevent the impudent jurist and the ignorant physician from practicing their professions because the former corrupts religion and the latter destroys lives. A saying that emerged from this concept states that, "Religion is corrupted by uneducated jurists, just as bodies are harmed by uneducated physicians."

In my opinion, a physician who lacks good morals, regardless of his medical knowledge, is no less dangerous to people than an ignorant physician. Whereas an ignorant physician must be prevented from practice, a corrupt physician, on the other hand, must be severely punished.

In order to further explore the objectives of Sharia associated with ethics, particularly those that are connected to and impact the field of medicine, the following sections will discuss two main principles in Islamic ethics:

- God-consciousness;
- Mercy.

As these two principles are discussed, the impact of the different moral behaviors emerging from each principle, on human conduct in general and medical practice in particular, will be explicitly elaborated on.

2.1.1. *God-Consciousness is the Source of Ethics*

The practice of God-consciousness in Sharia entails a moral, spiritual, and psychological state of self-accountability. It requires that an individual be fully aware and considerate of the consequences of his actions whether in regards to himself, God, or any of God's creations.

A person who maintains a state of God-consciousness is one who is appreciative of God's blessings and thus is pious towards Him. He reveres

God and is apprehensive of His vigilance and thus fears disobeying Him. He is fearful of God's anger and is wary of His punishment. He is also cognizant of immoral behavior and its negative impact on himself and others and therefore refrains from committing any sinful actions.

Hence, God-consciousness is a source of self-discipline and self-improvement. As 'Umar bin Abdul-Aziz explains, "A God-conscious person is restrained; he does not behave as he wishes",[25] meaning that a person willingly chooses to restrain himself with God-consciousness. Talq bin Habib, may God have mercy upon him, further elaborates saying, "God-consciousness (*taqwá*) is obeying God, under the guidance of God, with the hope of gaining God's mercy. God-consciousness is also abstaining from sin, under the guidance of God, out of fear of God's punishment."[26]

God-consciousness induces one to be vigilant and cautious regarding all his actions and behaviors. A man once asked Abu Hurayrah, may God be pleased with him, to explain the meaning of God-consciousness. Abu Hurayrah asked the man, "Have you ever walked along a thorny path?" The man replied in the affirmative. Abu Hurayrah then asked, "How did you walk along it?" The man replied, "Whenever I came across any thorns, I avoided them, bypassed them, or turned away from them." Abu Hurayrah, in turn, asserted, "That is God-consciousness (*taqwá*)."[27]

(a) God-Consciousness in the Qur'an and Prophetic Tradition

The religious texts that address the principle of God-consciousness are abundant and diverse, particularly in the Qur'an. These texts all reinforce the centrality and pivotal role of God-consciousness in Islam and Sharia as outlined earlier in this chapter. Further, God-consciousness is also found to be central across the messages of all God's prophets and messengers. In the Qur'an, God the Almighty says, "So have God-consciousness

[25] Narrated by Al-Bayhaqi in *Shu'ab al-īmān*, vol. 5, 63, no. 5788 and *Al-zuhd al-kabīr*, 357, No. 925, 929. It was also narrated by Al-Baghawi in *Sharḥ al-sunnah*, vol. 14, 341.

[26] Narrated by Ibn Al-Mubarak in *Al-zuhd wal-raqā'iq*, no. 1343; by Ibn Abi Shaybah in *Al-Muṣannaf*, vol. 15, 599, No. 30993 and vol. 19, 357, No. 36308; by Abu Nu'aym in *Al-ḥilyah*, vol. 3, 64; and by Al-Bayhaqi in *Al-zuhd al-kabīr*, 367, No. 963.

[27] Narrated by Al-Bayhaqi in *Al-zuhd al-kabīr*, 367.

(*taqwá*) towards God and obey me" (Qur'an 26:108).[28] This order was admonished by several Messengers[29] emphasizing that God-consciousness is a common purpose and a consistent tenet across all divine religions.

In an extensive *hadith*, Abu Dharr, may God be pleased with him, was reported to have said, "I said, 'O Messenger of God, advise me.' He said, 'I advise you to have *taqwá* towards God, because doing so is the core issue.'"[30] In other words, God-consciousness is the source of all good and a source of protection from all evil.

(b) The Impact and Effectiveness of God-Consciousness

As described earlier, God-consciousness is an ongoing, internal process of self-accountability that takes place in both public and private settings. Often, a person may be able to escape monitoring, pressure, and reproach by those around him or avoid accountability, especially if he possesses power due to a position of authority or some rank due to his knowledge and status. However, in the event of God-consciousness, for one who observes this principle, it is a constant presence that monitors and guides his actions day and night, across all locations and settings.

Given the comprehensive, positive impact of observing God-consciousness, there is no doubt that those who are most in need of maintaining this principle are those individuals who are entrusted with the souls, bodies, and dignity of others. The beneficial impact of a physician observing God-consciousness and sincerity in his practice, on the protection of souls and bodies, alleviation of suffering, and conservation of money and effort, is no less effective than the beneficial impact of a physician's extensive knowledge and expertise. This is because a God-conscious physician monitors himself and holds himself accountable ensuring his integrity whether internally or externally. Hence, the integrity of a God-conscious physician does not arise from nor is contingent upon a medical oath, just as the integrity of a God-conscious ruler does not

---

[28] Translator's note: Muhsin Khan translation has been modified to better reflect the context of the text.

[29] See Qur'an 3:50; 26:108, 110, 126, 131, 144, 150, 163, 179; and 43:63.

[30] Narrated by Ibn Hibban, *Kitāb al-birr wal-iḥsān*, vol. 2, 78; Abu Nu'aym, in *Al-ḥilyah*, vol. 1, 168.

emerge from a constitutional oath. Rather, those individuals who lack the internal virtue of God-consciousness and self-accountability will fail any oath, be it Greek or Islamic.

2.1.2. *Mercy and Compassion in Medicine and Sharia*

Mercy, as an ethical principle, is a cornerstone of both Sharia and medicine. Some scholars encapsulate the objectives and obligations of Sharia with two concise statements: "glorifying the Creator and being merciful towards creation."

In summary, the term "mercy" encompasses gentleness, compassion, kindness, forgiveness, sympathy, affection, and all associated actions, including preventing harm, promoting benefit, providing advice, alleviating pain, or offering assistance. It also represents countering acts of cruelty, severity, vulgarity, and harm.

(a) Mercy in the Qur'an and Prophetic Tradition

The prevalence of the term "mercy" and its derivatives in the Qur'an and Prophetic Tradition, covering various aspects of life, can be enumerated in the hundreds. This explicitly emphasizes mercy as a major principle in religion and a general objective of Sharia. Below are some examples of verses and narrations from the Qur'an and Prophetic Tradition respectively:

(i) In the Qur'an

(1) The divine books are sources of mercy:

- "O mankind, there has come to you instruction from your Lord and healing for what is in the breasts and guidance and mercy for the believers. Say, 'In the bounty of God and in His mercy — in that let them rejoice; it is better than what they accumulate'" (Qur'an 10:57–58).
- "Say, 'I only follow what is revealed to me from my Lord. This [Qur'an] is enlightenment from your Lord and guidance and mercy for a people who believe.' So when the Qur'an is recited,

then listen to it and pay attention that you may receive mercy" (Qur'an 7:203–204).

- "And We had certainly brought them a Book which We detailed by knowledge — as guidance and mercy to a people who believe" (Qur'an 7:52).
- "So there has [now] come to you a clear evidence from your Lord and a guidance and mercy" (Qur'an 6:157).
- "Then We gave Moses the Scripture, making complete [Our favor] upon the one who did good and as a detailed explanation of all things and as guidance and mercy that perhaps in [the matter of] the meeting with their Lord they would believe" (Qur'an 6:154).
- "So is one who [stands] upon a clear evidence from his Lord [like the aforementioned]? And a witness from Him follows it, and before it was the Scripture of Moses to lead and as mercy" (Qur'an 11:17).

(2) Familial and marriage relationships should be characterized with mercy, affection, and peace:

- "And of His signs is that He created for you from yourselves mates that you may find tranquility in them; and He placed between you affection and mercy. Indeed in that are signs for a people who give thought" (Qur'an 30:21).
- "And [mention] Job, when he called to his Lord, 'Indeed, adversity has touched me, and you are the Most Merciful of the merciful.' So We responded to him and removed what afflicted him of adversity. And We gave him [back] his family and the like thereof with them as mercy from Us and a reminder for the worshippers [of God]" (Qur'an 21:83–84).
- "And We granted him his family and a like [number] with them as mercy from Us and a reminder for those of understanding" (Qur'an 38:43).

Mercy is integral within all of God's ordinances, and His obligations serve as a pathway to mercy: "The believing men and believing women are allies of one another. They enjoin what is right and forbid what is wrong and establish prayer and give zakāh and obey God and His Messenger. Those — God will have mercy upon them. Indeed, God is Exalted in Might and Wise" (Qur'an 9:71).

(ii) In the Prophetic Tradition

(1) It was narrated on the authority of Abdullah bin Amr, may God be pleased with them, that the Messenger of God (PBUH) said, "The Compassionate One has mercy on those who are merciful. If you show mercy to those who are on the earth, He Who is in the heaven will show mercy to you."[31]

(2) It was narrated on the authority of Jarir bin 'Abdullah that the Messenger of God (PBUH) said, "God will not be merciful to those who are not merciful to mankind."[32]

(3) Imam Al-Bukhari allocated several chapters in his *Ṣaḥīḥ* for topics of mercy, including chapter 27 in the "Book of Manners" named, "chapter of showing mercy to people and animals." One of the *hadiths* included in this chapter was narrated on the authority of Abu Hurayrah that the Messenger of God (PBUH) said, "A man felt very thirsty while he was on the way, there he came across a well. He went down the well, quenched his thirst and came out. Meanwhile he saw a dog panting and licking mud because of excessive thirst. He said to himself, 'This dog is suffering from thirst as I did.' So, he went down the well again and filled his shoe with water and watered it. God thanked him for that deed and forgave him." The people said, "O God's Apostle! Is there a reward for us in serving the animals?" He replied, "Yes, there is a reward for serving any animate (living being)."[33]

[31] Narrated by Ahmad in *Al-musnad*, no. 6494 on the authority of 'Abdullah bin 'Amr; Abu Dawud in *Al-adab*, no. 4941; and Al-Tirmidhi, *Al-birr wal-ṣilah*, no. 1925 and he said: "This is a fair authentic *hadith*." Translator's note: translation of Professor. Ahmad Hasan (Abu Dawud, book 41, No. 4923).

[32] Narrated by Al-Bukhari, *Al-adab*, no. 6013 and Muslim, *Al-faḍā'il*, no. 2319. Translator's note: translation of Muhsin Khan (USC web, Bukhari, vol. 9, book 93, No. 473).

[33] Narrated by Al-Bukhari, vol. 3, 132–133, No. 2466 and vol. 8, 9–10, No. 6009 and by Muslim, vol. 4, 1761, No. 2244. Translator's note: translation of Muhsin Khan (USC web, Bukhari, vol. 3, book 43, No. 646).

It was narrated on the authority of Abu Hurayrah that the Prophet (PBUH) said, "A prostitute saw a dog moving around a well on a hot day and hanging out its tongue because of thirst. She drew water for it in her shoe and she was pardoned (for this act of hers)."[34]

Al-Hasan bin Battal, generally commenting on *hadiths* included in this chapter of *Ṣaḥīḥ Al-Bukhārī*, says,

> These hadiths urge showing mercy toward all people, including believers and disbelievers, and toward animals. Doing so is a way to expiate one's sins. Therefore, sagacious believers should have mercy upon people and animals, which were not created for no purpose. Everyone is responsible in front of God for everyone he is entrusted with, be it a person or an animal that cannot speak of the pain they suffer from. Mercy needs also be shown toward animals that one does not own. There was a man who watered a dog in the desert, although the dog was not his own, and God forgave him as he descended a well and brought water in his shoe to the dog. This also applies to feeding animals, as the Prophet, may peace and blessings of God be upon him, said, "If any Muslim plants any plant and a human being or an animal eats of it, he will be rewarded as if he had given that much in charity."[35] In addition to watering and feeding animals, it is also recommended not to burden them beyond their capacity out of showing mercy toward them. Animals should not be beaten up, harmed, or used at night or out of work time. We have been forbidden to put servants to work at night because night is their time of rest, as they work during the day to their masters. The same applies to using animals.[36]

Al-'Izz bin 'Abd Al-Salam indicated how the two attributes of mercy and compassion of God should be applied by people: "Mercy

---

[34] Narrated by Muslim, No. 2245 and by Ahmad in *Al-musnad*, No. 10583. Translator's note: translation of Abdul Hamid Siddiqui (USC web, Muslim, book 6, No. 5578).

[35] Narrated by Al-Bukhari, *Al-muzāra'ah*, no. 2152 and Muslim, *Al-musāqāh*, No. 2904 on the authority of Anas bin Malik. Translator's note: translation of Muhsin Khan (USC web, Bukhari, vol. 8, book 73, No. 41).

[36] Ibn Battal, *Sharḥ Ṣaḥīḥ Al-Bukhārī*, Riyadh: Maktabat Al-Rushd, vol. 9, 219–220.

should be observed as much as possible toward everything including even flies and ants."[37]

(b) Mercy and Euthanasia

One of the contentious medical debates associated with the ethic of mercy is that of mercy killing (euthanasia). Euthanasia involves the physician ending the life of a chronically-ill patient based on the patient's request or with permission from the patient's family in cases where the patient is in a chronic coma. The justifications often presented for this action involve arguments of mercy and compassion towards ending the patient's suffering.

This issue has been extensively explored within Islamic law. Muslim scholars unanimously agree on the prohibition of euthanasia, and it is considered to be a proscribed killing of a human being. However, it is neither the purpose nor focus of this chapter to present an in-depth discussion of this issue. The aim here is merely to focus on the ethical aspects of the debate so as to explore whether euthanasia is indeed a merciful solution to ending a patient's suffering.

Euthanasia, as a solution, is both superficial and shortsighted in its approach. Firstly, it increases the potential of taking risks with human life and undermining its sanctity. This is especially true when a probability of cure exists, however small it may be.

In addition, any level of pain could not be weighed against the cost of ending a human life. If we were to prioritize preventing pain over protecting life, then the act of suicide would be permissible in cases where individuals suffer from chronic pain and have no hope of recovery. Further, allowing euthanasia as an option may result in the hindrance of medical advancement that should not simply surrender to despair but rather endeavor to seek the cure.

Moreover, the concept of mercy in Islamic ideology encompasses mercy in the afterlife, which entails repentance, patience, forgiveness, and reward. There are several authentic Prophetic traditions reinforcing the concept that pain serves to erase sins and elevate one's status as a

[37] 'Izz bin 'Abd Al-Salam, *Shajarat al-ma'ārif wal-aḥwāl wa ṣāliḥ al-aqwāl wal-a'māl.* Bayt Al-Afkar Al-Duwaliyah: 40.

means of mercy and alleviation in the afterlife. This was expressed by the Prophet (PBUH) in his saying, "No fatigue, nor disease, nor sorrow, nor sadness, nor hurt, nor distress befalls a Muslim, even if it were the prick he receives from a thorn, but that God expiates some of his sins for that."[38]

The Prophet (PBUH) also said, "Calamities will continue to befall believing men and women in themselves, their children and their wealth, until they meet God with no burden of sin."[39] This is a great form of divine mercy. The purpose of all this being to encourage the patient to endure the pain of his illness, remain hopeful, and safeguard his life.

3. Conclusion

The following ethical principles serve as a summative outline of the concepts addressed in this chapter:

(i) The purpose and mission of medicine should be promotion of the physical, mental, and psychological health of all persons.
(ii) The main, essential objectives of medicine intersect with three of the objectives of Sharia; namely, preserving life, preserving offspring, and preserving intellect.
(iii) The two ethics, God-consciousness and mercy, are essential ethical principles for those professionals entrusted with the protection of people's lives and with maintaining public and private health for society and individuals.

---

[38]Narrated by Al-Bukhari, *Al-marḍá*, no. 5641 and Muslim, *Al-birr wal-ṣilah*, No. 2573 on the authority of Abu Hurayrah. Translator's note: Translation of Muhsin Khan (USC web, vol. 7, book 70, No. 545).

[39]Narrated by Ahmad in *Al-musnad*, No. 7859. It was also narrated by Al-Tirmidhi, *Al-zuhd*, No. 2399, and he said it is a fair authentic *hadith*, on the authority of Abu Hurayrah.

Response by Hassan Chamsi-Pasha to Raissouni's Paper

Hassan Chamsi-Pasha

I read with great interest the paper of Sheikh Ahmed Raissouni who laid down an approach to medical ethics based on the higher objectives of Sharia. Sheikh Raissouni is an authority in the field of the fundamentals of Islamic jurisprudence (*uṣūl al-fiqh*) and the higher objectives of Sharia; hence his paper reflects his deep knowledge and understanding of this subject. I would like to emphasize a few points in relation to the issues discussed in his paper.

1. Islam and Medicine

The relation between Islam and medicine is without doubt a close one, as stated by Sheikh Raissouni.[1] Islam supports the use of science, medicine, and biotechnology as ways to arrive at appropriate solutions that alleviate human suffering.[2] Thus, we find Muslims throughout the world are eager

[1] Hormoz Ebrahimnejad (2011). What is 'Islamic' in Islamic medicine? An overview, in Feza Günergun and Dhruv Raina (ed.). *Science between Europe and Asia*. Boston, MA: Springer: 259–270.
[2] Marcia C. Inhorn (2003). *Local Babies, Global Science: Gender, Religion and In Vitro Fertilization in Egypt*. New York, NY: Routledge.

to benefit from the latest medical advancements and in many cases prefer Western biomedicine to its alternatives.[3,4] Furthermore, Islamic religious authorities play an important role in encouraging techno-scientific developments through their *fatwas*, which permit some medical advances while they place limitations on other practices of medicine.

2. Roots of Medical Ethics in the Qur'an

As Western ethics has developed into a philosophical science, it has moved away from a Christian conception of good and evil to draw more upon human reason and experience as the arbiter between right and wrong action. This shifting of ethics to a more philosophical formulation does not have an equivalent in the Islamic intellectual discourse. While Islamic ethics does incorporate various philosophical traditions, it still mainly draws its sources from religious texts and holds a religious worldview.[5]

The discussion on medical ethics in Islamic law is but a branch of the high status ethics in general has in Islam as seen in the Qur'an, the Tradition of the Prophet Muhammad (PBUH), and the understanding of the Islamic Sharia. Sheikh Raissouni clearly emphasizes that the same standard of ethical values and principles should guide the physician in both his private and professional life.

A person who lacks moral values in his private life, no matter how knowledgeable and skilled he is in medicine, is dangerous and harmful to people and cannot be trusted in professional activities, even if he has the highest professional and technical qualifications. It is impossible for a person to live by two different ethical standards, adopting one set of ethical principles in his private life and contradictory principles in his

[3] Morgan Clarke (2009). *Islam and New Kinship: Reproductive Technology and the Shariah in Lebanon*. New York, NY: Berghahn.

[4] Marcia C. Inhorn and Gamal I. Serour (2011). Islam, medicine, and Arab-Muslim refugee health in America after 9/11. *Lancet* 378 (9794): 935–943.

[5] Aasim Padela (2007). Islamic medical ethics: A primer. *Bioethics* 21(3): 169–178.

professional life.[6] Truthful is God the Almighty when He says: "God has not made for a man two hearts in his interior..." (Qur'an 33:4).

The following verses from the Qur'an are most suited as a guide for the personal characteristics of the physician. God says,

> And [mention, O Muhammad], when Luqman said to his son while he was instructing him, "O my son, do not associate [anything] with God. Indeed, association [with him] is great injustice." And We have enjoined upon man [care] for his parents. His mother carried him, [increasing her] in weakness upon weakness, and his weaning is in two years. Be grateful to Me and to your parents; to Me is the [final] destination. But if they endeavor to make you associate with Me that of which you have no knowledge, do not obey them but accompany them in [this] world with appropriate kindness and follow the way of those who turn back to Me [in repentance]. Then to Me will be your return, and I will inform you about what you used to do. [And Luqman said], "O my son, indeed if wrong should be the weight of a mustard seed and should be within a rock or [anywhere] in the heavens or in the earth, God will bring it forth. Indeed, God is Subtle and Acquainted. O my son, establish prayer, enjoin what is right, forbid what is wrong, and be patient over what befalls you. Indeed, [all] that is of the matters [requiring] determination. And do not turn your cheek [in contempt] toward people and do not walk through the earth exultantly. Indeed, God does not like everyone self-deluded and boastful. And be moderate in your pace and lower your voice; indeed, the most disagreeable of sounds is the voice of donkeys." (Qur'an 31:13–19).

Sheikh Raissouni elaborated on the issue of mercy and stressed its importance in the field of medicine. God says, addressing His Prophet Muhammad (PBUH), "So by mercy from God, [O Muhammad], you were lenient with them. And if you had been rude [in speech] and harsh in heart, they would have disbanded from about you. So pardon them and ask forgiveness for them and consult them in the matter. And when you have

---

[6]Abdul Rahman Amine and Ahmed Elkadi (1981). Islamic code of medical professional ethics. *Journal of the Islamic Medical Association of North America* 13: 108–210.

decided, then rely upon God. Indeed, God loves those who rely [upon Him]" (Qur'an 3:159).

Based on the above, the Muslim physician must believe in God and in what Islamic teachings call for, regarding both his private and public life. He must be grateful to his teachers and respectful towards his elders. He must also be humble, merciful, patient, and forgiving. He should follow the path of the believers and always seek God's support and assistance.[7]

No doubt a physician with the above-mentioned virtues is capable of fulfilling the professional requirements of this noble occupation. The first professional requirement is having the appropriate knowledge. God says in the Qur'an, "...Say, 'Are those who know equal to those who do not know?'..." (Qur'an 39:9). God also says, "...Only those fear God, from among His servants, who have knowledge..." (Qur'an 35:28). Therefore the believer is expected to always seek knowledge and understanding. God says, "...and say, 'My Lord, increase me in knowledge'" (Qur'an 20:114). The physician must also abide by the legal rules regulating his profession provided they do not violate Islamic principles. The need to respect law and order is reflected in the following Qur'anic verse, in which God says, "O you who have believed, obey God and obey the Messenger and those in authority among you..." (Qur'an 4:59).

When entrusted with the life and care of a patient, the physician must offer the needed advice with consideration for both the patient's body and mind, always remembering his basic obligation to enjoin what is right and forbid what is wrong. The physician must respect the patient's confidentiality, reflecting God's description of the believers, "And they who are to their trusts and their promises attentive" (Qur'an 23:8).

3. Islam and Secularization

Sheikh Raissouni pointed out the fact that Islam rejects secularization; secularization here meaning humans ruling their lives with no regard or consideration to a religion or a higher spiritual authority. Some secular

---

[7] *Ibid.*

proponents believe following the divine law would lead to hardship.[8] This may be the basis as to why some societies have separated the church from everyday life and replaced God's rules with man-made laws and guidelines. This secular reasoning evolved when societies were faced with ethical and practical dilemmas. No doubt this reasoning can be contradictory as it lacks logical coherence when it is not based on an underlying coherent system of ethical values.[9]

Islam is not only a religion with rituals; it is a way of life. Once an individual accepts Islam, he is to live by its rulings in all of his affairs, in accordance with God's statement, "But no, by your Lord, they will not [truly] believe until they make you, [O Muhammad], judge concerning that over which they dispute among themselves and then find within themselves no discomfort from what you have judged and submit in [full, willing] submission" (Qur'an 4:65) and,

> And We have revealed to you, [O Muhammad], the Book in truth, confirming that which preceded it of the Scripture and as a criterion over it. So judge between them by what God has revealed and do not follow their inclinations away from what has come to you of the truth. To each of you We prescribed a law and a method. Had God willed, He would have made you one nation [united in religion], but [He intended] to test you in what He has given you; so race to [all that is] good. To God is your return all together, and He will [then] inform you concerning that over which you used to differ. And judge, [O Muhammad], between them by what God has revealed and do not follow their inclinations and beware of them, lest they tempt you away from some of what God has revealed to you. And if they turn away — then know that God only intends to afflict them with some of their [own] sins. And indeed, many among the people are defiantly disobedient (Qur'an 5:48–49).

[8]Shlomi Tal (2001). *Necessity and Primacy of Secularism.* Institute of Secularization of Islamic Society. Available online via http://www.secularislam.org/separation/tal.htm (retrieved 13 November 2013).

[9]Omar Hasan Kasule (2004). Ethics and Etiquette of Human Research. Paper presented at the International Scientific Convention jointly organized by the Jordan Society for Islamic Medical Studies, the Jordan Medical Association, and the Federation of Islamic Medical Association in Amman, Jordan 15–17 July 2004.

One might ask what is the relationship of such rejection of secularization in Muslim communities and biomedical research ethics for example? The simple answer is that certain research projects are considered unlawful under Sharia. The best example here is the use of surrogacy for the treatment of infertility and the use of tissue cloning and gene therapy with the aim of controlling the genetic characteristics of an embryo, which is tantamount to interfering with God's will.[10]

4. The Four Principles

Although Sheikh Raissouni did not discuss the principlist approach to medical ethics as it is out of the scope of his paper, I will discuss it very briefly. The principlist approach to biomedical ethics proposed by two American bioethicists, Tom Beauchamp and James Childress, has received some attention from Muslim scholars.[11] According to this approach, there are four general principles of biomedical ethics: (i) respect for autonomy, (ii) beneficence, (iii) nonmaleficence, and (iv) justice.

Several authors claim that the roots of the four principles presented by Beauchamp and Childress are clearly identifiable in Islamic tradition as well.[12,13] Beneficence is strongly connected to the principle of nonmaleficence, but it is so connected to other principles as well that we can say the principle of beneficence is the starting point of all kinds of human relations. PBUH said, "The best of you is the one who is most beneficial to others."[14] Similarly, Islam forbids all kinds of actions that may harm a person's health and life. In the Islamic tradition, many statements stress the avoidance of harm to others. The PBUH commanded that, "There should be neither harming nor reciprocating harm."[15]

[10] Raafat Y. Afifi (2007). Biomedical research ethics: An Islamic view: Part I. *International Journal of Surgery* 5(5): 292–296.

[11] Bagher Larijani and Farzaneh Zahedi (2008). Contemporary medical ethics: An overview from Iran. *Developing World Bioethics* 8(3): 192–196.

[12] Sahin Aksoy and Abdurrahman Elmai (2002). The core concepts of the 'Four principles' of bioethics as found in Islamic tradition. *Medical Law Review* 21: 211–224.

[13] Gamal I. Serour (1994). Islam and the four principles, in Raanan Gillon (ed.). *Principles of Healthcare Ethics*. New York: Chichester Wiley: 75–91.

[14] Muhammad Nasir Al-Din Al-Albani, comp., *Ṣaḥīḥ al-jāmi'* no. 3289.

[15] *Ṣaḥīḥ al-jāmi'*, no. 7517.

Islam does not permit man to act as he wishes without limits but instead outlines for him certain rules to abide by. These rules are derived from the Qur'an and the life of the PBUH. It is reported in various verses of the Qur'an that God revealed the Qur'an as a clarification for people and a guide for them so that they may lead the best life and that the PBUH is the best example and role model.[16]

Aksoy and Elmai cite many instances within Islamic texts that urge respect for a patient's autonomy.[17] Van Bommel says, "For a Muslim patient absolute autonomy is very rare, there will be a feeling of responsibility towards God, and he or she lives in a social coherence, in which influences of the imam and relatives play their roles."[18] Consequently, personal choices are recognized only if they prove to be the "right" ones. The Noble Qur'an gives great importance to the principle of justice; about 16 of its verses talk about this principle.[19]

According to these verses, the main purpose behind sending the prophets was to establish justice in the world. God says, "We have already sent Our messengers with clear evidences and sent down with them the Scripture and the balance that the people may maintain [their affairs] in justice..." (Qur'an 57:25).

5. Euthanasia

Finally, Sheikh Raissouni touched briefly on the subject of euthanasia. He stated that life is given by God and cannot be taken away except by Him or with His permission and that preservation of life is one of the five foundational objectives of Islamic Sharia.[20]

Human beings are considered to be responsible stewards of their bodies, which are viewed as gifts from God. The sanctity of human life is

[16] Sahin Aksoy and Ali Tenik (2002). The 'four principles of bioethics' as found in 13th century Muslim scholar Mawlana's teachings. *BMC Medical Ethics* 3: 4.
[17] Sahin Aksoy and Abdurrahman Elmai (2002). The core concepts of the 'four principles' of bioethics as found in Islamic tradition, *Medical Law Review* 21: 211–224.
[18] Abdulwahid van Bommel (1999). Medical ethics from the Muslim perspective. *Acta Neurochirurgica Supplement* 74: 17–27.
[19] Kiarash Aramesh (2008). Justice as a principle of Islamic bioethics. *The American Journal of Bioethics* 8(10): 26–27.
[20] Al-Shatibi (1997). *Al-Muwāfaqāt*, 2. Khobar: Dar Ibn Affan: 20.

affirmed in the Qur'an. No one can deprive another of his life: "...And do not kill the soul which God has forbidden [to be killed] except by [legal] right..." (Qur'an 6:151) and, "Because of that, We decreed upon the Children of Israel that whoever kills a soul unless for a soul or for corruption [done] in the land — it is as if he had slain mankind entirely. And whoever saves one — it is as if he had saved mankind entirely..." (Qur'an 5:32).

The physician therefore has no right to terminate any human life under his care. Taking away life is only the domain of the One who gives life, and He is God. True, there is pain and suffering [at the end of a terminal illness], but Muslims believe there is immeasurable reward from God for those who patiently persevere in suffering. "...Indeed, the patient will be given their reward without account" (Qur'an 39:10).

Script of Oral Discussions (Day 1, Session 2)

After **Abdul Sattar Abu Ghuddah** presented his paper, the following discussion took place.

Hassan Chamsi-Pasha

A number of papers have been published demonstrating that the four principles of biomedical ethics exist in Islam. Sheikh Abu Ghuddah mentioned a book earlier entitled *Ethics of the Physician* (*Akhlāq al-ṭabīb*) of Abu Bakr Al-Razi (known also as Rhazes). It mentions ethical issues, such as respecting the confidentiality of the patient, refraining from arrogance, treating the poor, and putting one's trust in God. All these principles were written about more than a 1,000 years ago, in the 9th century. Another important book in this matter is called *Practical Ethics of the Physician* (*Adab al-ṭabīb*) by Al-Ruhawi. It is believed to be the first known book about the practical ethics of the physician and one of the foundational books on the subject. Martin Levey translated it into English in 1967. Sahin Eksoy considers it the first book on ethics in Islamic medicine. Dr. Padela described it as an attestation to the ability of Islamic thinkers to integrate philosophical principles into Islamic methodology.

Al-Ruhawi's *Practical Ethics of the Physician* consists of 20 chapters addressing all sorts of medical ethics. Although we do not have the time to discuss them all, I would like to concentrate on the three tenets that Al-Ruhawi highlighted in his introduction.

The first tenet a doctor should hold true is that behind every created being exists the One Creator who is Most Wise and Able to do all things. The second tenet entails a doctor's believing in firm affection towards God and devoting himself fully to Him in mind and soul, by choice. Third, a doctor should believe that God sent messengers to mankind in order to guide them towards good.

It is for this reason that a doctor must believe the human mind alone is not sufficient, and so, before they begin examining a patient, Muslim doctors should say, "In the name of God, The Most Gracious, The Most Merciful." For the 30-some years I have practiced medicine, by the Grace of God, I cannot remember a single case of examining a patient — whether in Syria, England, or Saudi Arabia — except that I began by saying "In the name of God, the Most Gracious, the Most Merciful." I say it out loud, even in England, in English. Saying this phrase provides me with reassurance and helps me remain hopeful for success in my work. It reminds the doctor that he is not the healer but rather God Almighty is. When the doctor says, "In the name of God," it gives the patient spiritual energy and makes him feel a connection to God.

As Sheikh Raissouni and Sheikh Abu Ghuddah mentioned, God likes for a person, if he does work, that he does it with meticulousness and precision (*itqān*). When somebody suffers from a heart problem, within hours the entire area dies. So here is an instance where seeking excellence is incredibly important. The doctor must take into account that time is a key factor and so should carry out the diagnosis and start treatment within minutes if possible.

There is no medical intervention that does not carry a risk for medical complications. We must clarify any possible complications to the patient before starting any medical or surgical intervention. Indeed, anything could happen during a surgical intervention that the patient would not be able to foresee. Of course, ultimately it is only God who knows what will happen.

We must also be truthful when we speak with the patient about undergoing any procedure such as gastric banding. Often the patient is made to believe that it is going to be a very easy procedure and that it will not have any subsequent complications. This is of course not the case, and this should be communicated to patients honestly. We distribute to patients before they undergo a medical procedure books that provide them with guidelines about the process and clarify the probabilities of various side effects and complications. As Sheikh Abu Ghuddah asserted earlier, the doctor has a responsibility to be truthful to the patient. He is held accountable not only before courts or medical authorities but also before God.

Another issue is that doctors need to smile more! Some doctors snarl in front of their patients. Many patients say that half of their cure involves their doctor smiling to them. Prophet Muhammad (PBUH) said it is a form of charity when you smile at another person. Also among the sayings of the PBUH are those that emphasize how people treat one another in general. Nowadays, the relationship between physicians and their colleagues is sometimes disappointing. A physician may negatively criticize a colleague due to jealousy, enmity, or another trait that contradicts with Islamic Sharia. Arrogance is also an unfortunate trait that many doctors are prone to exhibiting. Some doctors think they are so important that they will not talk to you unless you present them with your ID card! PBUH said that whoever has even the smallest trace of pride or arrogance cannot enter Paradise or would not be admitted to Paradise. These are the ethical concepts and ideals by which we should abide.

We should also strive to be true role models in all our actions. In England, we had a consultant respiratory physician who was a heavy smoker. His ashtray would fill up with more than 30 or 40 cigarettes by the end of each day, and yet he advised patients to quit smoking. In what way is this doctor being a good role model? It is likewise important for a physician to care about his appearance and not to visit a patient while he looks untidy. PBUH said that God is beautiful and loves beauty. This is a Prophetic principle that we should abide by in general and in particular with our patients.

Breaching patient confidentiality is prohibited as Sheikh Abu Ghuddah already mentioned. A doctor has access to many personal details about his or her patients. In addition, medical files are no longer only paper files; they are recorded on computers and databases. We once had a nurse who entered the system and saw all of her colleagues' medical records and lab results. As soon as this was found out, she was expelled from work immediately because this was an infringement of others' right to confidentiality. The point is that a patient's file of information comes from different parts of the hospital — it is not just between him and his doctor — and could be available to anyone who has access to this file. As a result, respecting confidentiality becomes even more significant. Certain doctors reveal confidential information simply to show off their knowledge about what happens in certain cases. These are all things that Islam prohibits. The PBUH said that for he who conceals (the faults of) a Muslim, God would conceal his faults in this world and in the Hereafter.

Mohammed Ghaly

In order to create a path for our discussion, I will attempt to draw a link between the paper presented by Sheikh Abu Ghuddah just now and the paper presented by Sheikh Raissouni that was discussed in an earlier session. Sheikh Raissouni addressed the question of principles and the search for them. He spoke to us about the attempts of Islamic scholars to find the core values (*ummahāt al-faḍā'il*). He then detailed to us what he had personally arrived at, which are the two principles of God-consciousness (*taqwá*) and mercy (*raḥmah*). Sheikh Abu Ghuddah took us in a different direction, one that involved the etiquettes of the physician. He mentioned that among Islamic scholars' search for the etiquettes of the physician was Abu Bakr Al-Razi and Dr. Chamsi-Pasha mentioned Al-Ruhawi. So it is apparent that a search has been taking place for centuries, whether it was for general ethics like in the case of Ibn Miskawayh and Al-Ghazali or for more specific ethics concerning the medical field. So this subject is not new to Islam and has been a topic of research for a long time.

Second, in their search for these ethical issues, Islamic scholars were not closed-minded. They did not limit themselves to looking only at Islamic texts; they also integrated related works from the traditions of other peoples. Ibn Miskawayh, for example, and others looked into the works of Greek philosophers. The books of Al-Ruhawi and Al-Razi are replete with quotes from Galen, Hippocrates, and others. However, they tried to frame these principles within the context of Islam and its principles. So in our present efforts to discuss a universal perspective on biomedical ethics and to answer the question of how to interpret them from an Islamic perspective, we are not coming up with something new in principle. Instead, it is the continuation of the constant communication across cultures that began long ago.

Sheikh Abu Ghuddah mentioned an important term in the title of his paper: the "governing principles" (*al-mabādi' al-ḥākimah*). It was translated into English as just "principles," but it is important to include the adjective, "governing." Another interesting point about Sheikh Abu Ghuddah's paper was that in the body of the paper itself, when he introduced the 12 main items, he called them "Islamic ethics in medicine" and not "governing principles." Furthermore, while Sheikh Abu Ghuddah detailed 12 ethics, Sheikh Raissouni specified only two. The two Sheikh Raissouni included also show up in Sheikh Abu Ghuddah's paper, directly or indirectly. So we have both commonalities and differences between the two papers that necessitate discussion so as to agree on some conclusions.

Jasser Auda

Among what we concern ourselves with in this center is how Islam can contribute to the world when it comes to the field of ethics, in order to serve humanity and civilization in general. There is no doubt that Islam has a lot to offer when it comes to biomedical ethics specifically. However, as Dr. Ghaly pointed out, this discipline is built on an inherited tradition that is not only Islamic but includes other nations and schools of thought, and Islam contributed or added to it. My question to Sheikh Abu Ghuddah is: Can Islamic Sharia give or present something to non-Muslims? As we are speaking about universal biomedical ethics, is it possible to speak of the universality of Islamic Sharia in this regard?

Abdul Sattar Abu Ghuddah

Islamic Sharia encompasses many areas, including belief or creed, acts of worship, daily transactions between people, the legal system, rules and regulations, and consequences for crime. Apart from the creed and acts of worship that are specific to Muslims, these areas are universal and are derived plainly from the principle of justice. They come from the attempt to preserve the rights of all and avoid that which causes disputes such as ignorance, betrayal, deception, and taking money fraudulently as is the case with usury and gambling. These ideals are expected of all of humanity, Muslims and non-Muslims alike.

It is interesting that we find many occasions in history when non-Muslims resorted to Muslim courts to deal with their cases, especially when they involved matters of inheritance. This is because many legal systems outside the Islamic tradition lacked elaborate processes in this area. For example, in the West, a person could leave his estate or money to literally anyone, including an animal if he so chose, and deprive from his money whomever he chose. In Islamic Sharia, however, there are clear criteria for how inheritance money is to be distributed. It is a structure that Muslims are proud and grateful to have. We have seen many Christian families request from a Muslim judge to divide their inheritance amongst them according to Islamic principles.

In addition, the world's recent financial crisis revealed how Islamic banking institutes that maintained Sharia standards did not suffer as much as non-Islamic banks. This left people considering why the Islamic system survived with fewer negative impacts, and it put Islamic banking in higher demand. There was more interest in knowing what exactly the Islamic principles of financial transactions are and how they work. For example, Islam prohibits the charging of interest on loans.

This drew attention of all people, not just Muslims. Accordingly and more generally, if others do seek our contribution or guidance in certain matters, we try to help. However, needless to say, we do not interfere with the freedom of other people or nations to choose whichever systems they desire. We do not impose our methods on them, and we always respect their freedom of choice regarding their religious beliefs. This is my view on the universality of the Islamic Sharia, apart from acts of worship and matters of creed that each person chooses for him or herself.

Ali Al-Qaradaghi

I have some clarifying questions. In his paper, Sheikh Abu Ghuddah mentioned the balance between when a doctor should guard his patients' secrets and when he should disclose them in specific cases, according to the resolution arrived at by the International Islamic Fiqh Academy. I believe this balance is what we were looking for earlier this morning and the resolution answers our questions in this regard.

I noticed the words "governing principles" (*al-mabādi' al-ḥākimah*) in the title of Sheikh Abu Ghuddah's paper and was under the impression that Sheikh Abu Ghuddah would specify to us what the governing principles actually are. I was also hoping he would clarify the distinction between governing principles, non-governing principles, and what are not considered to be principles at all. In fact, the title of his paper, "The Governing Principles of Islamic Ethics in Medicine," is comprises two main points. We need to understand the current usage of the word *principles* (*mabādi'*) in its meaning both as "comprehensive principles" (*kullīyāt*) and as "fundamentals" (*uṣūl*), contrary to its usage in previous generations.

The traditional definition of the term *principle* (*mabda'*) in Arabic has historically been the "beginnings" or "introductions," according to scholars of the Arabic language. Therefore, the terms "comprehensive principles" and "fundamentals" are in fact not far from the traditional meaning. I come now to my point. It is imperative that we distinguish principles from that which are not principles as Dr. Beauchamp did when he distinguished between the criteria (*mi'yārīyah*) of ethics on the one hand and the individual ethics themselves on the other hand. When he defined ethics in four elements, he clarified that he is not talking about the categories or types of ethics; instead, he is talking about the criteria [or ways of measuring]. So we are in need of these criteria, and I hope our discussion will address this point. This is the first remark.

My second point concerns the 12 items that Sheikh Abu Ghuddah included in his paper. They all are of course based on Sharia, but I did not find them all to be issues of ethics, strictly speaking. For instance, in regards to acquiring the appropriate medical knowledge and experience, that is a practical and legal matter since no physician will be certified without this knowledge. While it is consistent with ethical considerations, it is not necessarily an ethical issue in and of itself. The same can be said about four more of the items: a doctor's conformity with standard occupational principles, religious (Sharia-based) knowledge of rulings in medical practice, respecting medical specializations, and abiding by professional laws and regulations.

Mohammed Ghaly

We will gather all questions and comments and allow Sheikh Abu Ghuddah the chance to respond afterward.

Annelien Bredenoord

What strikes me about what I have heard thus far regarding Islamic medical ethics is that it is an ethics of the physician. It is much about the virtues of being a good physician and about the principles guiding the conduct of a physician. The difference in Western bioethics, and also in the four principles, is that we are more focused on medical ethics in society and on the patient's ethics. What I have heard so far about professional ethics, or the ethics of the doctor, is almost the same as the ethics we teach our medical doctors, and they are rooted in the principles of beneficence and nonmaleficence.

However, our other two universal principles, autonomy and justice, are not physicians' ethics, but they are more on the societal level. Furthermore, autonomy is more about the virtue of a patient, of being a good patient, of what we can expect from the patient regarding responsibilities, and so on. I would be interested to hear whether there is similarly extensive scholarly work on that aspect as well.

Also, I think we would not call the 12 principles presented by Sheikh Abu Ghuddah a common morality but rather a particular morality. As Dr. Beauchamp would say, there is the common morality, which is the universal principles shared by all of us, and there are particular moralities that can be plural and different.

Hassan Chamsi-Pasha

I will comment very quickly on the issue of certification and degrees. It seems that very often the ministry of health in some Arab country, especially in the Gulf, discovers individuals pretending to be doctors who have presented forged degrees. I think this is what Sheikh Abu Ghuddah meant in his paper when he highlighted this as a fundamental ethical issue. Alternatively, some doctors do have proper medical certification but occasionally practice outside of their specialization(s). Although this may be a technical aspect, it also has a large ethical element to it. Take as an example an individual with proper certification to perform general surgery. It is allowed for him to perform some types of orthopedic surgery, for example, because it falls within the umbrella of general surgery. However, there are other types of orthopedic surgery that he is not allowed to perform because of their professional requirements. This is how an ethical issue intersects with professional and technical issues.

Mohammed Ghaly

Do you think this falls under the scope of God-consciousness?

Hassan Chamsi-Pasha

We may place it within the scope of God-consciousness, but it is certainly within the scope of honesty.

Mohammed Ali Al-Bar

I will make some brief comments. First, I would like to clarify that Al-Razi lived about a hundred or more years before Al-Ruhawi; there are often misconceptions about this. Second, scholars are unsure as to whether Al-Ruhawi was a Muslim, Christian, or Jew. Most opinions indicate he was a Christian. He might have converted to Islam later as many non-Muslim doctors did at the time, but we do not know for sure. In the Arab medical legacy, it is difficult to distinguish between doctors who were Muslim and those who were Christian. They used many of the same phrases, such as, "praise be to God" and, "blessings be upon the messengers of God," and so forth. The Islamic civilization was inclusive of all, and the language was shared among all.

Mohammed Ghaly

Do you see this as an indicator of the universality of what was written in that time period?

Mohammed Ali Al-Bar

Yes. There was a culture within the Islamic civilization in which everyone spoke a common language, so distinguishing between members of different religions was difficult. Even their names were very similar. Names such as Abu Ali, Abu Al-Hassan, and Hebatullah may seem to belong to a Muslim and yet we discover that a person with such a name is Christian or Jewish. This similarity extended to writing styles, appearance, attire, and other areas. So this gives us insights into the civilizational dimension of this period of time.

Throughout history and across civilizations, medical practice has been founded on the two ethical principles of doing good and preventing harm. The physician was to treat his patients as a father would treat his children. Islam introduced the emphasis on the principle of justice in the physician's practice of medicine and in the distribution of services.

The principle of autonomy was also alluded to in Islam during its very early stages. Muslim jurists wrote about the topic about 1,200 years ago. They introduced two conditions that needed to be met. First, an individual must seek the permission of the concerned authorities to become a doctor and practice medicine. Second, the patient or the guardian of the patient must grant the doctor permission to treat the patient. A doctor who treats a patient without meeting these two conditions could be penalized and potentially prevented from practicing even if he made no medical mistakes. What is new to us and what has developed only more recently is the notion that the patient should have all the relevant information when he or she consents. This is called informed consent. Other than that, the idea of consent was there, and in Islam even veterinarians were not allowed to treat an animal without the consent of the animal's owner.

Therefore, there were two principles in the history of Islamic medicine that are worth mentioning. The first is justice and the equal distribution of services. The caliph would send medical care to even the most remote areas and even to prisons. This was not included in Hippocratic medicine. The second is the freedom of the patient to accept or refuse treatment. The Prophet (PBUH) rebuked his companions when they force-fed him medicine after he had refused treatment.

We must acknowledge there are differences in certain understandings. The Islamic civilization's notion of the patient's autonomy, for example, does not reach the excess that is present in the Western understanding. According to the Western concept, the understanding of the patient's autonomy is that it is absolute. This restricts the doctor's actions to a large extent. For example, a patient has the right to request from a doctor to change his gender from male to female, and I do respect this right. However, as a Muslim doctor, I may not agree with this procedure, and I have the right to refuse to perform it. In the Western system, the doctor does have the right to refuse the procedure, but he or she must refer the patient to another doctor. The same goes in matters of abortion without a medical reason: although in the Western system a doctor may refuse to perform this procedure, he or she must refer the patient to another doctor who will.

The question is, to what extent does the patient have the freedom to do as he or she chooses? If a patient is taking drugs or abusing alcohol, to what extent am I as a doctor allowed to tell the patient that this is right or wrong? The term that is often used in these situations is "paternalism." This was previously understood as wanting the best for someone or trying to save a person from harm. Now it is considered an insult in the Western medical context. Of course, I am not saying there is no limit to how much a father or doctor should advise his child or patient. I am not against the principle of autonomy. Islam advocates for an individual's freedom to choose his or her own religion. We see this in the Qur'anic verse, "There shall be no compulsion in [acceptance of] the religion…" (Qur'an 2:256). By extension, there should be no compulsion in medical care. However, the aversion to the concept of paternalism should not reach to the point that it almost becomes a crime in and of itself. Nevertheless, the differences I have outlined lie in the details, not in the foundational principle.

Tariq Ramadan

I have a question regarding Dr. Bredenoord's comment that we are not talking about ethics of the physician but rather about the ethics of medicine more generally. Does it suffice for us to simply mention the higher objectives (*maqāṣid*) of Sharia and the necessities (*ḍarūrīyāt*) among them? Or is there more to be explained? For example, when you talk about behavior (*sulūkīyāt*), the last point talks about equality (*musāwāh*). Equality could mean justice (*'adl*). Where do we draw the line of autonomy or independence? These are important matters, and there are never responses. We always go back to the higher objectives of Sharia and the necessities alone. Does this suffice as a response to what comes from the West? Can we offer something from Islam and its understandings, principles, and objectives?

Mohammed Ghaly

Dr. Ramadan, do you mean that we should expand the understanding of the higher objectives of Sharia so they may be used in the scope of medicine?

Tariq Ramadan

No, I do not mean expansion in this way. I mean we need to be more precise about our goals. Sheikh Raissouni mentioned three of the five objectives of Sharia (the preservation of life, offspring, and the intellect) that he thought have a connection to medicine. In my opinion, it is not enough to simply repeat these words [i.e. these higher objectives] without going back to some of the principles and really talking about their meanings. We need to really talk about autonomy and other principles and how they relate to practices on the ground (*sulūkīyāt*). Can these points be considered in the Islamic response?

Mohammed Ghaly

So the question is, can we rely exclusively on the higher objectives of Sharia to create the governing principles in medicine?

Abdul Sattar Abu Ghuddah

The higher objectives of Sharia are high principles from which practical applications are derived. We cannot confine them to just the three that were mentioned — preserving life, the intellect, and offspring — even though they are the most important and relevant to medicine. We can also include other higher objectives like preserving religion or preserving wealth. These are all principles to pay attention to when considering relevant practical applications. Some scholars have also added other objectives to these original five, both long ago and in modern times. For example, preserving the environment was recently added.

We do not limit ourselves to the higher objectives of Sharia alone; rather, they direct our interpretations of texts so we do not go outside of them when engaging in independent legal reasoning (*ijtihād*) and so we do not cling to literal interpretations of texts. It seems to me that the higher objectives of Sharia are not these five alone. We may add to them anything that realizes sound behavior and the safety of human beings, societies, and the environment. Dr. Al-Najjar wrote a book about this, in which he added several other higher objectives and provided evidence for these additions. The higher objectives of Sharia that we have been talking about were articulated by Imam Al-Haramayn and then Al-Ghazali, but their contributions were only the beginning, and we are of course allowed to add to them.

When I used the phrase "the governing principles for ethics," I wanted to highlight two issues. First, when talking about governing principles we must clarify what is being governed, which in this case are the ethics. Some principles are indeed governing, and I started with them: the need for acquiring medical experience, conforming to standard occupational principles, respecting specializations, abiding by rules and regulations, and obtaining knowledge of Sharia rulings. These five are governing principles for all the actions the physician does. After this come ethical values such as God-consciousness (*taqwá*), excellence (*iḥsān*), sincerity (*ikhlāṣ*), honesty (*ṣidq*), trustworthiness (*amānah*), humility (*tawāḍu'*), and compassion (*rifq*).

It is worth mentioning that compassion includes mercy. The Prophet (PBUH) said, "Indeed, compassion is not in something except that it beautifies it, and compassion is not removed from anything except that it blemishes it."[1] In fact, the physician has been called *rafīq* (the compassionate one). Needless to say, I could not talk about the governing principles

[1] Narrated by Muslim (No. 2594).

without explaining in detail what they govern, and I could not talk about ethics without explaining the higher principles from which those ethics are derived.

As for focusing on the ethics of the physician, this is because the patient submits to the physician. Sufis or ascetics say that a disciple before his or her teacher should be like a patient in the presence of his or her doctor, doing as the teacher or doctor wishes. Therefore, we do not need ethics for the patient, except in some rare cases. Some patients behave poorly towards their doctors because of arrogance, pride about their wealth, or social standing. A poet once wrote,

> Indeed neither the teacher nor the doctor offers their counsel
> If not respected or given due credit,
> So bear with your illness if you degrade its healer
> And bear with your ignorance if you forsake a teacher.

So a student and a patient should behave appropriately with their teacher and doctor if they seek benefit from them. The issue of confidentiality is an example of a two-way ethical expectation: the patient should provide the doctor with all relevant information so the doctor has a complete picture, while the doctor should not divulge information about the patient outside the examination room. Other examples of ethical values that are expected of both parties are God-consciousness and humility.

In regards to the four principles, I think they are included within the ethics that have been mentioned in my chapter and in the chapters of my colleagues but perhaps with different names. For example, being compassionate is the same as showing mercy. The same applies to the terms *autonomy* and *consent*. Likewise, enjoining what is good and refraining from harmful deeds are different names that can have similar meanings. The related concept of *iḥsān* (excellence) exists in the Qur'an and the Prophetic tradition.

Annelien Bredenoord

I am thinking about your last comment that you recognize the four principles of bioethics from Islamic ethics. You say that they are the same but that you use different names. My question is, are these four principles enough?

Is everything confined to these four principles, or do we need to have more? Because Beauchamp and Childress argue that the four are enough.

Abdul Sattar Abu Ghuddah

These four principles are what we would call innate principles (*dhātīyah*) [i.e. principles innate to a human being]. What we need to add are acquired principles such as God-consciousness, which involves vigilance and self-monitoring and is not captured by the four principles. We also have to add humility, which is not included in the four principles. Sometimes when doctors excel in their work, they may become arrogant and stop respecting other specializations. Doctors must also be both conscious and fearful of God or, if they do not believe in God, at least fear their reputation among other people. Trustworthiness (*amānah*) is also not included in the four principles. So I would say the four principles can be considered seeds for the universal principles, but we need to add to the set of four principles from the Islamic perspective what would complete it and increase it in applicability.

Jasser Auda

I would like to clarify that Dr. Abu Ghuddah is talking about the doctor's ethics. He is not talking about legislation, policy, or — in your words — something related to the society. The realm of society or law is the Islamic law or Sharia, and that realm is directly induced from the [religious] texts rather than something that is tied to or based on the ethics that you are talking about. So it seems that the ethics in this sense is virtues and morals rather than law.

Annelien Bredenoord

As I said before, Islamic medical ethics seems to focus exclusively on the ethics of the doctor. I think there is a big difference between it and Western bioethics, which is an ethics of the patient as well as an ethics of how medicine is distributed in society, which is related more to policy. If it is exclusively an ethics of what the professional is doing, then there might be difficulties in stating some universal principles.

Tariq Ramadan

I think we are touching upon something essential. This is why I wanted Dr. Bredenoord to be quite clear on her understanding of what is being said. She talked about the four principles as principles for the society. The question Sheikh Al-Qaradaghi raised was exactly in light of the four principles: Do we have something in Islam to contribute to that field, not only for the doctor but also for the society? Sheikh Abu Ghuddah said he does not have a problem with the four principles but rather we have a problem of wording and also that maybe other aspects are missing, such as God-consciousness. In this context he is using the term *God-consciousness* not only in reference to God but also in terms of one's consciousness or self-conscience as a doctor or as a human being. When you listen to this, Dr. Bredenoord, do you think we are talking about something different, or do you find that there is common ground beyond the words?

Annelien Bredenoord

There is common ground. I understood it differently, but this helped to clarify. The interesting point of discussion is whether the four principles are necessary and sufficient or whether they need elaboration and even expansion.

Tariq Ramadan

Sheikh Abu Ghuddah argues that they are not enough. He argues that all the principles might amount to nothing if there is no conscience as an integral part of the whole process. Do you agree with this, or are we talking about different issues?

Annelien Bredenoord

In my opinion, the concept of consciousness or even self-consciousness is a part of autonomy. Autonomy is not only concerned with the patient's autonomy but also with the physician's autonomy. Autonomy is understood in many different ways. In fact, there are bookshelves full of books written by philosophers about the concept of autonomy, so it is a difficulty that we have different interpretations of autonomy. Taking a more rich interpretation, for example that of Isaiah Berlin, would give more positive accounts of autonomy. They are about consciousness, self-consciousness, authenticity, and taking responsibility. I think this concept may be part of our concept of autonomy. It might be that you think it is not the same or it is not sufficient.

Ali Al-Qaradaghi

Both my commentary and Sheikh Abu Ghuddah's research indicate that we accept these four principles but maintain that some principles may need to be added. I have said before that Islam includes practical ethical principles that can be adopted by all of humanity, including non-Muslims and non-Christians. This is because we have scriptures indicating that Islam was sent as a healing for all people. I was in France once with a group of scholars, and the French Minister of Economy asked us, "Do you Muslim religious scholars want, through [achieving] an Islamic economy, for everyone to be Muslim?" I answered, "Of course not," and explained that we want mercy for all of humanity and that this can be of benefit to everyone. Ultimately, everyone takes of it what he or she wills. If people want to benefit they are most welcome to do so, but it does not mean they have to be Muslim.

Mohammed Ghaly

I received a question from the audience. Dr. Ramadan asked Sheikh Raissouni three questions, but Sheikh Raissouni only answered two of them. The third question was: Is there a difference between the ethics of the medical profession in general and the ethics of the doctor? If so, what is it?

Ahmed Raissouni

The physician is the backbone of the medical profession. It is perhaps for this reason that Sheikh Abu Ghuddah's paper and mine focused on the physician's practice and behavior as an embodiment of medical practice. The process of applying the four principles as laws in society is a different issue. We do not have a problem with applying these four principles to economics for instance or even to marital issues. They still apply perfectly well. Where is the singularity of medicine? The singularity of medicine comes when we address the practice, behavior, ethics, and attitude of the physician.

I am still unsure as to why these principles are considered specific to medicine. As I understand it, once these principles are expanded to the rules, habits, and policies of society, then they are no longer exclusive to medicine. Justice is required in everything. Similarly, a human being is entitled to own property and do what he likes with it. This is considered autonomy. So the way I understood the task at hand was putting our focus on physicians and other medical professionals like nurses, pharmacists, etc. According to the way the four principles have been expressed, it seems they can be expanded to everything in society. My focus was on doctors because this was the task at hand.

Mohammed Ali Al-Bar

I have a comment in regards to the principle of justice and distributing medical services. Societies today are complex. The relationship is no longer only between the doctor and the patient. It has expanded to the scale of an entire society whose members either receive medical services or do not. For example, a country like the United States is very advanced in medical care and possesses excellent hospitals and doctors. Yet there are some 50 million people who have no medical insurance and do not have access to medical care. Beauchamp himself admits that in the latest edition of his book. There are another 30 million who occasionally may get medical insurance for about 6 months and then spend the following year or two without any. This means about one-third of the entire population of the United States does not have proper medical insurance.

I will give a simpler example. Malaysia spent $680 per capita on healthcare in the year 2010 while the United States spent $7,800 per capita in the same year. That is almost 12 times the amount Malaysia spends. In comparison though, the mortality rates of children (one of the standards for health used by the World Health Organization) in Malaysia was 3 out of 1,000, and in the United States the rate was about 5.5 out of 1,000 in the same year. In other words, the United States spends 12 times as much as Malaysia on healthcare and yet by the standards of the World Health Organization, Malaysia is doing better. Singapore's mortality rate of children is 1 out of 1,000, the lowest rate in the world. If we look at countries in northern Europe like Sweden and Norway, they spend about one-third of the amount spent by the United States, and their rates are much better than the United States'. In fact, the United States ranks last among the 28 industrial countries. The United States ranks below even Cuba and perhaps ranks around the same level as Sri Lanka with regards to the large portion of the population without medical insurance.

Therefore, if the principle of justice encompasses all these considerations, then medical care and health issues are no longer about the doctor–patient relationship but rather address an entire system. This system calls for comprehensive policies. Despite being the strongest country with some of the world's best medical advancements, doctors, and hospitals, large amounts of money are spent and yet their ranking remains low. This leads to a clear conclusion, that there is a major flaw in their system. The expenditure of large sums of money and yet failing to achieve the required levels of medical care should raise a lot of eyebrows. Clearly, the United States system needs extensive re-evaluation.

Achieving justice certainly extends beyond the doctor–patient relationship nowadays, and the West is right to consider justice at a broader societal level with associated political issues. In addition, these are not issues exclusive to countries like the Netherlands, Britain, or the United States. The issues of injustice and discrimination from a medical perspective are issues of concern for the global community as a whole. Our colleagues in the West are talking about these issues while we have yet to pay much attention to them.

Mohammed Ghaly

This is a central point: in Western academic research that addresses guiding principles of medical ethics, they are not merely concerned with the doctor–patient relationship. Rather, their focus encompasses the distribution of wealth, social justice, and the like. As a result, they lay down what we could call "fundamental virtues" (*ummahāt al-faḍā'il*) and "fundamental ethics" (*ummahāt al-akhlāq*) and then choose the most appropriate and most cohesive of them with regards to medical matters. So, it is not about matters specific to the doctor–patient relationship. Rather, they are more concerned with broad ethics and guiding principles and then after that they choose what is most relevant with regards to the problems that exist in medicine. This may be a good discussion point for us in the future.

Abdul Sattar Abu Ghuddah

It is true that the question of justice was not dealt with elaborately in the history of Islam. The reason for this is that medical care used to be free of charge and its costs were covered through endowments (*waqf*). Dr. Ahmed Issa wrote a book on the history of what is called the *bīmāristān*, which in Islamic history was a medical city in which people would receive medical care free of charge. Anyone could visit it and stay as long as he or she wished. Some people would even choose to remain there after being treated because there were good meals and other services. So justice was present automatically because of the system of endowments. There were no hospitals making profit, fairly or unfairly, from providing medical care to sick people. It was a comprehensive medical system where medical care and medication was free of charge.

Tariq Ramadan

This is an important point because it is not only related to economy and justice; it is also associated with culture. I was in Morocco and spoke with some doctors about issues surrounding cancer. I noticed that when the doctor would speak to the patient, the entire family would urge the doctor to remain silent and not disclose information about the patient's illness to the patient. This may seem like a detail, but it is actually a crucial point regarding autonomy and independence of choice. This silence is characteristic of the Arab culture, but it is not correct according to Islam. Surely, it is not acceptable for a cultural trait to overrule an Islamic principle.

Ahmed Raissouni

All in all, if the principle of justice includes issues concerning society, then it applies to education, employment, transportation, and all areas — not only medicine. Hence, my question is, why do we call it medical or biomedical ethics? Everything we have been talking about applies to so many areas of life. If indeed this is our discussion, then let us open the door for all our morals, values, ethics, principles, priorities, and objectives. In Islam for instance, things such as justice, freedom of choice, and principles like, "there should be neither harming nor reciprocating harm" can apply to everything. Medicine need not be distinguished from other fields in this regard. Thus, I propose we focus on those things that have a direct application in medicine.

Governing Principles of Islamic Ethics in Medicine

Abdul Sattar Abu Ghuddah

Abstract: This chapter is divided into three main sections. In the first section, the focus is on the great attention paid by Islamic Sharia to ethics as compared with schools of law from outside the Islamic tradition, which are usually exclusively concerned with rights and obligations from a judiciary perspective. The second section is dedicated to terminology and especially the distinction between two types of ethics, namely philosophy-based ethics and religion-based ethics. The third section introduces a list of the basic Islamic ethics in medicine, extracted from Islamic sources including the Qur'ān, the Sunna, and the writings of early Muslim physicians, especially the work of Abu Bakr Al-Razi *Akhlāq al-ṭabīb* (The Ethics of the Physician). The list consists of nine items: developing medical experience; the conformity of the physician's practices with the professional standards; having knowledge of Sharia-based rulings related to practicing medicine; God-consciousness (*taqwá*) and fear of Him; sincerity and dedication to work; modesty towards God and compassion towards the patients; truthfulness and honesty; practicing medicine within the limits of one's own medical specializations; and confidentiality.

In the name of God, the Most Gracious, the Most Merciful.
Praise be to God, The Lord of the worlds, and peace and blessings be upon our Prophet Muhammad, his household, and his companions.

Our contemporary world has been overwhelmingly immersed in material matters and preoccupied with worldly discoveries and achievements. There is a dire need to regulate the directions of this rapid progress through adherence to the ethics and behaviors encompassing each field. This is especially true for medicine, in light of the significant and widespread impact of its outcomes, be they positive or negative. Hence, it is necessary to intensify efforts in clarifying the fundamentals of ethics, linking them to firmly established and constant principles, and avoiding any influences arising from the potential of commercial gain and/or individual interests. The best principles that one can rely on in this regard are those embraced by Islam, the religion that God has perfected and through which He completed His favor to the last nation, enjoining it as a creed, legislation, and way of life.

God is the Granter of success.

1. Morality in Islamic Sharia

Islamic Sharia enjoys certain unique characteristics that differentiate it from other schools of law and intellectual doctrines. Among these characteristics is its great concern with moral behaviors, which are ranked in Islamic Sharia among the legal rulings (*al-aḥkām al-taklīfīyah*) that include those classified as obligatory, recommended, permissible, reprehensible, and forbidden acts. This concern with moral behaviors is apparent in both general prescriptions and prescriptions specific to different societal sectors:

- In regards to the general legal prescriptions, we find within the diverse chapters and topics of Islamic law (*fiqh*) considerable sections dedicated to issues of moral behavior. For example, in chapters addressing prohibition and permissibility or those addressing recommended and abhorred acts, jurists have highlighted numerous moral issues related to different professions and specializations. These moral issues are classified in an independent category, as they neither belong to the prescribed obligations nor to the absolute prohibitions.

- Some authors writing about Islamic law used the title *Al-jāmi'*, meaning "the comprehenesive," for the section dedicated to moral issues and would place it as the last chapter in juristic manuals. Further, in cases where the content of this chapter was found to be extensive, it was developed into a separate, independent book. Examples of these books include *Al-jāmi'* by the Maliki jurist Ibn Abi Zayd Al-Qayrawani and *Al-jāmi'* by Ibn Rushd (the grandfather of Averroes), while other authors used titles that explicitly identified the book's content such as *Sharia-Based Etiquettes* (*Al-ādāb al-shar'īyah*) by the Hanbali jurist Ibn Muflih and the famous *Revival of the Islamic Sciences* (*Iḥyā' 'ulūm al-dīn*) by Abu Hamid Al-Ghazali.
- In addressing legal prescriptions within professional fields, scholars from different specializations and disciplines explicitly emphasized the moral behaviors associated with each field of knowledge and/or specialty. In their books, jurists (*fuqahā'*) differentiated between legal rulings, for which the judiciary system can be consulted for guidance, and those behaviors that are not within the scope of judicial obligation but rather are subject to a person's morality. They termed this latter scope of behaviors "religiosity" (*diyānah*), meaning those behaviors that are ordained by religion but remain between God and His servants. Scholars have authored numerous books on diverse areas of morality such as the etiquettes (*ādāb*, singular *adab*) of learning and teaching, the etiquettes of the physician, the mufti, the merchant, the traveler, princes and ministers, the accountant, and the banker, etc. In these contexts the word *ādāb* encompasses moralities or behaviors.

It is worth mentioning that, half a century ago, morality was taught to students as a distinct subject using modern, specialized texts as well as classical, traditional texts such as summaries of *Revival of the Islamic Sciences*. However, this practice was temporarily discontinued until contemporary scholars, once again, revived the focus on behaviors and codes of conduct as they recognized the necessity of these issues in achieving the desired purposes of diverse professions and scientific research, especially within the medical field. This renewed attention was extended to numerous professions and resulted in the issuance of several professional protocols particularly for those fields with serious social impacts.

It is also worth noting that law schools are not concerned with — and even do not acknowledge — moral standpoints. Instead, they focus exclusively on rights and duties that can be settled through the judiciary system. As mentioned earlier, jurists, on the other hand, have emphasized the dual importance of both moral obligations and judicial obligations. This alienation between laws and moral values is not surprising; rather, it is quite expected from disciplines and systems that choose to isolate religion from daily life and focus on the utilitarian aim of actions while excluding the religious perspective on these actions.

On the other hand, Islamic moral values, emerging from the Islamic belief (the doctrine of human succession on earth, *istikhlāf*) and deduced from the Sharia (the criterion for what is lawful and unlawful), are meant to achieve superior aims. These superior aims may encompass immediate, materialistic objectives, or their objective may be retained for the Day of Judgment. Therefore, values must be observed and maintained even if they may seem to be detrimental to people, as this perceived detriment is compensated for through the real benefit of satisfying God's mandates.

There is insufficient space in this chapter to list the various texts from the Qur'an and Prophetic Tradition that prove Islam's great interest in and concern with moral values as reflected in its approach to God-consciousness and self-monitoring. God says, "Nay! Man will be a witness against himself [as his body parts (skin, hands, legs, etc.) will speak about his deeds]" (Qur'an 75:14).

2. Definition of Ethics

Ethics are the foundational principles employed by Sharia, legislation, and custom (*'urf*) within the regulatory frameworks governing different specialties and professions. They enjoy a constructive characteristic with the intention of regulating behavior through identifying right from wrong across actions, relationships, and policies.

2.1. *Definition of Values, Ethical Values, and Behaviors*

Values are those high ideals which direct the mindset and actions of a person or a society. They are the standards according to which the behaviors of one's self or others are judged.

2.1.1. *Values are categorized as follows*

- Intellectual, belief-based, and faith-based values such as the principle of human succession on earth.
- Ethical values such as truth and honesty. Ethical values are often referred to in short as "ethics" (*akhlāq*). Linguistically, the singular term "ethic/virtue" (*khuluq*) means habit and instinct. It refers to a person's natural disposition or an acquired habit that becomes part of a person's nature. Hence, ethics are similar to habits; they are a person's second nature.

The difference between intellectual (belief-based) values and ethical values is at the relative and absolute levels. Belief-based values govern one's ideology and behaviors and serve as a reference base for more than one ethical value. Meanwhile, ethical values are derived from intellectual values. Each of the two categories has its own particular scope.

Thus, the discipline of ethics, or "morality," is divided into:

- Philosophical morality, which relies on the mind and absolute philosophical methods in the analysis of moral dilemmas.
- Religious morality, which relies on divine revelation and derives moral principles from religion, given that the righteous application of religion ensures striving for good and virtue and avoiding evil and vice. This is due to God being *Al-Laṭīf* (The Subtly Kind), *Al-Khabīr* (The All Aware), whose superior knowledge of His creatures outweighs any inferior theories which may be influenced by a person's environment or personal biases.

However, the theological nature of religious morality does not eliminate the role of the mind and human reasoning in the exploration and analysis of a practical procedural framework that is committed to good moral behavior and avoids harmful behavior. Although these explorations and analyses are means towards an end, they fall under the legal ruling for objectives (*maqāṣid*) due to their significant impact. This is contingent upon the means being lawful and that they do not overshadow or neglect the higher goal under which they are functioning.

Ethical values — just like creed, religious law, and intellectual values — aim at achieving superior goals. These goals may be accompanied by an immediate materialistic objective, or the objective may be retained to the Day of Judgment. Therefore, as mentioned earlier, it is imperative that one strongly commits to ethical values, even if they disadvantage a person, as this is compensated for by the ultimate benefit, namely the pleasure of God Almighty.

2.1.2. *Definition of behaviors*

Behaviors are external, visible human actions. Values, whether intellectual or ethical, are ideals which guide internal aspects of the human being such as mental reasoning or psychological processes. Behaviors are the external indicators for a person's internal attributes. Hence, any consistent behavior exhibited by a person reflects his or her intellectual and moral values.[1]

Ethical values (ethics) within the field of medicine have been addressed from multiple perspectives. Several researchers have identified certain principles of biomedical ethics that they found to be common across different regions of the world. These include[2]:

(i) Respect for human life, dignity, and one's right to confidentiality.
(ii) Acknowledgment of an individual's right to choose, whether to accept or reject treatment.
(iii) Adherence to the principle of providing benefit and preventing harm to the patient as much as possible.
(iv) Equality and justice in the treatment of all patients.

---

[1] Ashraf Yahya Abdul-Hadi (1995). *Moral and Behavioral Aspects of Judgment* (*Al-jawānib al-akhlāqīyah wal-sulūkīyah lil-muḥāsabah*). Cairo: Faculty of Commerce, 3–9, 27–31.
[2] Mubarak Sayf Al-Hashimi (n.d.). *Muslim Physician Ethics* (*Akhlāqīyāt al-ṭabīb al-Muslim*), n.p., 5–6.

The subject of Islamic ethics for physicians has been extensively addressed within literature dealing with the topic of preserving morality and public order (*al-ḥisbah*).[3] One example to cite is the book titled *The Restorer of Favors and the Restrainer of Chastisements* (*Mu'īd Al-Ni'am*)[4] by Imam Taj Al-Din Al-Subki in which he outlined that a physician has the right to:

- Provide advice.
- Act with kindness and compassion towards the patient.
- Appropriately allude to the writing of a will if he observes indicators of the patient's imminent death.
- Examine sensitive body parts when and as deemed necessary.
- Common blameworthy traits of a physician include:

  (a) A lack of understanding of the disease.
  (b) Making a hasty diagnosis.
  (c) A lack of understanding regarding the patient's psychological health.
  (d) Practicing medicine prior to completing all requirements and earning the necessary credentials.
  (e) Further, he must believe that his medical treatment does not prevent divine predestination. Rather, he is acting in accordance with Sharia law and acknowledges that both the disease and cure are ultimately in the hands of God.

2.2. *Properties of Islam, Objectives of Sharia, and their Relationship to Ethics*

One of Islam's most significant properties is that it is a complete, comprehensive, and balanced religion. This is due to Islam's divine origin from God who has created mankind, knows their nature and their dynamic

[3] Among them are: Ibn Al-Ukhuwa (1937). *Rulings for Controlling Public Market* (*Ma'ālim al-qurbah fī aḥkām al-ḥisbah*). Cambridge: Dar Al-Funun; Al-Shayzari (1946). *The Ultimum in the Rulings for Controlling Public-Market* (*Nihāyat al-rutbah fī ḥalab al-ḥisbah*). Cairo: Matba'at Lajnat al-Buhuth wal-Ta'lif wal-Tarjamah wal-Nashr.

[4] Taj Al-Din Al-Subki (1993). *The Restorer of Favors and the Restrainer of Chastisements* (*Mu'īd al-ni'am wa-mubīd al-niqam*). Cairo: Maktabat Al-Khanji, 133.

needs, and thus knows best how to fulfill these needs: "Should not He Who has created know? And He is the Most Kind and Courteous (to His slaves), All-Aware (of everything)" (Qur'an 67:14).

The objectives of Sharia (*maqāṣid al-sharīʻah*) arise from the above-mentioned properties of Islam. The five objectives of Sharia are preserving religion (*dīn*), life (*nafs*), intellect (*ʻaql*), offspring (*nasl*), and wealth (*māl*). Some researchers have also included preservation of the environment as a sixth objective.[5]

The objective "preservation of life" refers to safeguarding a person's right to live. This includes provision of basic necessities for survival and safety as well as prevention of murder, suicide, or infliction of harm on oneself or on others.

In order to uphold these objectives, particularly "preservation of life," the Sharia outlines well-known checks and balances such as retribution, blood-money (*diyah*), and disciplinary punishment. Authorized rulers are delegated to make these decisions so as to ensure the protection of human life from its enemy or from any harm that is a result of aggression, negligence, or malpractice in a profession concerned with the well-being of the body.

Following this, jurists, through a process of deduction from legal texts, formulated numerous legal principles (rules) to address the field of ethics.[6]

3. Types of Medical Ethics

The categories of medical ethics vary according to origin and nature as follows:

- Vocational ethics, those specific to the practice of medicine as a profession.
- Religio-legal ethics.
- Professional ethics related to medical licensing and certification.

[5] See Abdul-Majid Al-Najjar (2006). *The Objectives of Sharia, with New Dimensions* (*Maqāṣid al-sharīʻah bi-abʻād jadīdah*). Beirut: Dar Al-gharb Al-Islami, 207.

[6] See Abdul Sattar Abu Ghuddah (1982). "*Al-mabādi' al-sharʻīyah lil-taṭbīb*" (*Buḥūth fī al-fiqh al-ṭibbī*). Second International Conference on Islamic Medicine: Islamic Medical Organization, Kuwait.

This chapter will address the second category despite the fact that some of these ethics arose prior to the advent of Islam while others emerged from the West with the introduction of professional protocols and codes of conduct.

The focus in this context will be limited to that which has relevance to Sharia-based religioethical character, directly or indirectly, given that wisdom is the believer's stray camel that he is always searching for (*al-ḥikmah ḍāllat al-mu'min*) wherever he finds it, it becomes his.

Common ethics, such as absolute Islamic ethics, shall be presented through both classical literature that is based on legal texts from the Qur'an and Prophetic Tradition as well as other writings which cannot be alleged to have been extracted from Western literature. One example of these writings is the book *Physician Ethics* (*Akhlāq al-ṭabīb*) by Abu Bakr Al-Razi which, as acknowledged by several impartial Western scholars, preceded all Western writings.[7]

4. Islamic Ethics in Medicine

4.1. *Acquiring Medical Experience*

Any medical practitioner must obtain sufficient theoretical knowledge and practical experience in his field. In addition, he must constantly remain informed of the latest advances and discoveries within the various medical fields so as to ensure that his treatment is consistent with the best and latest medical discoveries, theories, and cures.[8] In a situation in which two physicians were recommended to the Prophet Muhammad — peace and blessings of God be upon him (PBUH) — to cure a patient, he asked, "Which one of you is more skillful?"[9] Also, as narrated in another *hadith*, the Prophet Muhammad (PBUH) said, "Anyone who practices medicine when he is not recognized as a practitioner will be held responsible."[10]

---

[7] See the introduction of Al-Razi (1980). The edited version of *Physician Ethics* (*Akhlāq al-ṭabīb*) Ed. 'Abdul-Latif Muhammad Al-'Abd. Beirut: al-Maktabah al-'Asriyah.

[8] Yusuf Abdullah Al-Turki (n.d.). *Muslim Physician: Significance and Attributes* (*Al-ṭabīb al-muslim: tamayyuz wa-simāt*), n.p.; Al-Razi (1980), *op. cit.*

[9] Quoted by Malik in *Al-muwaṭṭa'*, vol. 4, 328.

[10] Narrated by Abu-Dawud in *Al-dīyāt*, no. 4586; Al-Nasa'i in *Al-qasāmah* , no. 4830; Ibn Majah in *Al-ṭibb*, no. 3466; and Al-Hakim in *Al-mustadrak*, vol. 4, p. 236.

Abu Bakr Al-Razi said, "Know that thieves and bandits are better than those who pretend to be physicians because the latter steal money and may even take lives, and they often do this to good humans. They do all this just so people would say, 'This person is a reliable reference in medicine.' However, if they had stopped doing this, it would have been better for their lifer and afterlife. It is very dangerous to treat humans without knowledge or to give orders and prohibitions without insight."[11]

Today, medical degrees and licenses are necessary conditions for the practice of medicine. Previously, the chief physician in major renowned hospitals (*bīmāristānāt*) was responsible for issuing medical licenses.[12]

Abu Bakr Al-Razi, and of course Galen and Hippocrates before him, condemn those who claim to have medical knowledge merely through experimenting on patients. Al-Razi says, "Neglect what the ignorant say when they claim that someone is skillful only by means experimentation. This never happens even if he lives the longest life. If such a person gives effective treatment, it is just good luck (coincidence). The best among those who do not study the foundations of their fields are those who read books and use treatments therein while not knowing that things included in books are not meant to be used in and of themselves but rather are essays written to be guiding and teaching." He then quoted from Galen that, "I prevent all those who consult me in medicine from undergoing medical treatment that is still in the phase of experimentation."[13]

4.2. *Conformity with Standard Vocational Principles*

In exercising his profession, the physician must uphold standard vocational principles. Given that he is dealing with the human body, if his aim

---

[11] Al-Razi (1980), *op. cit.*, p. 81. He listed some of his observations about those who pretend to be doctors.

[12] Ali Al-Muhammadi and Ali Al-Qaradaghi (1980). *Jurisprudence of Contemporary Medical Issues* (*Al-qaḍāyā al-ṭibbīyah al-mu'āṣirah*). Beirut: Dar Al-Basha'ir Al-Islamiyah, 110. Also see Ahmad 'Isa (1938). *The History of the Bimaristans in Islam* (*Tārīkh al-bīmāristānāt fī al-Islām*). Damascus: Jam'iyyat al-Tamaddun al-Islami.

[13] Al-Razi (1980), *op. cit.*, 77.

is not to cure, his actions would be deemed a crime or an act of aggression against another person's soul, limbs, or organs.

Arising from this premise, jurists established certain conditions that serve to regulate the physician's liability in circumstances when treatment leads to harmful outcomes. Among these conditions is the physician's compliance with standard vocational principles acknowledged by medical sciences and the experts in these sciences. Actions that contradict these principles are religiously and legally prohibited, and the physician must be held accountable for any such violations.

In their justification for regulating the burden of liability in professional practice, jurists explained that the purpose of the physician's action is to cure, not harm. The evidence indicating this purpose is conformity with the recognized principles and standards within the profession.

4.3. *Sharia-based Knowledge of Rulings Related to the Medical Practice*

Physicians must be fully aware and knowledgeable of all legal rulings associated with the practice of medicine. This is considered to be binding on every physician (*farḍ 'ayn*) — and not a collective obligation (*farḍ kifāyah*) — as stated by Abu Hamid Al-Ghazali in his identification of individual duties and obligations. Al-Ghazali did not limit personal obligations to prayer, fasting, almsgiving (*zakāh*), and pilgrimage (*ḥajj*); he also included any necessary type of knowledge that professions may require. Professionals are obligated to exert all efforts in becoming knowledgeable about legal requirements and rulings within their fields and should not claim that this responsibility falls exclusively on jurists. This is particularly critical in situations when there is insufficient time to inquire and obtain a jurist's opinion.

This legal knowledge protects both the physician and his patients from any possible errors that they may fall into. In addition, such knowledge may benefit the physician by enabling him to invest his medical practice in inviting people to get closer to God: "…So ask the people of the Reminder [Scriptures — the *Tawrāt* (Torah), the *Injīl* (Gospel)] if you do not know" (Qur'an 21:7).

Some researchers have put forth a suggestion of assigning one or more jurists to individual hospitals so as to guide patients in jurisprudential rulings regarding their medical circumstances. Alternatively, hospitals could coordinate with religious institutions that may be contacted and referred to when needed.

4.4. *God-Consciousness (taqwá) and Watchful Contemplation (murāqabah) of God*

Linguistically, *taqwá* in Arabic is the protecting shield between you and what you have fear of. In the Islamic tradition, it is the fear of God which is reflected through a Muslim's compliance with His orders and abstinence from His prohibitions. *Taqwá* (God-consciousness) is the approach that enables individuals to make the best decisions and maintain integrity in their actions: "O you who believe! If you have *taqwá* towards God, He will grant you *furqān* [(a criterion to judge between right and wrong), or (*makhraj*, i.e. a way for you to get out from every difficulty)]..." (Qur'an 8:29).

God-consciousness prevents the physician from committing any immoral actions and induces him to comply with legal rulings in his practice. Furthermore, if the physician is consciously aware of being seen by God while treating his patient, this will protect him from falling into negligence or taking advantage of the patient's weakness and submission to his doctor. God-consciousness and engaging in mindful contemplation of God consequently lead the physician to hold himself accountable before being judged by external authorities, not mentioning that it is far more effective given that self-monitoring encompasses all mistakes, even those that may not have been discovered. God says, "Nay! Man will be a witness against himself" (Qur'an 75:14) and, "...And God is Ever a Watcher over all things" (Qur'an 33:52).

It was narrated that the second caliph, 'Umar, may God be pleased with him, said, "Hold yourselves accountable [in this life] before you are held accountable [before God in the Hereafter]. Also, critically evaluate your work before it gets evaluated."[14]

[14] Narrated by Ibn Abi Shiba in *Al-muṣannif* in the book *Al-Zuhd*, vol. 7, 96.

Some researchers of professional ethics have attributed all morals and behaviors required in the different professions — including medicine — to this concept of God-consciousness. They argue that it establishes an attitude of self-monitoring that, in turn, leads to a voluntary commitment on the individual's part to ensure that his actions and performance are in alignment with Sharia. Thus, one will be characterized with personal reproach in case of negligence of obligations or in case of ignorance of legal rulings associated with medical principles, ethics, and practice.[15]

4.5. *Sincerity in Work*

Al-Razi agreed with the following quote from Galen:

> The physician must be sincere to God. He must lower his gaze when he approaches beautiful women and should avoid touching their bodies. In the process of treating them, he should examine only the diseased area of their body.[16] The physician must be dedicated to his work, respect the rights of others, and pursue excellence and innovation in all his efforts.[17] Dedication to work requires that the physician abstain from practicing any other profession that may conflict with his medical practice, such as pharmacy, through which the physician may prescribe medication to his patients in order to receive undue profit.

4.6. *Modesty towards God and Compassion for Patients*

God says, "And by the Mercy of God, you dealt with them gently. And had you been severe and harsh-hearted, they would have broken away from about you..." (Qur'an 3:159). It is related that Prophet Muhammad (PBUH) said, "God has revealed to me that you must be humble, so that no one oppresses another and boasts over another."[18]

---

[15] *Mas'ūlīyat al-murāji' fī al-sharī'ah*, p. 123.

[16] Al-Razi (1980), *op. cit.*, 28–29.

[17] Ali Al-Muhammadi and Ali Al-Qaradaghi (2006), *op. cit.*, p. 110. For more information, see the *International Islamic Fiqh Academy Journal*, 3(8): 407–410; and Ahmad Kan'an (2006). *Medical Jurisprudential Encyclopedia*. Beirut: Dar al-Nafa'is: 651–655.

[18] Narrated by Muslim in the book *Al-jannah wa-ṣifat na'īmihā wa-ahlihā*, no. 2865; Abu-Dawud in the book *Al-adab*, no. 4895; Ibn Majah in the book *Al-zuhd*, no. 4179, on the authority of 'Iyad bin Himar.

Modesty diverts the physician from arrogance and self-adulation. It enjoins him to thank God for the gift of knowledge through which he is able to benefit others and gain God's pleasure. This quality ensures the physician's acknowledgement that the cure is ultimately in the hands of God and that his work or intelligence is but a means intended to execute God's will.

Al-Razi also transmitted the following quote from Galen: "I saw some physicians who, once they visit with kings and gain their pleasure, become arrogant with the public, deny them cure, and interact with them in an aggressive manner. Thus, these persons are deprived from blessings."

Following this, Al-Razi added, "Know that modesty in this profession (medicine) is an ornate and beautiful quality that does not imply weakness or humiliation. Modesty is practiced through eloquence, compassion, and avoiding vulgarity and insolence towards others… I saw some physicians who, in instances when they managed to treat a patient from a dangerous ailment, became arrogant and boastful. These persons will never be successful."[19]

Modesty requires reliance on and trust in God (*tawakkul*) in addition to the belief that God is the source of the cure and any efforts exerted by the physician are only a means through which God provides the cure.

Abu Bakr Al-Razi said, "The physician must rely on God in all his actions and expect the cure from Him. He must never presume that his efforts and abilities are the source of the cure, otherwise, God shall prevent him from arriving at the cure."[20]

4.7. *Truthfulness (ṣidq) and Trustworthiness (amānah)*

Truthfulness (*ṣidq*) requires the correct explanation of a disease's complications so that the patient, or his relatives, can make the right decision regarding the acceptance or rejection of treatment. If the patient discovers that the physician is lying, the doctor will lose credibility and the patient will doubt the physician's knowledge, experience, and reports.

[19] Al-Razi (1980), *op. cit.*, 36, 38.
[20] *Ibid.*, 37.

The physician must always be truthful about himself and his clinic. Further, he must never award a medical license or attendance certificate except to those who deserve it.

However, the manner in which to inform the patient of the truth about a dangerous illness he is suffering from is a matter of debate. The lawful approach to informing the patient with the truth is in a manner that does not exacerbate his illness or cause him to lose hope. Therefore, the physician should abide by the following guidelines:

- Conveying the truth gradually, without implying a sense of finality.
- Communicating through the appropriate person and avoiding direct statements, particularly if the patient is young, as well as emphasizing the possibility of being cured, etc.

Trustworthiness (*amānah*) refers to the conviction that medicine is a sort of trusteeship and responsibility. Thus, the physician may not refrain from treating patients, especially if their condition requires urgent intervention. This also entails that the physician must be punctual and immediately show up whenever there is an emergency. In brief, trustworthiness requires the fulfillment of duty, the treatment of patients, and earnestly seeking their cure that is to take place by God's will.

Abu Bakr Al-Razi said, "The physician must provide equal treatment to the rich and poor; hence, we should follow the approach of Galen the Sage."[21]

4.8. *Respecting Medical Specializations*

The field of medicine includes diverse specializations. The physician should practice within the limits of his specialization only. However, he should have basic knowledge of the other branches of medicine so as to refer the patient to the appropriate specialization whenever needed. This is particularly important in the area of psychology as stated by Ibn Al-Qayyim.[22]

---

[21] *Ibid.*

[22] Ibn Al-Qayyim (1993). *Prophetic Medicine* (*Al-ṭibb al-nabawī*). Beirut: Dar Maktabat Al-Hayat: 117.

This moral value also entails that a physician exhibits respect towards his colleagues of different specializations and refers patients to them without any hesitation or arrogance. He may not insult or humiliate them or undermine their scientific credibility.

Further, respect for other disciplines includes refraining from the practice of any specialization that may conflict with the physician's medical practice, especially if this may pose a physical or religious risk. An example of this is a physician issuing legal rulings (*fatāwā*) to his patients. Instead, the physician should ask the relevant experts (professionals) within each medical branch or other fields, particularly in issues of jurisprudence and Sharia rulings.

4.9. *Confidentiality*

The physician should safeguard secrets that he comes to know because of the nature of his work. He is not entitled to disclose these secrets except in special cases regulated by Sharia and professional laws. The physician may not divulge a patient's secret, his personal history, or his private relationships which the physician may deduce based on conversations with the patient. The breaching of confidentiality is considered to be a negative quality, an abuse of trust, and an action that must be subjected to legal, professional, and religious accountability.

The physician's oath, in all its forms, strongly emphasizes the obligation of confidentiality.

It was narrated that the Prophet Muhammad (PBUH) said, "When a man tells someone something and then departs, it is a trust (*amānah*)."[23] Similarly, a well-known idiom asserts, "Gatherings are characterized by trustworthiness,"[24] [i.e. when people meet in an assembly, they expect mutual trustworthiness]. Given this significant weight placed on confidentiality within regular circumstances, accordingly, this weight is augmented under medical circumstances that often require full disclosure by the patient.

Abu Bakr Al-Razi states, "The physician should treat people with decency, respect them in their absence and safeguard their secrets. Often,

[23] Narrated by Ahmad in *Al-musnad*, no. 15062.
[24] *Ibid.*, 14693.

individuals do not share their illness with their core family such as parents and children, and yet they share this information with their physician out of necessity."[25]

In issues of confidentiality, Al-Razi reproaches patients who withhold secrets from their physician. He states, "It is a major error to withhold secrets from a doctor for fear of being blamed. The patient has thus committed two crimes as the doctor will be unable to find the appropriate cure without full disclosure."[26]

See further Appendix A for the resolution of the International Islamic Fiqh Academy (IIFA) on confidentiality.

4.10. *Experimentation Cannot Be Done without Patient Consent*

As mentioned earlier in this chapter, patient consent is a condition for the administration of treatment. Hence, the prescription of any new medication or drug must be approved by both the patient and relevant authorities. In addition, research regulations must be adhered to when conducting any experimentation such as gaining patient consent prior to extracting any sample that exceeds regular requirements.

Consent given by the patient will not be considered if it relates to an experiment that involves a definite risk, but it will be considered once it relates to experimenting with medicine whose benefit is likely. This rule does not apply for patients only but also for those who volunteer to undergo experiments for trying a new medicine. After getting the official license, they can give their consent to participate in experimenting a new medicine as long as it is expected that it will yield benefit. Necessary precautions should also be taken such that in case the experiment produces side effects, the costs of treating the volunteer should be afforded.

4.11. *Abiding by Professional Laws and Regulations*

As with all professions, the physician must abide by Sharia and operative laws in addition to any resolutions and regulatory frameworks stipulated by relevant authorities as long as they do not conflict with Sharia laws.

---

[25] Al-Razi (1980), *op cit.*, 27.
[26] *Ibid.*

This also entails cooperation with public health institutions and authorities when addressing epidemics and other societal health risks.

This falls under the religious obligation of adhering to higher authorities as long as this adherence does not contradict with any Sharia laws.

4.12. *Excellence (Iḥsān) in the Sense of Quality and Perfection*

There are numerous Sharia laws that emphasize the importance of striving for excellence in the performance of any work. In the Qur'an, God states, "Verily, God enjoins justice and excellence (*iḥsān*)" (Qur'an 16:90). Justice in this context refers to maintaining the rights of all parties. Excellence, on the other hand, refers to providing the highest quality of service, above and beyond basic obligations. As narrated in one *hadith*, "Verily God has enjoined exclellence (*iḥsān*) in every action…"[27] and another *hadith* further emphasizes that, "God loves from you that when you do something, you do it with excellence."[28]

The physician must fulfill his commitment to the patient or hospital in performing a full diagnosis of his patient's case. He must ensure accuracy through conducting a full review of his patient's file; otherwise, any ignorance or negligence of even the slightest details may lead to misdiagnosis. This, in turn, could result in the physician prescribing wrong medications and treatments that may cause harm to the patient. Hence, the physician must exert sufficient time and effort in diagnosing and treating his patients, as most medical mistakes occur due to inaccurate examinations and rash actions.

It is worth noting that a large volume of patients neither justifies a physician's heedlessness nor excuses imprecision. In cases of imprudent diagnosis and negligent treatment, the physician must be held legally liable for any errors and harmful consequences that may have occurred.

In general, the physician must avoid any potential risks associated with his practice and diligently take all necessary precautions in every situation.

See Appendix B on Ethics of Biological Scientific Research.

[27] Narrated by Muslim, no. 1955, on the authority of Shidad bin Aws.

[28] Narrated by Abu Ya'la in his *Musnad*, vol. 7, 349.

See Appendix C on The Medical Oath and the Codes of Medical Ethics.

5. Breach of Medical Liability (Medical Malpractice)

5.2. *Definition of Liability (mas'ūlīyah)*

"Liability" in this sense refers to a person's commitment. Imam Al-Shafi'i articulated a synonymous expression using the term *ma'khūdhīyah.*[29]

Liability is defined as the commitment made by a person regarding his ability to perform an assigned task or duty under specific conditions (standards of performance) and being accountable to any breach of this liability on his part. In a situation of violating professional standards, the physician is held responsible for any harm he causes the patient as a consequence of this violation. As narrated by the *hadith,*[30] "Anyone who practices medicine although he is not recognized as a practitioner will be held accountable."[31]

5.3. *Medical Malpractice*

Imam Abu Hanifa declared that legal restrictions (*ḥajr*) must be placed on the following three types of people:

- An irreverent *mufti*, who issues excessively lenient *fatwas* to the extent that he contradicts Sharia in order to increase worldly gains.
- An ignorant physician, who practices medicine without earning the required qualifications and training.
- A bankrupt leaser, who deals with people for the purposes of renting from him but has nothing to rent.[32]

It is no secret that an unqualified physician has the status of an ignorant physician, who is inconsiderate in the matter of providing correct

[29] Al-Shafi'i (1990). *The Message* (*Al-risālah*). Beirut: Dar Al-Kutub Al-'Ilmiyah: 20–21.
[30] The source of this *hadith* has been mentioned earlier.
[31] Mahmud Shaltut (n.d.). *Al-mas'ūlīyah al-madanīyah wal-jinā'īyah fī al-sharī'ah al-Islāmīyah.* Cairo: Azhar University; Husayn Shihatah (n.d.). *Al-ittijāhāt al-mu'āṣirah fī al-murāja'ah*: n.p.
[32] Al-Kasani (1950). *Al-badā'i'.* Beirut: Dar Al-Kutub Al-'Ilmiyah: vol. 5, 200.

information. The point here is not — as Hanafi scholars said — that *ḥajr* means halting and invalidating their actions. Rather, the point is preventing them from practicing and dealing with people, and such prevention is considered an act of enjoining good and forbidding evil since an ignorant physician corrupts health and wealth. Sharia has ordained the preservation of health and wealth, by consideration of its objectives, and prohibiting an ignorant physician from practicing is obligatory on the ruler and everyone with authority over such matters.

Islamic Sharia prohibits both perpetrating harm and assisting in the perpetration of harm, and it considers the one who does so as coperpetrator. This includes failing to speak out against harmful acts. God enjoins, "Help you one another in *al-birr* (virtue, righteousness) and *al-taqwá* (God-consciousness); but do not help one another in sin and transgression. And fear God. Verily, God is Severe in punishment" (Qur'an 5:2).

If a physician practices medicine while lacking the adequate training and experience or failing to abide by professional standards (i.e. practicing without a medical license), he will be liable and must be held accountable for any harm resulting from his error, incompetence, or negligence.

Thus, the physician's liability is both contractual and criminal. When dealing with an independent physician, contractual liability means that the patient is hiring the physician's medical services and the physician is committed to providing treatment to those who hire him. However, if the physician works in a hospital, he is contracted by the hospital to provide specific medical services. Thus, liability shall arise initially against the hospital, before final settlement with the physician (from the resolution of IIFA on Liability).

As for criminal liability, in principle the physician should not be liable because he is performing a collective duty (*farḍ kifāyah*) and the Sharia-based rule stipulates, "[Performing] a duty is not conditioned by a guarantee for safety." However, because *the way* in which this duty is to be performed is the physician's choice alone — bearing in mind his extensive power and authority to choose the method of performance based on his best judgment — it becomes necessary to examine the possibility of the physician's criminal liability when his work results in damage. This is because, in this case, the position of the physician is closer to the possessor of a right rather than someone who is performing a duty, and the possessor of a right can be held accountable in case he exceeds his right.

As mentioned earlier, there is unanimous agreement on the exoneration of the physician if he possesses knowledge and experience, acts in good faith and for the purpose of treatment, adheres to the principles of medical practice, and gains consent from the patient or legal guardian.[33]

6. The Sharia-Based Deterrents Concerning the Breach of Medical Liability

6.1. *The Ruler's Role in Implementing Penalties*

Islamic legislation classifies crimes under two categories. The first category is crimes with prescribed penalties, referred to as *ḥudūd*. The second category is crimes with non-prescribed penalties, namely "disciplinary crimes." These include all crimes for which a definitive punishment has not been specified within scriptural sources of legislation. This second category encompasses all transgressions against God's rights or human rights whose penalties have not been divinely ordained. The determination of the appropriate punishments for these crimes was left, by the Wise Legislator, to the discretion of the ruler so as to ensure consideration for the conditions of time and place. This reinforces the comprehensive nature of Sharia and its assured compatibility with the ongoing changes and developments of life.[34]

Professional malpractice that results in apparent or hidden damage, especially amongst professions based on trust and honesty, poses a threat to public interest, or as coined by jurists, "right of God," which in this context denotes the right of society. Jurists affirmed that the

[33] Abdul Sattar Abu Ghuddah (n.d.). *Physician's Jurisprudence and Etiquettes* (*Fiqh al-ṭabīb wa-adabuh*). Kuwait: University of Kuwait: 10.

[34] Ibn Taymiyah (1992). *Al-siyāsah al-shar'īyah*, Beirut: Dar Al-Fikr Al-Lubnani: 120–133; Ibn 'Abidin (1889). *Ḥāshīyat Ibn 'Abdīn*, Istanbul: Dar al-Tiba'ah al-'Amirah: vol. 3, 184; Abdul-Qadir Auda (2001). *Al-tashrī' al-jinā'ī fī al-Islām*. Cairo: Dar al-Shuruq: vol. 1, 63, 704.

harmful impact of malpractice must be eliminated in accordance with the Sharia-based rule stating, "There should be neither harming nor reciprocating harm," as quoted in the *hadith* narrated by Ibn Majah.[35]

The responsibility of ensuring accountability for malpractice falls upon the ruler. Further, imposed punishments should not be limited to the request put forth by the victims. This is because the harmful impact of malpractice extends to all people even if the direct victim was only one individual. A jurisprudential rule states that "Anyone who commits an offense for which there is no prescribed penalty (*ḥadd*), s/he may be liable to a discretionary punishment (*ta'zīr*)."[36] In regards to forms of punishment, Sharia law has defined physically deterring corporeal sanctions as well as sanctions restricting freedom (jail), which Ibn Al-Qayyim explains as, "This does not include restricting the person and preventing him from free action."[37] Sharia law also recognizes financial sanctions, such as the confiscation of money to the State's treasury, or sanctions that discredit the perpetrator in order to condemn this action and warn people against committing it. Sanctions may also be in the form of excommunication including revoking the physician's license to practice and all associated benefits. In some cases, sanctions may require psychological retribution through issuing advice, notices, warnings, or even ostracizing (boycotting, etc.) him.

More Readings

Al-Razi (1977). Ethics of the physician (*Akhlāqīyāt al-ṭabīb*), Dr. Abdul-Latif Al-Abd (ed.). Al-Turath.

Muhammad Lutfi Al-Sabbagh and Al-Maktab Al-Islami (1988). Ethics of the physician (*Akhlāq al-ṭabīb*).

Dr. Ali Al-Jaffal. Ethics and liability of the physician and the rulings related to some of those who have incurable diseases (*Akhlāq al-ṭabīb wa ḍamānuh wal-aḥkām al-muta'alliqah bi-ba'ḍ dhawī al-amrāḍ al-musta'ṣiyah*). *International Islamic Fiqh Academy Journal* 8(3): 363–406.

[35]Narrated by Ibn Majah in *Al-Aḥkām*, no. 2340.

[36]Mahmud Hamza (1880). *Al-fawā'id al-bahīyah fī al-qawā'id*, Damascus: Maṭba'at Ḥabib Khalid: 134.

[37]Ibn Al-Qayyim (1899). *Al-ṭuruq al-ḥukmīyah*. Cairo: Matba'at Al-Adab: 102.

Mubarak bin Sayf Al-Hashimi. Ethics of the Muslim physician (*Akhlāqīyāt al-ṭabīb al-muslim*). Available online via www.scribd.com (retrieved 18 October 2014).

Dr. Muhammad Sulayman Al-Ashqar. Revealing the secrets in Islamic Sharia (*Ifshā' al-sirr fī al-sharī'ah al-Islāmīyah*), in *Al-ru'yah al-Islāmīyah li ba'ḍ al-mumārasāt al-tibbīyah*, 86–106.

WHO. Electronic code of health ethics (*Dustūr akhlāqīyāt al-ṣiḥḥa*). Middle East Regional Office.

Dr. Ahmad Raja'i Al-Jindi. Medical profession secret between confidentiality and publicity (*Sirr al-mihnah al-ṭibbīyah bayn al-kitmān wal-'alānīyah*).

Dr. Amin As'ad Khayr Allah (1946). Arabic medicine (*Al-ṭibb al-'arabī*). Beirut: Catholic Press.

Dr. Zuhayr Ahmad Al-Suba'i and Dr. Muhammad Ali Al-Bar. The physician: Etiquettes and jurisprudence (*Al-tabīb, adabuh wa fiqhuh*). Dar Al-Qalam.

Dr. Yusuf Abdullah Al-Turki. Muslim physician: Distinguishing characters (*Al-tabīb al-Muslim: Tamayyuz wa simāt*). Dar Al-Watan Publication Press, no date.

Dr. Shawkat Al-Shatti. The Science of medical ethics (*'ilm ādāb al-ṭibb*). Damascus University Press, no date.

Dr. Abdul Sattar Abu Ghuddah (1981). Physician's jurisprudence and etiquettes (*Fiqh al-ṭabīb wa adabuh*). *Majallat al-Muslim al-mu'āṣir* 28: 145–165.

Dr. Ali Al-Qaradaghi, Dr. Ali Al-Muhammadi and Dar Al-Basha'ir (2008). Jurisprudence of contemporary medical issues (*Fiqh al-qaḍāyā al-ṭibbīyah al-mu'āṣirah*).

Rulings for controlling public market (*Ma'ālim al-qurbah fī aḥkām al-ḥisbah*). Ibn Al-Ukhuwwah (1938). London, Luzack.

Ahmad Muhammad Kan'an (2000). Juristic medical encyclopedia (*Al-mawsū'ah al-ṭibbīyah al-fiqhīyah*). Dar Al-Nafa'is.

WHO. *International Islamic Code of Medical and Healthcare Ethics*. Middle East Regional Office.

Al-Shayzari (1981). The ultimum in the rulings for controlling public market (*Nihāyat al-rutbah fī ṭalab al-ḥisbah*). Dar Al-Thaqafa li Al-Tiba'ah wal-Nashr wal-Tawzi'.

Kuwait Document on the Islamic Code for the Medical Profession, Kuwait Islamic Organization for Medical Sciences, 1981.

Appendix A

Below is the resolution no. (79) 10/8 issued by the IIFA addressing the question of confidentiality in the profession of medicine during their 8th conference held during the period 1–7 Muharram, 1414 AH (21–27 June 1993)[38]:

First: Confidential information is whatever someone tells another with a request, beforehand or afterwards, to keep it secret. This includes matters conventionally known to be of a confidential nature, *per se*, as well as a person's private matters or defects which he loathes to make public.
Second: Confidential information is a trust in the hands of the person who is asked to keep it secret, as enacted by the Islamic Sharia and the ethics of magnanimity and proper conduct.
Third: The general rule is that divulging confidential information is proscribed and divulging it without a genuine motive warranting it makes the person liable to punishment from the perspective of Sharia.
Fourth: Secrecy is even more of a duty for individuals working in professions that are adversely affected by indiscretion such as the medical professions. Those in need of advice and assistance usually resort to medical professionals and communicate to them all (intimate) affairs that may help them fulfill their vital tasks properly. This may include information one keeps from all others, including one's own kin.
Fifth: On exceptional basis, the duty of secrecy is not binding in cases where keeping the secret may entail damage for the concerned person greater than the one that ensues from divulging it or when divulging the secret may entail a benefit that exceeds in importance the risks of keeping it. Such cases are of two categories.

(a) Cases where the confidential information *must* be revealed on grounds of the rationale of committing the lesser evil in order to avoid the greater one, and the rationale of achieving the public interest which may entail enduring an unavoidable private harm so as to prevent a public one. These cases include two types:
  - What involves protecting society from harm.
  - What involves protecting an individual from harm.

(b) Cases where where the confidential information *can* be broken:
  - To achieve a public interest.
  - To prevent a public harm.

---

[38]Translator's note: this section is taken verbatim from http://islamicstudies.islammessage.com/Fatwa.aspx?fid=100 (retrieved 25 February 2016).

In all such cases, one should be committed to the objectives and priorities as set out by Sharia in terms of preserving religion, human life, the intellect, offspring, and wealth.

Sixth: Exceptional cases in which revealing the confidential information will be permissible or obligatory must be clearly mentioned in the codes of medical and professional practice. Such cases must be clearly defined and enumerated along with all the details as to the manner in which the secret would be divulged, and to whom. The relevant authorities need to familiarize each and every one with these cases.

Then the IIFA issued a recommendation of incorporating this topic in the programs and curricula of medical faculties.

Appendix B: Resolution of IIFA no. 161 (10/17) Concerning Sharia-Based Standards of Conducting Biomedical Research on Human Subjects

The IIFA, affiliated with the Organization of Islamic Conference (OIC) holding its 17th session held in Amman (Kingdom of Hashemite Jordan) from 28th Jumadah-al-Uwla to 2nd Jumadah-al-Akhirah, 1427 Hijri (24–28 June 2006).

Having reviewed research papers received by the IIFA regarding the Sharia-based standards of conducting biomedical research on human subjects as well as the document issued by the Islamic Organization for Medical Sciences in its seminar held in Kuwait from 29th Shawwal to 2nd Dhul-Qi'dah 1425 Hijri (11–14 December 2004) concerning "International Ethical Guidelines for Biomedical Research Involving Humane Subjects: An Islamic Perspective," and after hearing relevant discussions, the IIFA has resolved the following:

(a) First: Endorsing the General Principles of the Document

The Academy ensures approving the general principles and foundations upon which the ethical standards which regulate biomedical research are based, according to the following:

(i) Respecting individuals and honoring the human being have strongly-rooted, well-established foundations in Islamic Sharia as God says, "And indeed We have honored the Children of Adam, and We have carried them on land and sea, and have provided them with *al-ṭayyibāt* (lawful good things), and have preferred them above many of those whom We have created with a marked preference" (Qur'an 17:70).

Thus, the autonomy of a person with full competence who volunteers to participate in medical research must be respected. He must be enabled to choose and take proper decisions with full satisfaction and free will without any compulsion, deception, or exploitation in accordance with the Sharia-based rule, "No one can interfere with a right assigned to a human being without his/her permission."

Likewise, an incapacitated person or one whose capacity is incomplete must be protected from injustice that may come even from his sponsor or guardian. According to a general jurisprudential rule, "The one whose actions are not legally valid (from a Sharia perspective) [e.g. a person whose judgment is impaired because of mental illness] has no say." Sharia provides for such a person a sponsor or guardian to take care of his affairs in a way that nurtures his personal interests without acting in an any harmful or potentially harmful way.

(ii) Achieving interest (*maṣlaḥah*) has its origins in Islamic Sharia by bringing benefits to and preventing evils from the servants [of God]. In the case of unavoidable evil, it is better to eliminate the bigger evil by committing the lesser one.

(iii) Justice is the moral commitment to treat everybody in accordance with what is right and good from a moral perspective. It is to give each person his/her right, whether the person is male or female. Justice is an established principle in Islamic Sharia, whose rules have been laid out by Islam and which Islam has made the foundation and basis of success and goodness in life.

(iv) Excellence (*iḥsān*): It is mentioned in the most comprehensive verse in the Noble Qur'an to induce all benefits and prohibit all evils:

> Verily, God enjoins *al-'adl* (justice) and *al-iḥsān* (excellence), and giving (help) to kith and kin and forbids *al-faḥshā'* (i.e. all evil deeds),

and *al-munkar* (i.e. all that is prohibited by Islamic law: polytheism of every kind, disbelief and every kind of evil deeds, etc.), and *al-baghi* (i.e. all kinds of oppression), He admonishes you, that you may take heed (Qur'an 16:90).

(b) Second: Standards of Biomedical Research on Human Subjects

The Academy asserts endorsing the standards of biomedical research on human subjects that were included in the document referred to in the introduction of this resolution, recognizing that they organize biomedical research within the framework of Islamic Sharia principles and provisions. We call for the Islamic Organization for Medical Sciences to hold a large-scale meeting that includes physicians and jurists to deepen the knowledge of such standards.

Recommendations:

(i) The Academy recommends to the officials in Islamic countries that they take concern in supporting research and researchers by allocating sufficient budgets, providing researchers with suitable conditions, and meeting their scientific and material needs in order to enable them to dedicate themselves to fulfilling their national duties.

(ii) The Academy recommends to the Islamic countries that they benefit from Muslim scientists abroad "as they are a great asset to the Muslim community (*ummah*)." The Academy recommends that Islamic countries open channels of communication with these scientists and encourage them to collaborate with their peers in Islamic countries to establish solid bases for research in Islamic countries.

(iii) The Academy recommends to the Islamic Organization for Medical Sciences in Kuwait along with the Ministries of Health in Islamic countries to organize training sessions for those working in medicine and healthcare sectors regarding medical and healthcare jurisprudence (*fiqh*), professional ethics — especially scientific research ethics — and the standards that have been referred to in this resolution.

God, though, knows best.

Appendix C: The Medical Oath and the Codes of Medical Ethics

C.1. *The Medical Oath Drafted by Ibn Abi Usaybi'ah*

A physician named Muwaffaq Al-Din Ahmad bin Al-Qasim, known as Ibn Abi Usaybi'ah,[39] formulated the following oath:

"*I do hereby swear in God, Lord of life and death, Granter of health, Creator of recovery and every cure, I call upon God's friends, men and women, to witness that I will fulfill this oath and condition. I believe that he who taught me this profession is like a father to me. I should help and support him from my own money. His children are like my brothers and sisters. I shall teach them this profession if they need to learn it, without payment or condition. I shall engage my teacher's children and my students, to whom I do set this condition, and I do hereby swear by this medical code in recommendations, sciences, and all what is included in this profession.*

I shall not give lethal medicine if I was asked to do so and will not advise anybody to do likewise. I shall never carry out an abortion. I shall keep my action and profession based on charity (*zakat*) *and purification. I shall never perform surgery for someone who has stones in the bladder but shall leave this to those specialized in this practice.*

I enter all houses for nothing but to help patients. I refrain from all injustice and intentional corruption. Anything I see during examination of patients or hear beyond the times of medical examination that should not be publicly communicated I shall keep confidential and will never disclose."

C.2. *The Medical Oath for the Islamic Organization for Medical Sciences*

The First International Conference of Islamic Medicine established a code of ethics for the medical profession,[40] and it included the following

[39] Ibn Abi Usaybi'ah (1965). *The Best Accounts of the Biographies of Physicians* ('*Uyūn Al-anbā' fī ṭabaqāt Al-aṭibbā*'). Beirut: Maktabat al-Hayat: 17ff.

[40] Researches and works of the First International Conference of Islamic Medicine (1981). Kuwait: Ministry of Public Health: National Council of Culture, Arts, and Morals: 700; Also see Kan'an (2006), *op. cit.*, 784–785.

medical oath: "*In the name of God, the Most Gracious, the Most Merciful: I do hereby swear by God the Greatest to regard God in my profession; to protect human life in all stages and under all circumstances; to do my best to save it from death, illness, pain, and anexiety; to protect people's dignity, cover their private parts* ('awrah), *keep their secrets; to be always an instrument of God's mercy, extending my medical care to close and strange persons, to the righteous and the sinner, and to friends and enemies; to steadfastly seek knowledge and to use it for the benefit of humans and not to harm them; to honor my teachers and teach my juniors; to be brother to every colleague in the medical profession joined in goodness and God-consciousness; to make my life a reflection of my faith, both in private and in public and make it pure and free from any evil that blemishes towards God, His Prophet, and His Believers. God is witness to what I say.*"

C.3. *Codes and Agreements of the Medical Profession*

The first manifestation of the idea of medical ethics was developed in the form of "codes" or "documents" that included laws and regulations. Some of these were just proposals, whereas others assumed formally-approved and official status. Given the focus of this chapter, below are references to international documents that are Islamic in nature:

1. International Islamic Code of Medical and Health Ethics

This code was issued by the World Health Organization (WHO) — Middle East Regional Office. It includes 10 chapters and 108 articles.

2. E-Health Code of Ethics

This code was also issued by the WHO — Middle East Regional Office. It includes an introduction and definitions followed by detailed explanations.

3. Islamic Code of Medical Ethics — Kuwait

This code was issued at the First International Conference on Islamic Medicine held in Kuwait during the period 12–16 December 1981. It includes 12 chapters. This document focused on the principles of Sharia as evidenced in Qur'anic verses and *hadiths*.

Response by Hassan Chamsi-Pasha to Abu Ghuddah's Paper

Hassan Chamsi-Pasha

I read with great interest the paper of Sheikh Abdul Sattar Abu Ghuddah entitled "The Governing Principles of Islamic Ethics in Medicine." It is very well written and reflects the high scholarly standing of Sheikh Abu Ghuddah.

For several centuries, the Islamic world has witnessed the great achievements of Muslim physicians in the area of medicine and health sciences. These advances were not based on technical skill or intellectual prowess alone. They were equally founded on a clear understanding of the role of the Muslim physician as derived from Islamic teachings and philosophy.[1]

1. Practical Ethics of the Physician (*Adab al-ṭabīb*)

Sheikh Abu Ghuddah clearly demonstrated the role of Islamic scholars in laying down the principles of medical ethics and referred to the book of Abu Bakr Al-Razi entitled *Ethics of the Physician* (*Akhlāq al-ṭabīb*) as

[1] Abdul Rahman Amine and Ahmed Elkadi (1981). Islamic code of medical professional ethics. *Journal of the Islamic Medical Association of North America* 13(July): 108–110.

one of the earliest books in medical ethics, preceding all Western writings on the subject. In addition, one of the earliest comprehensive works on medical ethics is entitled *Practical Ethics of the Physician* (*Adab al-ṭabīb*) by Ishaq bin Ali Al-Ruhawi, who lived in the second half of the 9th century C.E. Al-Ruhawi's *Practical Ethics of the Physician* was translated to English by Martin Levy in 1967, and it contains 20 chapters:

(i) The beliefs that a physician should hold and the etiquettes he or she should abide by to improve his or her soul and moral character.
(ii) The measures that should be taken to maintain a healthy body and by which a physician should treat his own body and limbs.
(iii) That which a physician should avoid and beware of.
(iv) The recommendations a physician should give to the caregivers of the patient.
(v) The etiquettes of the patients' visitors.
(vi) What the physician should examine concerning single and compound medicines and their putrefaction.
(vii) Matters about which a physician should question the patient or the patient's caregivers.
(viii) On what healthy and sick people should all think of and believe about the physician during the times of health and sickness.
(ix) That both the ill and healthy should accept the counsel of the physician.
(x) The behavior of the patient towards his family and caregivers.
(xi) The behavior of the patient towards his visitors.
(xii) The dignity of the medical profession.
(xiii) That people should respect a physician according to his skill and that kings and other honorable people should respect him more.
(xiv) On anecdotes that happened to physicians, some of which have already been mentioned, so that the physician may be forewarned. Some of these [anecdotes] are entertaining which urge the physician to check the intelligence of his patient so that misconceptions will not be ascribed to the physician.
(xv) That not everyone may practice the profession of medicine but that it should only be practiced by those who have a suitable nature and moral character.

(xvi) Examination of physicians.

(xvii) Ways by which kings can combat corruption among physicians and can guide all people with regards to how they can get well through medicine and how this all was in ancient times.

(xviii) The necessity of warning against charlatans who call themselves physicians and the difference between their deceit and true medical practice.

(xix) Reprehensible habits to which people are accustomed but that may harm patients and cause physicians to be blamed.

(xx) Matters a physician should be careful about during periods of health in order to prepare for periods of illness, and also at the time of youth for the time of old age.[2]

As the chapter titles illustrate, *Practical Ethics of the Physician* is not merely a manual of professional ethics. It also contains important material about personal health and the relationship between the patient and the doctor. It even comments on the medical profession itself and how it relates to the governing authority. This monumental work demonstrates the complementarity of early medical principles and the moral framework of the Islamic tradition and culture. Al-Ruhawi's work attests to the ability of Islamic thinkers to assimilate different traditions and philosophies in the Islamic discourse.[3]

In the first chapter of *Practical Ethics of the Physician*, Al-Ruhawi writes about the beliefs a physician should hold and the etiquettes he or she should follow to better his or her soul and moral character. Al-Ruhawi describes three beliefs that a physician should hold:

(i) The first thing in which a physician must believe is that every created being should have a sole Creator who is Omnipotent, Wise and can perform all deeds wilfully.

[2] Martin Levey (1967). Medical ethics of medieval Islam with special reference to Al-Ruhawi's 'practical ethics of the physician.' *Transactions of the American Philosophical Society* 57(3): 1–99.

[3] Aasim I. Padela (2007). Islamic medical ethics: A primer. *Bioethics* 21(3): 169–178.

(ii) The second article of the physician's faith is to have true love for Allah the Sublime and to be devoted to Him with all his reason, soul, and free will.

(iii) The third article of faith which a physician must possess is that Allah sent His messengers to mankind in order to teach them what is good and beneficial since the intellect alone is not sufficient.[4]

Practical Ethics of the Physician is a beautiful illustration of the fact that problems of responsibility, ethical dilemmas, and needs of society are not new to the discipline of medicine. A review of this work makes us wonder if the physician of today is negligent of his responsibilities towards current ethical needs.[5]

2. Preserving Morality and Public Order (*ḥisbah*) and Medicine

In his paper, Sheikh Abu Ghuddah alluded to the topic of *ḥisbah*, and it is clear from the sources that addressed this topic that practicing medicine *in toto* has been subject to strict regulation since the 9th century up until the introduction of modern systems.

It is stated that when a physician visits a patient he should ask him about what is not apparent to the senses and what the reasons are for his health condition. He should then prescribe the appropriate medication and write it out for the patient's family or present relatives. The following morning, the physician should examine the patient, inspect his urine, and ask the patient about his health condition. Then he should prescribe for him whatever the condition requires and write a copy for the family.

The same routine should be repeated on the third and fourth days and so on until the patient recovers or dies. If the patient recovers, the physician should receive due payment. If the patient dies, the patient's close relatives should go to the chief physician and submit the copies of the

[4] Levey (1967), *op cit*., 1–99.

[5] Sharif Kaf Al-Ghazal (2004). Medical ethics in Islamic history at a glance. *Journal of the International Society for the History of Islamic Medicine* 3(5): 12–13.

prescriptions that the doctor had written for him. If the chief physician holds that the physician abided by medical standards and was wise in his decisions without practicing negligence or deficiency therein, then he should decide that death simply occurred at the termination of the deceased's allotted time. However, if the chief physician holds that the doctor was guilty, then he should ordain that blood money be paid by the doctor to the deceased's family because he killed the patient out of ignorance and negligence." Through these excellent procedures, it was made certain that no unqualified individual would intrude on the field of medicine and that medicine was only practiced by those who were well versed in its various specializations.[6]

The *ḥisbah* also carefully regulated the study of medicine. It determined the topics to be studied by the physician. It also determined the penalties to be paid by physicians and surgeons in case of negligence or carelessness resulting in malpractice. For example, those who performed circumcision were subject to liability if the operation caused the patient injury or death.[7]

3. Realistic and Evolving Jurisprudence in the Islamic Tradition

One of the intriguing aspects about Islam is that it has a realistic jurisprudence that is constantly evolving. This quality has paved the way in recent decades for the approval of laws pertaining to the field of medical ethics that address emerging issues in biomedical sciences and technologies.

Muslim scholars have determined a group of fixed Islamic principles to consider for ethical decision-making. These include: interest (*maṣlaḥah*), the principle of "there should be neither harming nor reciprocating harm" (*la ḍarar wa-lā ḍirār*), the principle of necessity (*ḍarūrah*), and the principle of "removal of hardship" (*raf' al-ḥaraj*).[8]

---

[6] Martin Levey (1963). Fourteenth century Muslim medicine and the *Hisba*. *Medical History* 7(2): 176–182.

[7] *Ibid.*

[8] Bager Larijani and Farzaneh Zahedi-Anaraki (2008). Islamic principles and decision making in bioethics. *Nature Genetics* 40(2): 123.

In the case of absolute necessity, where religiously lawful alternatives do not exist, it becomes possible to suspend the general ruling according to the jurists' assessment of the level of necessity. As an example, religious scholars permitted the use of porcine insulin and heart valves from pigs on the basis of the principle of necessity.[9]

Recent scientific and technological advances have resulted in a range of complex issues that have triggered ethical dilemmas for healthcare professionals regarding patients and society at large.

Responding to this challenge, many religious scholars have concluded that in situations requiring specialist knowledge (as is the case with the medical field), decisions and legal rulings should be made based on collective legal reasoning (*ijtihād jamā'ī*) and mutual consultation (*shūrá*).

For the *fatwas* pertaining to medicine, the bodies exercising collective legal reasoning should include a large group of scholars and experts from different disciplines relevant to the issue at hand in order to clarify the technical aspects related to their specializations.[10]

4. Confidentiality in the Context of Research

The Tradition of the Prophet (PBUH) incites us to learn and to conduct medical research. He stated that Allah has made for every disease a cure. Islam puts emphasis on seeking knowledge and making benefit therefrom. Islam also urges spreading knowledge and refraining from withholding it; as the Prophet (PBUH) said, "Whoever withholds knowledge, Allah on the Day of Judgment will bridle him with a bridle made of fire."[11]

Sheikh Abu Ghuddah emphasized the importance of maintaining confidentiality in the context of medical research as well as other fields. Protecting confidentiality is an essential value necessary in all human relationships, not only in medical practice and research. Doctor–patient and researcher–participant relationships are built on trust and recognizing

---

[9] Abdul Rashid Gatrad and Aziz Sheikh (2001). Medical ethics and Islam: Principles and practice. *Archives of Disease in Childhood*, 84(1): 72–75.

[10] *Ibid.*

[11] *Ṣaḥīḥ al-Tirmidhī*, No. 2649

the necessity of not disclosing the patients' secrets. However, there are exceptional cases in which secrets may be disclosed when it is necessary to meet a strong conflicting duty. Confidentiality has received much importance in Islamic Sharia and has received much interest by Muslim jurists, as can be seen in their works. There have been some legal rulings about this issue, and there have been constant efforts by both individuals and medical organizations to make use of the collective *fatwas* issued by institutions that practice collective *ijtihad* in the context of research.[12]

[12] Giath Alahmad and Kris Dierickx (2012). What do Islamic institutional *fatwas* say about medical and research confidentiality and breach of confidentiality? *Developing World Bioethics* 12(2): 104–112.

Script of Oral Discussions (Day 1, Session 1)

Day 1, Session 1

After **Ahmed Raissouni** presented his paper, the following discussion took place.

Mohammed Ghaly

Sheikh Raissouni mentioned two ethics, neither of which falls in the framework of the four principles. They are God-consciousness (*taqwá*) and mercy (*raḥmah*). Sheikh Raissouni, since you are known to be an expert on the identification of the higher objectives of Sharia, is it similarly possible to identify the fundamental ethics (*ummahāt al-akhlāq*)? How?

Ahmed Raissouni

Regarding the fundamental ethics, we should first look at the Sharia itself, wherein we find ethics that are very widespread. For example, when it comes to the issue of mercy, the Prophet (PBUH) said that when he would lead a prayer that he [originally] intended to prolong, and if he heard an infant crying, he would shorten the prayer out of consideration for the child. The concept of mercy was present with him in his prayer. The Prophet (PBUH) recommended to those leading prayers to be considerate in this regard and make the prayer short because within the congregation there may be those who are sick, children, weak, or needy.[1] The widespread presence of ethics in acts of worship, in one's dealings with others, and in everything else points to the centrality of this virtue in Islam.

One thing that points to the centrality of God-consciousness is that every prophet commissioned by God told his people to worship God and to have God-consciousness. The centrality here is clear. If we examine the matter from a practical point of view, God-consciousness is the only ethical value that is present with every person in every moment, in private and in public. The Prophet (PBUH) said, "Have God-consciousness wherever you are."[2] There are things a person does that nobody will ever find out about and nobody will be able to hold one accountable for. Nevertheless, a person has an internal accountability to himself that is present with him wherever he goes. Thus, when we come to the test of practicality of ethics, we can identify the ethical value of God-consciousness as a central and pivotal value. Similarly, we say that a doctor should be gentle and humble, but if both of these are included in the value of mercy, then [it suffices to say] mercy is the fundamental ethical value and the central moral. This is why we call for the doctor to exhibit the set of fundamental ethics.

The search for the set of fundamental ethics happens either by pursuing Sharia and looking at its texts that branch off into various legal domains, or by pursuing practicality. The broader we find an ethical value and the more prevalent we find it in a person's life regardless of the texts, the more evidence we have that this is a central ethical value. This is what was done by those who examined many ethical values and derived from them the four principles.

Mohammed Ghaly

To summarize what Sheikh Raissouni said, there are two ways or methods of identifying the set of fundamental ethics. The first is by examining

[1]Narrated by Bukhari in Al-Adhan (no. 703) and Muslim in Al-Salah (no. 467) on the authority of Abu Hurayrah.
[2]Narrated by Ahmad in *Al-Musnad* (no. 21354) on the authority of Abu Thar.

the texts and sources to determine how central a certain ethical value is therein and how much it has been mentioned. It is worth noting whether a particular ethical value was present in the legislations of prophets before the Prophet Muhammad (PBUH), as its presence would indicate that it is not exclusive to a specific era or a particular religious law but rather that it has existed throughout human history. The second way or method of identifying the set of fundamental ethics is to note the current reality, meaning a person's need of a particular ethical value at a particular time in a particular situation. The repeated need for an ethical value in this way leads to the conclusion that it should be counted among the fundamental ethics.

Tariq Ramadan

I have some questions. Firstly, when we talk about ethics and the set of fundamental ethics, are we talking about principles (*mabādi'*), fundamentals (*uṣūl*), or higher objectives (*maqāṣid*)? Even the word *principles* in English means both *mabādi'* and *uṣūl* in Arabic, so what is the correct understanding of ethics? Does it involve the higher objectives of Sharia or does it involve principles, and is there a difference between the two?

Secondly, in the first part of your paper you talk about ethics in general then you talk about ethics and medicine. Is there a difference between ethics in medicine and the ethics of the physician?

My last question is about God-consciousness. Is God-consciousness universal, such as when a doctor stays behind at the end of his shift for the sake of God or out of God-consciousness? There are many physicians who do not recognize God and are far from religion, so can we say that God-consciousness is indeed universal?

Ahmed Raissouni

Regarding terminology, the word *mabādi'* (principles) is a new term that does not exist in our Islamic heritage except to mean "the beginnings of" a science or discipline or "the introductions to" a science or discipline. Thus, I do not usually use the word *mabādi'* but rather use the words *uṣūl* (fundamentals), *akhlāq* (ethics), and *faḍā'il* (virtues), so these are the words about which I will answer.

Firstly, all ethics are higher objectives. Messengers were sent for the purpose of purification of the soul (*tazkiyah*). This means they were sent in order for ethics to be present, strong, and effective in the life of the people. In other words, the purpose was for ethics to be practiced and embodied by the people. Today people use the term "ethicizing" (*takhlīq*): the ethicizing of public life, of politics, of economics, etc. Ethics or ethicizing is a higher objective (*maqṣid*). It is a higher objective of religious codes of law to transform the human into an ethical being who exhibits judicious, ethical behavior. In this way, ethics are indeed higher objectives. This is affirmed by the words of the Prophet Muhammad (PBUH) in his famous narration, "I was only sent to perfect noble character (*makārim al-akhlāq*),"[3] where "to" here means "in order to," and thus perfecting noble character or perfecting ethics is clearly an objective.

Ethics are also virtues, albeit the Arabic word *akhlāq* (ethics) of course includes both virtuous ethics and reprehensible ethics. When we say this word we technically mean both kinds, but most of the time we mean to speak about the virtuous side, which is the more dominant side. One person's ethics can include bad morals such as being harsh towards others while another person's ethics can include good morals such as being merciful. Religious codes of law and scholars of ethics often introduce the positive side first because it automatically negates the negative side.

Ethical values are also starting points; they are virtues from which a person springboards, and they serve to guide a person's behavior and elevate his actions. Ethics are also fundamentals (*uṣūl*) because from ethics we can derive legislation and [decisions about] behavior. What counts as a "fundamental" (*aṣl*, singular of *uṣūl*) is that which gets built upon or from which something else branches off. The name of this center is the research Center for Islamic Legislation and Ethics. Ethics are the fundamentals for Islamic legislation. Yes, the fundamentals for Islamic legislation are indeed the Qur'an and Prophetic tradition, but ethics are fundamentals for it also. This is a point that scholars of

[3]Narrated by Al-Bazar in his *Musnad* (15/364) and by Al-Bayhaqi in *Al-Kubra* (10/191, no. 21301).

Islamic legal theory have not paid much attention to, but this center can renew consideration for ethics in the discipline of legislation. To be more accurate, ethics is a source for legislation if one cannot find a legal or legislative text.

With regards to God-consciousness (*taqwá*), its Islamic meaning is what we consider to be the most complete and comprehensive. However, regardless of the presence or lack of religion, God-consciousness is comparable to the human conscience. A person who has a conscience that is alive and well will hold himself accountable by it and will be guided by it. He does not need an external authority to watch him or punish him; rather, he monitors himself. This is a type of *taqwá*. However, there is a problem. When a person monitors his own self, after a while his whims and desires may get in the way and affect his actions, while he still thinks or claims his actions are compliant with the principles [he aspires to]. With religion, it is more objective than his desires or personal inclinations.

Furthermore, when a person's *taqwá* is based on faith and religion, God Almighty is never absent and never leaves the person. The person's awareness and fear of God in the presence of people is like his awareness and fear of God in their absence. So, he will act according to this awareness. Whoever does not have this awareness and instead acts according to his own self may go astray, especially in difficult situations. A person without *taqwá* based on faith and religion is susceptible to changing and switching states, so he may exhibit conscientiousness at a certain time but not at another. We all know this very well. When a doctor or politician deals with much wealth and is exposed to corruption, he may change and end up participating in it.

A person with a conscience based on faith — while we do not say he is free from the possibility of changing — is perhaps more immune and protected because of the internal monitor that he maintains. To conclude, conscience is at its best when a person maintains a personal, internal monitor that he does not separate from, and this is actualized if the conscience was based on faith and religion. If this is actualized without faith, the success differs according to the differences of people. We believe that conscience is most complete and lasting when it springs from faith and creed.

Jasser Auda

I have a question about considering higher objectives (*maqāṣid*) and ethics to be fundamentals (*uṣūl*). If we do consider them as fundamentals, then practical rulings should be based on them since this is the definition of fundamentals. Yet how can practical actions be based on fundamentals of higher objectives and ethics? You touched on this point when you said that if there is no basis in the text, then rulings should be based on the higher objectives and ethics. However, is the text in and of itself connected with these ethics? In other words, can we consider the higher objectives and the ethics — meaning the fundamentals — principles in the modern philosophical meaning of being that which, alone, practical rulings are built upon? And what are the conditions if so?

Ahmed Raissouni

When we examine and study the [religious] texts, we are led to conclude that they are all based on ethics. Exhibiting honesty and trustworthiness, maintaining gentleness, and taking into account the interests of people are all examples of higher objectives and ethics. For example, we learn from the Prophetic example that it is not acceptable for a person to surprise another with alarming news, even if it is true. So when someone has bad news to break to another, he should circumvent its harshness and try to put it as gently as possible. If we take the example of the penal law (*'uqūbāt*), which is seemingly far from our discussion, it is also built on ethics. The punishments for, for example, committing fornication, murder, or theft serve as deterrents to committing atrocious unethical acts. Similarly, for contracts and sales, we are required to be faithful and to honor the deals or contracts into which we enter: "O you who have believed, fulfill [all] contracts…" (Qur'an 5:1). Honoring contracts is a general fundamental (*aṣl 'ām*) and is first and foremost a part of ethics.

Similar to other scholars, the prominent scholar and author of *Aḍwā' al-bayān*, Muhammad Al-Amin Al-Shinqiti, in his commentary on the verse, "And indeed, you [O Muhammad (PBUH)] are of a great moral character" (Qur'an 68:4), inquired, what was the Prophet Muhammad (PBUH) upon such that he would be described as being of great moral character? He was upon Islam. Therefore, Islam in its entirety is ethics and the Prophetic Tradition in its entirety is ethics. So interpreters of the Qur'an explained the verse, "And indeed, you are of a great moral character" as meaning he was upon Islam. Furthermore, the Prophet's wife, 'A'ishah — may God be pleased with her — said that the Prophet Muhammad's (PBUH) ethics were the Qur'an. Therefore, the whole Qur'an is ethics; Islam in its entirety is ethics; ethics is what the Prophet Muhammad (PBUH) was upon; and it is to this end that he was sent. Therefore, when we follow the texts, we realize that they are based on ethics at both particular and general levels.

If we adopt the above understanding and acknowledge that the scholars — such as Al-Shatibi, Ibn Al-Arabi, and Al-Ghazali — deduced the "mother" of fundamentals (*ummahāt al-uṣūl*), then these fundamentals become governing upon human behavior, whether under the direction of a text or under the direction of ethics. Furthermore, it is important to note that a person's method of applying a text can vary. He can apply the text in a dry, legal way or in an ethical way that emphasizes mercy and compassion towards others. The latter method should be followed. We have an example in the famous Prophetic narration, "...Verily God has enjoined goodness to everything; so when you kill, kill in a good way and when you slaughter, slaughter in a good way. So every one of you should sharpen his knife, and let the slaughtered animal die comfortably."[4] So a person can kill in a way compliant with Sharia, or he can kill in an inhumane and atrocious way. Applying the texts with ethical considerations is one option, and applying the texts without ethical considerations is another one. When there is a lack of textual evidence, the matter is decided based upon (i) the ethics since the ethics are themselves higher objectives and (ii) the rest of the higher objectives of Sharia.

Ethical values in Islam are not confined to chapters and books dedicated specifically to them; rather, ethical values pervade all chapters, rulings, and Sharia-based obligations, including creed, ritual acts of worship, habits, contracts, dealings with others, criminal law, and politics. All of these domains have the stamp of ethics, are built on ethics, and are ruled by ethics.

---

[4]Narrated by *Muslim* (no. 1955) on the authority of Shadid bin Aws. Editor's note: The speaker quoted a shorter part of the narration (until "slaughter in a good way"); of the remaining part of the narration has been included here for elaborating the full context.

Jasser Auda

If there is a text that points to a particular ethical value, does this ethical value control how we interpret the text? Let us take as an example a text that points to the ethical value of mercy. Is it the case that mercy is the essential point of the text and that the particular manifestation of mercy present in the text is just a means that can change?

Ahmed Raissouni

I think this necessitates a more detailed discussion in the science of Muslim legal theory (*uṣūl*); it has to do with the relationship between connotations (*dalālāt*) and effective causes (*'ilal*). In this regard we can refer to what Al-Shatibi says and most Muslim legal theorists also agree with: we should respect what the text says outwardly and the text's particular wording. However, in parallel, we should pay attention to the meanings and the higher objectives of the text. As Al-Shatibi said, this is a difficult task but is the more rightly guided way. That is, how does one maintain a balance between respecting the text and its wording and taking into consideration the text's meaning alongside the more general meanings present in other texts and in our human natural disposition (*fiṭrah*)? To this last point, Ibn 'Ashur held the opinion that our human natural disposition itself can be taken as a reference. As a matter of principle we have to take this balance into consideration.

The natural question here is: What happens if when the wording of the text is applied, it seemingly contradicts the [relevant] higher objective in some cases? Here, we can limit the text's applicability to a particular situation or to special circumstances such that the application of the text would in fact lead to the avoidance of evil or hardship on people. This is what 'Umar bin Al-Khattab did in the Year of Ramadah, and Sheikh Bin Bayyah alluded to this by saying that there are some rulings we can place on a temporarily extended leave (in other words, we can choose to not apply them) because the conditions, challenges, and obstacles of the current situation necessitate that we operationalize another text for this situation.

We all know the famous *fatwa* of Ibn 'Abbas. While amongst his students, Ibn 'Abbas was asked by a man, "Can someone who intentionally kills a Muslim repent?"[5] Ibn 'Abbas looked at the questioner with scrutiny and replied with a no, stating that a person who commits this act would be condemned to Hell. After the questioner left, the students of Ibn 'Abbas then questioned their teacher, saying, "Didn't you used to give the *fatwa* that the repentance of someone who kills a Muslim intentionally can be accepted?" Ibn 'Abbas said, "I saw in this man's eyes evil, as if he desired to kill somebody. It seemed he was waiting for a *fatwa* from me so that he could go kill someone and then repent." Ibn 'Abbas found that his original *fatwa* would now, in this situation, lead to an act of killing. This is why Ibn 'Abbas told the questioner that such a person would be condemned to Hell.

Of course, the words of Ibn 'Abbas here are valid because the Qur'anic verse states, "But whoever kills a believer intentionally — his recompense is Hell, wherein he will abide eternally, and God has become angry with him and has cursed him and has prepared for him a great punishment" (Qur'an 4:93). But of course, due to the mercy of God and the intercession provided by belief in Him, there is the possibility of God accepting repentance for this act [as indicated by other Qur'anic texts]. In this specific case, with this particular questioner, it is as if Ibn 'Abbas suspended his original *fatwa* — or put a hold on the apparent meaning of the text — and issued a different ruling based on the conditions. This all goes back to the scholars, legal jurists, and trustees of Sharia.

Mohammed Ghaly

I had a comment about the issue of *taqwá*. First, I have noticed that *taqwá* is normally translated as "piety" or "fear of God." However, through the in-depth academic studies that have been carried out, we know the Arabic word encompasses more than piety and fear of God. In my opinion, the best translation that has been put forth so far is "God-consciousness." So if we consider *taqwá* to mean God-consciousness but we remove the word "God" and replace it with the word "self," that could make it universal since we would end up with the word "self-consciousness" or simply "conscience." This is a term that is perhaps more familiar in Western circles of bioethics and medical ethics.

[5] Narrated by Ibn Abi Shaybah in *Al-muṣannaf*, Book of *Al-diyyāt* (5/435).

Furthermore, in the West, the dependence on or incorporation of one's religion — whether it is the doctor's or the patient's — is considered potentially problematic from an ethical point of view. The doctor is expected to be neutral, meaning the issue of religion should not have an effect on his work. Of course, on the other hand, this does not imply the lack of accountability. Dr. Bredenoord, do you have anything to say about this?

Annelien Bredenoord

What strikes me is the similarity between what we call the concept of autonomy and the concept of *taqwá*. I would like to ask some questions about that. First, I would like to ask Sheikh Raissouni about what he called principles. I would like to know whether there is a hierarchy for these principles. Is there one principle more important than the other principles? In our principles approach, one major discussion is about whether there is a hierarchy. Is one principle more important than the others?

My second question is about *taqwá*. What is striking about the principle of autonomy, which is defined as self-rule, is that it is also defined as consciousness. It is about having discipline to achieve one's aims. It is about judging for yourself instead of being judged by authorities. It is about following your own moral rule. If you interpret it in this way, it has many similarities with the concept of *taqwá*. So if we define autonomy as some kind of consciousness, I would be interested to hear what other similarities it has with *taqwá*.

Ali Al-Qaradaghi

I would like to make a few comments about what Sheikh Raissouni has said. If we follow the methodology of the Muslim legal theorists (*uṣūlīyūn*) in the issue of *al-sabr wa-al-taqsīm* (examining all possible rationales and then selecting the appropriate one), especially in the scope of Islam and other religions, then we would find all these things refer back to God-consciousness. However, in my opinion, God-consciousness has a religious connotation because it is related to the idea of fear of God since it is the fear of God that makes you feel that you are being observed by

Him and thus should be conscious of Him, as Dr. Chamsi-Pasha has pointed out previously. If we link God-consciousness with this meaning then we will find, as Dr. Bredenoord has suggested, that some ramifications of God-consciousness are indeed present in human conscience and in autonomy. However, God-consciousness encompasses much more. Therefore, if we chose to restrict the scope of biomedical ethics to God-consciousness, I think this would be valid from the [theoretical] perspective of fundamentals (*uṣūl*). However, from a practical perspective, we would need to specify fundamentals and principles besides God-consciousness. We do not want to expand the number of ethical values to reach the hundreds, and we also do not want to limit them to just one ethical value that would need further detailing and elaboration.

The second point is about considering ethics as fundamentals on which legislation may be made. Someone touched upon the situation where there is no text [on which to base the legislation of a certain issue]. In my opinion, the ethical values and the higher objectives should be used as part of the measuring criteria one employs when issuing a *fatwa* and engaging in independent legal reasoning (*ijtihād*).

Muhammad Ali Al-Bar

There are a few issues to consider as we further our understanding of the concept of ethics in general. The first is about human natural disposition (*fiṭrah*), which is mentioned in both the Qur'an and the Prophetic Tradition. It is a basic and fundamental aspect of a person. Everybody knows that lying is wrong and telling the truth is virtuous. Everybody knows that killing an innocent person is a crime and that saving an innocent soul is morally commendable. God has made these ethics innately intuitive to us. Whether or not a person is conditioned in such a way that encourages or discourages him from these ethics is a different issue.

The second issue is reason or the intellect. God in the Qur'an addresses the reader's intellect and encourages him to use reason. He says, "...Then will you not reason?" (Qur'an 2:44) and, "...'Then will you not give thought?'" (Qur'an 6:50). The intellect is a scale by which a person knows truth as truth and falsehood as falsehood. For example, how do I know that a particular religion is true or false? The basis for answering such a question is the ability of sound thought and reasoning that God has bestowed upon us as human beings. Again, this is irrespective of whether that reasoning is tampered with at some point in a person's life.

The third issue is religion. As narrated in the Prophetic tradition, God sent 124,000 prophets and many messengers. They all came with one message, not differing except in the details [of legislation]. It has been one message from the time of Adam to that of the Prophet Muhammad (peace and blessings be upon them).

Islam and all religions have incorporated these three elements — human natural disposition (*fiṭrah*), reason or intellect, and the divine message — into their teachings. Indeed, these three elements are practiced by all of humankind, in both primitive and advanced civilizations, both ancient and modern ones. Over time, these positive ethical elements may be suppressed by the negative effects of the environment and other things. If you remove the negative effects, then human natural disposition (*fiṭrah*), reason or intellect, and the one true message become apparent. The three elements are present among all groups of people across humanity.

There is no doubt that the details may differ. Honesty, as Dr. Chamsi-Pasha previously pointed out, is a foundational principle at all times, and lying is considered a crime ethically speaking. So I must inform a patient of his illness, and if I do not inform him then I am a liar. People across civilizations do not differ on this; instead, they may differ in the method used or in the details.

A final point I would like to address is the relationship between ethics and interests (*maṣāliḥ*). In Islam, some interests have to be restricted. Utilitarianism on the other hand may consider selling cigarettes or alcohol an interest worth pursuing if it benefits a group of people. There is disagreement between our philosophies in this matter as well as in the matter of autonomy, which will be discussed later.

Abdul Sattar Abu Ghuddah

Sheikh Raissouni started by saying that all of religion goes back to ethics. In my opinion, religion is *'aqīdah* (creed), Sharia, and ethics. So when we restrict religion to ethics alone, we run the risk of neglecting revelation and the texts; of course, Sheikh Raissouni did not mean this. He mentioned a verse in which we are informed that God sent Prophet Muhammad (PBUH) to purify the people (*yuzakkīhim*) [of inclinations towards wrong-doing], and if we continue the verse, we find that it also says, "…and purifying them (*yuzakkīhim*) and teaching them the Book and wisdom…" (Qur'an 3:164). So we need both *tazkiyah* (purification), which represents ethics, and abiding by legislation in the Qur'an and the Prophetic tradition. Some have interpreted the word "wisdom" in the verse to refer to the Prophetic tradition.

I would like to refer here to Imam Al-Shatibi and his student Muhammad Al-Sheikh. They said the objective of legislation and religion is for a (morally responsible) person to exit the state of submission to his desires so that he may enter into a state of submission to God voluntarily, like he is in a state of submission to God necessarily.[6] Therefore, it is necessary to abide by the obligations ordained by God, some of which have purposes that are clear to us while others do not. The important thing is obeying His commands.

As for *taqwá* (God-consciousness), scholars of Sharia have defined it as doing the actions that God has commanded and avoiding the actions that God has forbidden. From where do we derive these commandments and forbidden acts? We derive them from religion. That is why we need to focus on the fact that Sharia is a reference for ethics and not vice versa. Likewise, creed (*'aqīdah*) is a reference for ethics. For example, the idea of succession (*istikhlāf*) on earth is a matter of creed, and it prompts a person to realize this succession through abiding by the rulings of Sharia. For a believer, God-consciousness comes about in this way.

For a non-believer, how does God-consciousness come about? As you know, there are traders who perform their work properly, do not cheat others, and are committed to the morals of their trade while their goal is materialistic: they want to gain customers and do not want customers to lose trust in their business. This is also considered *taqwá*: such a person fears something that is, in his opinion, high. This applies in medicine as well. The physician who wants to preserve his reputation in order to have more also exhibits a kind of *taqwá*. This type of *taqwá* is in isolation from the religious element that involves the concept of being observed by God

---

[6] Al-Shatibi, *Al-Muwāfaqāt* (2/282).

and being held accountable to Him. If such a doctor had the opportunity, without anyone noticing, to do something wrong that benefited him, he may take that opportunity because he has no concept of being observed by or held accountable to God.

Regarding fundamentals (*uṣūl*), we cannot say that the fundamentals are based on ethics. Rather, ethics are based on the fundamentals. The fundamentals permit us to follow the "absolute benefit" (*al-maṣlaḥah al-mursalah*), which is defined as something that the religious texts are silent about but that is in itself beneficial. If something is established as an "absolute benefit," then it is considered to be among the general [ethical] principles. Ethics in general can be derived from interests (*maṣāliḥ*) that have benefits for people. I hope we do not focus on one side at the expense of the other.

Ahmed Raissouni

Regarding Dr. Bredenoord's question about whether principles and ethics exist in a hierarchy, I would say in principle, the answer is yes. Islam in its entirety, as it has been detailed by scholars, is built upon the concept of hierarchy. This concept exists in the verse, "Have you not considered how God presents an example, [making] a good word like a good tree, whose root is firmly fixed and its branches [high] in the sky? It produces its fruit all the time, by permission of its Lord…" (Qur'an 14:24–25). In Islam, everything is built starting from a word and grows from there to become bigger and bigger.

Turning now to the higher objectives of Sharia, it is well known how they were organized and how the five necessities (*ḍarūrīyāt*) were categorized and how the rest followed. The same thing applies to ethics. There is a prioritization such that some ethics are ordered above others and some ethics branch off of others, etc. In principle, this usually is taken by default. However, personally, I have never attempted to set this kind of hierarchy apart from what pertains to the topic of God-consciousness. I quoted in my chapter and am convinced by the words of Muhammad Abdullah Draz. God-consciousness is the most comprehensive ethical value, and it is the ultimate source and fountainhead of ethics.

We heard many perspectives and comments on the religious and non-religious interpretations of God-consciousness. Sheikh Abu Ghuddah suggested it is striving to obey God's commands and avoid God's prohibitions. Perhaps this is not God-consciousness but rather the fruit of God-consciousness. As for God-consciousness (*taqwá*) itself, one companion of the Prophet (PBUH), 'Umar bin Al-Khattab, asked another, Obayy bin Ka'b, "What is *taqwá*?" He replied, "Have you walked along a thorny path before?" He said, "Yes." He asked him, "How did you do so?" He replied that he would walk carefully, vigilant of where he stepped and turning this way and that [so the thorns did not hurt him]. He answered, "This is *taqwá*." In other words, God-consciousness means that a person must always be vigilant of where he is going to set his foot and hold himself accountable before being held accountable by God. These are the traits of a person who practices God-consciousness. However, as I said before, God-consciousness is achieved sustainably and completely only through revealed religion.

Regarding a physician's practice of religion or lack thereof and regarding the religiosity of ethics, I think the fundamental fountainhead of ethics is religion, whether that of Muslims, Jews, Christians, Buddhists, or others. Even those who reject religion use religious ethics but strip them of their religious source or background. As the saying goes, they took the fruit and ignored the tree. Yet they must know that the fruit is bound to be eaten or to rot and the tree is more lasting and thus is what we have to go back to. It is true there are those who have adopted ethics without adopting religion and those ethics are valid; my point is that the source of those ethics is religion. I believe that without religion these ethics will come to an end or will be faced by many obstacles such as obstacles of trade or other interests. Each doctor of course does as he wishes, but from a purely scholarly or academic perspective, ethics without religion will eventually be distorted and come to an end.

Formulating Ethical Principles in Light of the Higher Objectives of Sharia and Their Criteria

Ali Al-Qaradaghi

Abstract: This chapter is divided into three main sections. The first section is an attempt to explain how the higher objectives of Sharia can be utilized to draft an Islamic version of biomedical ethics. Besides the well-known six higher objectives (*viz.*, protecting religion, life, intellect, wealth, offspring, and honor), the author adds two others, namely preserving the integrity of the legitimate state and the integrity of society. The second section is dedicated to a number of legal maxims and rules by which the objectives-based approach for the principles of biomedical ethics can be specified and applied with a considerable degree of precision. In this context, reference is made to legal maxims like, "There should be neither harming nor reciprocating harm," and "Certainty cannot be overruled by doubt." The author also makes reference to the so-called "jurisprudence of balances (*fiqh al-muwāzanāt*)" by which the possible clash between benefits and harms in specific cases can be avoided or resolved. The third section provides a list of virtues and etiquettes to which physicians should adhere, most of which can be summed up into two, namely professionalism (*ikhtiṣāṣ*) and sincere devotion (*ikhlāṣ*). The percept of confidentiality and the duty to keep all information between physician and patient private are also underscored.

In the name of God, the Most Gracious, the Most Merciful.
Praise be to God, The Lord of the worlds, and peace and blessings be upon our beloved example Prophet Muhammad, who was sent as a mercy to the worlds, upon his brothers the prophets and messengers, his virtuous household, his blessed companions, and those who follow them in excellence until the Last Day.

1. A Well-constructed Formulation of Effective Ethics in Light of Tremendous Medical Advancements

The world we live in today constantly witnesses immense developments and discoveries in areas of science, technology, communication, and travel. The field of medicine is no exception: it has undergone tremendous revolutions in specialties such as biology, optics, and genetic engineering. The ground-breaking discovery of the genetic code in May 2001 has led to incredible progress in biomedical knowledge and has been accompanied by impressive research and discoveries in the fields of genetics, embryo cloning, *in vitro* fertilization, artificial insemination, human genome projects, gene therapy, organ transplants, stem cells, and numerous others.

In light of this considerable progress and these remarkable discoveries, it becomes incumbent upon us to pay due attention to the nurturing and ingraining of ethics in the hearts of those practicing within these fields. No effort should be spared to ensure a full commitment to ethical principles, as the separation between ethics and scientific advancement often leads to consequences that endanger humanity and potentially result in unknown harm in the long term.

The separation of ethics and law has existed since the development of Roman legislation. This was followed, throughout the last four centuries, by the European revolutions against despotism and the Church. As a result, religion was separated from the state, and even from life itself, leading to a spiritual vacuum accompanied by dangerous consequences. In time, several wise and rational individuals highlighted the enormity of this issue, especially in light of the rapid progress achieved in science and technology. Consequently, several positive efforts took place, and the field of ethics received the undivided attention of philosophers, scholars, and researchers. Ethical issues, both general and medical, dominated scientific journals in order to emphasize the criticality of identifying the advantages and disadvantages of biotechnology and to ensure the application of ethical principles so as to minimize harm or completely avoid it wherever possible.[1] Moreover, specialized academic centers with international committees and associations were established with the purpose of regulating ethical issues and establishing authoritative sources of reference for scholars and researchers. The most prominent amongst these committees are the International Bioethics Committee (IBC), the International Union of Biological Sciences (IUBS), and the Eubios Ethics Institute.[2]

Arising from their recognition of the importance of ethics, European and American scholars have exerted noteworthy efforts in addressing this issue through several ethical theories, including:

(i) Utility theory, which is based on promoting benefit. It aims to achieve maximum advantage with the least disadvantage possible. However, the weakness of this theory lies in the fact that it accepts ethical violations as long as there is a benefit to be gained. This theory emerges from the well-known philosophy of utilitarianism, which has been adopted by many people.

(ii) Immanuel Kant's categorical imperative and deontology theories. According to Kant, the justification for moral action should be based on duty and commitment, not merely arising from emotions and conscience. The problematic issue in this theory is how to ensure compliance with ethics.

(iii) The rights-based theory. This theory is based on an individual's right to life, property, and freedom. Contention in this theory arises when individual rights occasionally contradict with the rights of the larger group.

(iv) Communitarianism, which is based on promoting general welfare and community-based objectives and preserving community norms. The problem with this theory lies in the fact that it often neglects individuals' rights.

---

[1] Talal Al-Zoabi (2008). "Al-mabādi' al-akhlaqīyah allatī yastanid ilayhā ṭalabat kulliyat al-ṭibb fi al-Jāmi'ah al-Urdunīyah fi iṣdār ḥukmihim 'alā al-qaḍāya al-akhlāqīyah wa mā madā ta'thīrihā bi-kul min al-jins wal-mustawā al-dirāsī wa mustawā fahmihim li ṭabī'at al'ilm". *Al-Najah University Journal for Researches* (*Human Sciences*) 22(4): 1191–1215.

[2] *Ibid.*

(v) The theory revolving around familial relationships and the physician–patient relationship. However, this theory does not address ethical problems in general.

(vi) The theory of casuistry, where decisions are made based on the specific conditions surrounding each case. This can be problematic when there are several contradictory decisions and when personal bias is involved.[3]

(vii) The Four Principles of Biomedical Ethics developed by Beauchamp and Childress, which is the focus of this chapter. In my opinion, this last theory is the most comprehensive. However, it is not free of remarks made by myself and others.

2. Ethics in Islam: An Overarching Purpose, Not a Means

As one explores the Sharia texts, ranging from those related to creed and the revelation of divine books, sending prophets, worship, and rituals to those concerned with interpersonal relationships, economics, legal punishments, family affairs, politics, and *jihād*, it becomes evident that the primary focus is on attaining virtue, reinforcing noble values, and maintaining excellent behavior so as to enable society to lead a happy life. Ethics do not form a separate branch of Islam but rather are a fundamental objective that pervades all elements of life. Ethics are essential to a person's survival just as a soul is to human life, blood is to a human body, or water is to the life of plants. In this sense, the Noble Qur'an summarizes the objectives of sending the Prophet Muhammad (PBUH) by referring to the concept of mercy — namely a mercy for all humans, animals, and inanimate creatures — and he is considered the epitome of ethics and values. God says, "And We have not sent you, [O Muhammad], except as a mercy to the worlds" (Qur'an 21:107). The Prophet (PBUH) similarly summarizes the objectives of his message as the perfection and application of noble behavior, stating, "I was only sent to perfect noble character (*makārim al-akhlāq*)."[4] Furthermore, God the Almighty, in describing the

[3] Omar Hasan Kasule (n.d.). *Al-akhlāqīyāt al-ṭibbīyah min al-maqāṣid al-shar'īyah*. Available online via http://forum.makkawi.com/showthread.php?t=29311 (retrieved 11 November 2013).

[4] Narrated by Al-Bazzar in his *Musnad*.

Prophet (PBUH), chose to highlight the best of his attributes, proclaiming, "And indeed, you are of a great moral character" (Qur'an 68:4).

One of the most important objectives of believing in God and the Last Day is for the believer to attain a level of God-consciousness enabling him to abstain from immoral behavior. The Qur'an includes a multitude of examples in this regard that would be difficult to sufficiently elaborate on in this chapter.

3. The Foundations of Ethics and their Status in Islam

In Islam, the concept of ethics encompasses the whole set of values and ideals that had been previously established by all divine religions as well as those values towards which the natural disposition (*fiṭrah*) of human beings has been inclined throughout history. As such, Islamic ethics are rather expansive, numerous, and diverse, as made evident by their dominance across most Qur'anic verses and Prophetic narrations (*hadith*). Throughout these verses and Prophetic narrations, a strong emphasis is placed on the human individual as the initiator and agent of these ethics. Islam then guides us to focus on nurturing the foundations that are the core of a person's ethical conduct, namely the heart, soul, mind, and spirit. Prophet Muhammad (PBUH) advises us, "Beware! There is a piece of flesh in the body that if it becomes good (reformed), the whole body becomes good but if it gets spoilt the whole body gets spoilt, and that is the heart."[5] Likewise, God the Almighty stresses the importance of these internal elements for genuine change and reform and in achieving happiness and progress (and vice versa), stating that, "Indeed, God will not change the condition of a people until they change what is in themselves..." (Qur'an 13:11). Countless experiences, events, and realities have reinforced the fact that internal transformation (of the soul and the heart) can best be attained by connecting them to God the Almighty and the Last Day. This is because there is no temporal law with the authority or ability to regulate or monitor a person's soul and heart. These laws are only capable of judging external behavior, while internal motivations are known only to the One Who sees them, namely, God the Almighty.

[5] Narrated by Bukhari, *Iman*, no. 52.

This is the approach adopted by Islam (and all true, divine religions) towards a person's internal reform and development. It is an approach that has proven successful in the reform of individuals, which in turn leads to the reform of families, communities, and nations. Based on this, the foundations of ethics can be traced back to the original concept of God-consciousness.

4. Delineating Ethics According to their Origins

Islamic ethics and values are abundant. An investigation of the books of Prophetic traditions will unequivocally reveal hundreds of chapters that address ethics directly or indirectly.[6] One perspective through which ethics may be delineated involves linking them to the eight higher objectives (*maqāṣid*) of Sharia as will be demonstrated later in this chapter. A second perspective involves associating them with the following moralities:

- A positive relationship between a person and his Lord.
- A positive relationship between a person and other people.
- A positive relationship between a person and animals.
- A positive relationship between a person and the environment.

These ethics, values, virtues, and ideals can also be delineated from a third perspective, which involves ranking them in terms of strength, outcomes, impacts, and associated punishment. For instance:

(i) Islam categorizes some ethics as obligations and duties whereby their violation entails legislative action and punitive measures.
(ii) There are other ethics that have been ordained by God, but worldly punishments were not set for those who violate them.
(iii) Ethics such as altruism are categorized in Islam as virtues and ideals to which one should aspire.

[6] See the books of *hadith*, especially *Ṣaḥīḥ Bukharī*, *Ṣaḥīḥ Muslim*, *Al-Sunan al-arba'ah*, *Al-muwaṭṭa'*, and *Sunan al-Dārimī*; where we find hundreds of sections about ethics.

5. The Theory of Drafting Ethical Principles in Light of the Higher Objectives of Sharia

As clarified earlier, ethics and morals are not merely peripheral ornaments of the Muslim character but rather are considered fundamental goals for all divine religions, which the Qur'an came to complete and perfect. Those ethics that are paramount were categorized as obligations and duties, while contemptible behaviors were classified as major sins and prohibitions. Other behaviors that do not negatively impact others were categorized either as recommended acts such as altruism, excessive generosity, or excessive courage (given that it is not recklessly excessive), or as reprehensible acts such as refusing to offer regular assistance given that no harm comes of it, etc.

Given this comprehensive nature of ethics in Islam, it is best that they are framed in alignment with the higher objectives of the Sharia, its purposes, philosophy, and types of wisdom. This is the methodology I will attempt to follow. As is commonly induced, Sharia is aimed towards the fulfillment of necessities (*ḍarūrīyāt*), needs (*ḥājīyāt*), and luxuries (*taḥsīnīyāt*) in five or six areas (or perhaps more). This has been reiterated by scholars ranging from the time of Imam Al-Haramayn, Al-Ghazali, Al-'Izz bin 'Abd Al-Salam, Ibn Taymiyah, Ibn Al-Qayyim, and Al-Shatibi, up to contemporary scholars such as Ibn 'Ashur and others.[7] The six objectives of Sharia have been identified as the preservation of religion, life, intellect, wealth, offspring, and honor. In a previous research project[8] of mine I suggested adding two other objectives: the security of the legitimate state and the security of communities and societies. The combination of these eight objectives encompasses the preservation and promotion of the individual's objectives, as well as those of communities, societies, and nations.

---

[7] For more information, see Al-Shatibi (1994). *Congruencies in the Fundamentals of the Revealed Law* (*Al-muwāfaqāt fī uṣūl al-sharī'ah*), Muhammad Abdullah Draz (ed.). Beirut: Dar Al-Ma'rifah; Ibn 'Ashur (2004). *Maqāṣid al-sharī'ah al-Islāmīyah*, Qatar: Ministry of Endowments and Islamic Affairs; Ahmed Raissouni (1995). *Naẓarīyat al-maqāṣid 'ind Al-Shatibi*. Herndon, Virginia: International Institute of Islamic Thought; and Yusuf Al-Qaradawi (2006). *Dirāsah fī fiqh maqāṣid al-sharī'ah*. Cairo: Dar al-Shuruq.

[8] See Ali Al-Qaradaghi (2010). *Ḥaqībat ṭālib al-'ilm al-iqtiṣādīyah*. Beirut: Dar Al-Basha'ir Al-Islamiyah, vol. 1, 188.

According to the perspective put forth by this theory of objectives, each objective is consists of three levels — necessities (*ḍarūrīyāt*), needs (*ḥājīyāt*), and luxuries (*taḥsīnīyāt*) — and also incorporates two elements. The first is an element of actualization (*wujūd*) or positive obligation, i.e. the promotion and development of interests and benefits, through the provision of necessities, followed by needs and then by luxuries. The second is an element of elimination (*'adam*) or negative obligation, i.e. eliminating or preventing harm, malevolence, and corruption. These objectives and rules are central to both the physician and to the morally accountable patient (or his or her guardians if the patient is a minor). This theory can be applied to ethics or principles of biomedical ethics as follows:

5.1. *The Preservation of the Higher Objective of "Religion"*

The preservation of religion in this context refers to two issues. The first issue is concerned with the preservation of Islam's principles and rulings, as Islam is the last of all divine religions. Since our discussion is focused on medical ethics, all divinely established ethics, values, ideals, and virtues are verily categorized under medical preservation and care according to their respective levels of strength, obligation, and so forth. Medical preservation and care likewise includes all common ethical principles and virtues such as abstaining from murder and theft; preventing evil and harm; honoring promises and contracts; saving those at risk; exonerating the innocent; and practicing honesty, integrity, sincerity, altruism, truthfulness, kindness, generosity, and empathy, in addition to all other morals as identified in the Qur'an and Prophetic tradition. The general principles of Islam are similarly included, such as justice, equality, seeking counsel, and respecting human rights. It is imperative that the concept of preservation and care in medicine incorporates both elements of positive and negative obligations, whereby people's interests and benefits are promoted and any harm or corruption is prevented from coming to them.

The second issue is the preservation of the patient's religion and avoiding any practices that may undermine it. Therefore, the physician should not attempt any experiment or prescribe a cure that conflicts with the patient's religious beliefs except in cases of extreme necessity or unequivocal need. In such cases, a physician may only use a proscribed treatment in the absence of alternative permissible treatments. This is in accordance with the Islamic principles, which read, "Necessity overrides religious prohibitions," and, "Dire need for medical treatment can acquire the status of necessity."[9]

A physician's ethical conduct entails that he respects the patient's beliefs and does not exploit a patient's vulnerability to impose other beliefs. For example, this is often practiced by Christian missionaries who exploit the dangerous triad of disease, ignorance, and poverty to proselytize religion. On the other hand, the patient is also responsible for maintaining his or her religion. The patient must adhere to the legal rulings of Sharia when seeking treatment, especially given that undergoing treatment may often be obligatory if rejecting it would lead to definite harm. Similarly, treatment may be prohibited if it utilizes forbidden means, except in cases of necessity.

It is important to note that preserving this higher objective also entails abstinence from everything that is deemed religiously forbidden and prohibited by Sharia in regards to a person's life or physical body (both externally and internally). This includes allowing a fetus to be killed, donating vital organs, altering natural appearance, human cloning, abortion, and all similar practices that God has forbidden. Likewise, these are all considered unethical actions if practiced by a physician and are simultaneously categorized under the preservation of life as is explained below.

5.2. *The Preservation of the Higher Objective of "Life"*[10]

This higher objective refers to a person's physical body, including all internal and external organs. Ethical principles in this regard entail that the physician and the patient prevent any malevolence and harm from coming

[9] See Ali Al-Qaradaghi, *Jurisprudence of Contemporary Medical Issues* (*Fiqh al-qaḍāyā al-ṭibbīyah al-mu'āṣirah*). Beirut: Dar Al-Basha'ir Al-Islamiyah: 225.
[10] For more details, see entry on nafs in: Al-Asfahani (1991). *Sharḥ al-mufradāt li-gharīb al-Qur'ān*, Damascus and Beirut: Dar Al-Qalam & Al-Dar Al-Shamiyah.

to a person's life and that they promote a person's welfare and interests. Consequently, the use of any medication, treatment, or experiment that harms one's body, organs, or internal systems or does not result in benefits is considered unethical, and both the physician and the patient are forbidden from utilizing it. This is because, in Islam, a person does not own his or her life, organs, internal systems, or any other part of the body; instead they all belong to God the Almighty.

The issue of organ donation during one's life is tied with this Islamic principle. The primary ruling for this issue is prohibition, unless it has been categorically proven that donating the organ will not result in any harm to the donor and that it is in the best interest of the patient. It is similarly for this reason that the donation of unpaired vital organs like the heart or liver is absolutely forbidden. Likewise, killing a patient for the sake of relieving him from an incurable disease (euthanasia) is considered unethical in Islam and in all divine religions, even if permitted by the patient, as it is not a right he has. In fact, it is considered a transgression against one of the rights of God the Almighty. Plastic surgeries that alter a person's original attributes also fall into this category, as do issues of cloning, abortion, and genetic manipulation.

In the case where a patient has passed away, organ donation is considered lawful given that consent has been provided through the patient's will or by his or her heirs and that it is in the best interest of the recipient. Resolutions in regards to these rulings have been issued by the International Islamic Fiqh Academy (IIFA), the Islamic Fiqh Academy (IFA), and the European Council for Fatwa and Research (ECFR).[11]

It is worth mentioning that the term *life* in this context may also refer to a person's soul, which could either be at peace (content, self-assured, and unwavering) or unsettled due to psychological diseases. Once again, the preservation of this higher objective may require a balancing of both positive and negative obligations and refraining from the use of any treatment or medication that may have negative psychological or emotional effects. In these cases, the physician must attempt to balance between informing the patient of all necessary details regarding the disease and

[11] See Group of Scholars (1990). *International Islamic Fiqh Academy Journal* (6/3): 1739, 1791, 1975, 2161.

treatment and withholding any information that may lead to the patient losing hope or rejecting treatment.

5.3. *Ethical Principles Associated with Preserving the Higher Objective of "the Intellect"*

Owing to the utmost significance and role of the intellect (*'aql*) in a person's life, a distinct higher objective is dedicated to it. Linguistically, the word *'aql*, is defined as the cognition and realization of matters as they are in reality and the ability to distinguish between them.[12] The technical definition, however, has stimulated extensive philosophical debates. According to Muslim scholars, it is defined as the instinct through which God has distinguished man from the rest of creatures. In its absence, there can be no accountability (*taklīf*) placed on a person.[13] It also refers to the process of grasping theoretical knowledge. In his definition, Al-Ghazali explained that, "*'Aql* can encompass a number of meanings…amongst them are two meanings that are relevant to our discussion: the first refers to the awareness and recognition of reality…and the second refers to the grasp of knowledge…in other words, comprehension."[14] Intellect in Islam holds a high status. It is an indispensable condition for affirming belief and mandating accountability, the comprehension of knowledge, juridical reasoning (to deduce legal rulings), and the development and progress of civilizations.

The ethical principles associated with intellect, in terms of positive and negative obligations, require that the physician exert his or her utmost efforts to preserve and advance intellect, while also preventing any harm from coming to it. Consequently, it is unethical to use any medication that may potentially damage a person's intellectual abilities. The patient must likewise avoid anything that harms his or her intellectual capacity and must exert effort towards intellectual development and prosperity.

Freedom and independence are central to the intellect. The patient should not be denied the right to freely decide whether to undergo

---

[12] *Al-qāmūs al-muḥīṭ*; *Lisān al-'Arab*; and *Al-mu'jam al-wasīṭ* for the entry of *'aql*.
[13] Abu Hamid Al-Ghazali (1939). *Iḥyā' 'ulūm al-dīn*, (3/4) (Cairo: Matba'at Al-Halabi); Ibn Al-Qayyim (n.d.). *Miftāḥ dār al-sa'ādah*. Beirut: Dar al-Kutub al-'Ilmiyah, 1/117.
[14] Al-Ghazali, *Iḥyā'*, (3/4).

treatment or participate in research experiments, provided that his or her decision does not conflict with an explicit legal text or public interest. Such cases include when a patient suffers from a serious contagious disease or when another person may be directly harmed, such as the enforcement of pre-marital medical check-ups that takes place in certain countries.

5.4. *Principles of Medical Ethics Associated with the Higher Objective of "Wealth"*

These principles are evident in the physician's or the medical institution's requirement to charge patients reasonable fees. Needless to say, exploiting a patient in order to gain extra money is unethical behavior. Similarly, the patient should not squander his or her money on extravagant, superfluous medication. It is also considered unethical for a terminal patient to offer the physician or other persons money with the purpose of depriving his or her heirs from their rightful inheritance.

5.5. *Principles of Medical Ethics Associated with the Higher Objective of "Offspring"*

The purpose here entails protecting the patient from harm, realizing the patient's welfare and interests, and doing our best to avoid any possible distortion of lineage. Arising from this, abortion is considered an unethical act with the exception of some cases in which the mother's life is in danger. In addition, it is the physician's ethical duty to preserve lineage during artificial insemination and any other similar procedures.

5.6. *Principles of Medical Ethics Associated with the Higher Objective of "Honor"*

It is not permitted for a physician or institution to act in any manner or disclose any secrets in regards to the patient that may potentially be disparaging of his or her honor, dignity, or character. On the contrary, the physician must protect and preserve the patient's honor and dignity (this objective is also related to preserving the patient's psychological and emotional well-being).

5.7. *Principles of Medical Ethics Associated with the Preservation of Communities and Societies*

This refers to the protection and preservation of public welfare and interests along with individual interests. It requires the protection of a society's political, social, economic, and environmental security from any potential harm or malfeasance. It also requires that medical insurance be distributed equally and justly among members of society without any form of discrimination. This has been firmly established as a basic legal right for all individuals.

Based on this, any practices performed by the physician (or the medical institution), whether for treatment or research, must be intended to increase benefit, not harm. Therefore, any action that results in the overall corruption of the society and the environment or leads to injustice and inequality is considered an unethical act. For this reason, the resolutions issued by the *fiqh* academies stipulated that DNA fingerprinting, gene therapy, or the like is permissible only if it does not cause any harm to humans, animals, or the environment.[15] In fact, the preservation of public interests is prioritized over individual interests. Hence, a patient's independent will in rejecting treatment is discounted if he or she suffers a contagious disease that poses a danger to society.

5.8. *Principles of Medical Ethics Associated with the State*

This involves the obligation of adherence to the laws and regulations that have been transparently issued by the state. It includes preserving the state's medical and rehabilitation institutions, maintaining its security, advancing its interests, and protecting it from harm or corruption. Consequently, any action practiced by the physician that contradicts the

---

[15] See Al-Qaradaghi (2010). *Ḥaqībat ṭālib al-'ilm.* Beirut: Dar al-basha'ir al-Islamiyah, 1/190ff.

state's established laws and regulations or that places its security at risk is considered unethical.

6. A Summary of the Link between the Principles of Biomedical Ethics and the Higher Objectives of Sharia

This chapter has made evident that the theory of drafting principles of biomedical ethics based on the higher objectives of Sharia is a comprehensive theory and successfully integrates the four principles of biomedical ethics. As explained, maintaining any of the eight higher objectives requires two elements: preventing harm and malfeasance and preserving interests and benefits. These represent two of the four principles in the principle-based approach. I also found that the principle of respect for autonomy falls under two of the higher objectives of Sharia, preserving religion and preserving life. We further found that the principle of justice falls under the higher objectives of preserving communities and societies as well as preserving religion.

This theory also encompasses the principle of equality through the two higher objectives of preserving communities and societies and preserving religion. Likewise was the protection of a person's psychological and emotional well-being through the higher objective of preserving honor and finally the principle of freedom and similar rights through the higher objective of preserving the intellect. It also covered the internal attributes of both the physician and the patient such as sincerity, altruism, and parental compassion, all of which fall under the higher objective of preserving religion.

There remain three aspects that are needed in order to complete this theory. They are the binding obligation (*ilzāmīyah*), normativity (*mi'yārīyah*), and coherence (*ḍabṭ*). Obligation and commitment have been addressed through the higher objective of preserving religion, which makes mandatory the adherence to beneficial medical ethics and prohibits immoral conduct, as ordained throughout numerous Qur'anic verses and Prophetic traditions. In turn, it becomes the responsibility of the individual to abide by these ethics and the responsibility of the state to decree binding legislations in order to regulate those medical ethics that impact other persons.

7. Normativity and Coherence

Although the aforementioned eight objectives and the principles of biomedical ethics already have a coherent relationship, this coherence may be enhanced and a more comprehensive framework can be developed through utilizing a set of legal maxims that serve to outline issues of harm, interest, and the balance between them. These rules are as follows:

7.1. *Governing Legal Maxims for Issues of Harm*

Islamic law provides a set of governing legal maxims or rules, deduced from the legal texts (the Qur'an and Prophetic tradition), that facilitate our development of a consistent framework in this regard. These governing rules include the following:

(i) *The rule, "There should be neither harming nor reciprocating harm"*[16]

This rule is a Prophetic narration (*hadith*) whose chain of narrators was deemed "acceptable" (*ḥasan*) by many scholars and "authentic" (*ṣaḥīḥ*) by others.[17] This *hadith* indicates that it is prohibited to cause any harm and that harm is not to be removed by way of another harm. A set of rules has been derived from this Prophetic narration such as: harm is to be removed, harm is not to be removed by way of harm, necessity renders the prohibited permissible, need is treated as necessity, necessities and needs must only be assessed and answered proportionately, hardship begets facility, and if a matter is difficult, ease it.[18]

[16]The *hadith* reads, "Let there be no harm or reciprocating harm." It was narrated by Malik in *Al-muwaṭṭa'* from Abu Hurayrah.

[17]Ibn Rajab (2001). *Jāmi' al-'ulūm wa-al-ḥikam*. Mu'assasat al-Risāla, 2/211.

[18]See Al-Suyuti (2004). *Al-ashbāh wa-al-naẓā'ir*. Cairo: Dar al-Salam, 1/210–218; Ahmad Al-Zarqa' (1989). *Sharḥ al-qawā'id al-fiqhīyah*. Damascus: Dar al-Qalam, 525–830.

There are some other maxims related to this *hadith* or general rules, including "Whatever is permissible because of a certain excuse ceases to be permissible with the disappearance of that excuse", "When what makes something forbidden no longer exists, what is forbidden shall return [to permissibility]", "A private harm is tolerated in order to ward off a public harm", "Minor damage will be endured to get rid of major damage", "In the presence of two evils, the one whose harm is greater is to be avoided by the commission of the lesser", "The lesser of the two evils is tolerated", "Warding off harm should always take priority over the accruement of benefit", "Harm is to be removed as much as possible", "Necessity does not invalidate the right of others", "Harm is to be warded off whether intended or not", "Harm is to be warded off as much as possible", and "Necessity is only considered when it is real and certain and not when it is conjectured."[19]

(ii) *The rule, "Certainty cannot be overruled by doubt"*

In the case of treatment, if there is certainty, positively or negatively, this certainty should not be dispelled by doubt, and it is not allowed to neglect such certainty. For example, if there is definite evidence that a particular treatment will be of no avail for a particular disease, it is not allowed to neglect this certainty unless we reach a different conclusion based on another certainty, which would in turn be based on proofs that impart certainty.

The following rules are related to this maxim: "The basic principle is: what has once existed is [deemed] as continuing," and, "The basic nature of things is permissibility." Imam Al-Shafi'i once said, "The fundamental principle upon which I base my decisions is that I use certainty, abandon doubt, and do not make use of conjecture."[20] We also have the following rules: "The basic principle is to ascribe the event to the nearest time of occurrence," and, "The original rule for all things is permissibility."[21]

---

[19] Al-Suyuti, *Al-ashbāh wa-al-naẓā'ir* (1/173); Al-Zarqa', *Sharḥ al-qawā'id al-fiqhīyah*, 113–164; Ali Ahmad Al-Nadwi, *Mawsū'at al-qawā'id wal-ḍawābiṭ*, (2/220–223).
[20] Al-Suyuti, *Al-ashbāh wal-naẓā'ir*, (1/156).
[21] *Ibid.* (1/151–168); Al-Zarqa', *Sharḥ al-qawā'id al-fiqhīyah*, 35–64.

8. How Should a Physician or Patient Decide Regarding Treatment or Research Experiments?

As discussed earlier, medication must be used with the purpose of advanc ing interests or preventing harms. This raises the question: Is certainty in regards to resulting benefits and/or harms a condition for decision-making? The answer is as follows:

The second rule mentioned above ("Certainty cannot be overruled by doubt") refers to situations of absolute certainty, which may only be negated by opposing absolute certainties. However, in cases lacking absolute certainty, the required condition is ensuring the existence of a predominant hypothesis based on professional principles as to whether treatment should be pursued or not. According to Al-'Izz bin 'Abd Al-Salam: "Efforts exerted to achieve the interests of this world and the Hereafter and warding off their evils are usually based on a preponderant presumption."[22] He also stated, "Because the preponderant presumption comes true in most cases, the interests of this world and the Hereafter have usually been estimated by this means ...So, it is not allowed to disrupt the interests that will most likely come true for fear of any banes whose occurrence is not guaranteed."[23] He then asserted that it is not permissible to act based on arbitrary assumptions. Rather, assumptions are classified into three categories: low-ranking assumptions, high-ranking assumptions, and middle-ranking assumptions.[24] Furthermore, Islamic law established a firm rule that explicitly erroneous assumptions are to be disregarded.[25]

It is not difficult to arrive at an acceptable level of assumption. In fact, it is quite possible to attain this through knowledge, experience, experimentation, and consultation. Imam Al-'Izz claims that, "Most of the elements of benefit and harm in this world can be identified by means of human discretion."[26] He continues, "Some beneficial and harmful issues can be recognized by both intelligent and unintelligent individuals,

[22] Ibn ʿAbd al-Salām (n.d.). *Al-qawā'id al-kubrá* (Qatar Ministry of Religious Endowments) (1/6).
[23] *Ibid.* (2/35).
[24] *Ibid.*
[25] Al-Suyuti (2004). *Al-ashbāh wal-naẓā'ir* (1/343).
[26] Ibn ʿAbd al-Salām (n.d.). *Al-qawā'id al-kubrá* (1/7,13).

while others are only discernible to intelligent individuals."[27] Hence, the formation of specialized committees that are qualified to make appropriate decisions for complicated situations is imperative.

9. Applying *Fiqh* of Balances in Decision-Making for Contradicting Cases

The *fiqh* of balances (*fiqh al-muwāzanāt*) plays a central role in cases where a conflict arises between benefits and interests themselves, damages and harms themselves, or between benefits/interests on one hand and damages/harms on the other hand. In these cases, decisions should be made by balancing between the quest to achieve the best, strongest, and most effective benefits and to prevent the most and worst harm and detriment.[28] For situations in which the benefits of a certain action are equal to those of inaction, after consultations and recommendations from relevant committees, the final decision is up to the physician's discretion. If equality, however, is not determined, the issue should be referred to another committee for the decision to be made, while practicing caution and emphasizing potential harm and detriment as much as possible.

The Muslim Physician's Oath adopted by the Islamic Organization for Medical Science (IOMS) during its first conference held in Kuwait in 1401 A.H. (1981 C.E.) emphasized the importance of promoting interests and preventing harms as illustrated below.

In the name of God, The Most Gracious, The Most Merciful,

> I swear by God … The Great
> To regard God in carrying out my profession
> To protect human life in all stages and under all circumstances, doing my utmost to rescue it from death, malady, pain and anxiety
> To keep people's dignity, cover their privacies, and lock up their secrets
> To be, all the way, an instrument of God's mercy, extending my medical care to near and far, virtuous and sinner and friend and enemy

---

[27] *Ibid.* (1/38).

[28] Ibn ʿAbd al-Salām (n.d.). *Al-qawāʿid al-kubrá* (1/8, 87).

To strive in the pursuit of knowledge and harness it for the benefit but not the harm of Mankind
To revere my teacher, teach my junior, and be brother to members of the Medical Profession joined in piety and charity
To live my Faith in private and in public, avoiding whatever blemishes me in the eyes of God, His apostle and my fellow Faithful.
And may God be witness to this Oath.[29]

10. The Broad Scope of Medical Ethics that Includes Physicians, Patients, and Others

Medical ethics must primarily stem from the physician himself. These ethics should be inherent qualities in his relationship with the patient since medicine is a means, not an end, for healing a patient. The healing of a patient is the principal end. Therefore, a physician's care for his patients must be unparalleled in its excellence. Likewise, the physician must maintain positive relationships with his colleagues, institution, and society. Given the significant role played by a physician, maintaining the following fundamental ethics and guidelines are crucial:

10.1. *The Ethics of a Physician*: *Guidelines and Behaviors*

Islamic Sharia has established a set of distinguished ethics (guidelines, rules, and behaviors) for the physician who treats people whether physically, psychologically, or otherwise. Below is a brief outline of these ethics:

First: The physician must be knowledgeable, experienced, and proficient in his or her medical profession. In our present day, it is also necessary for him or her to obtain a medical degree and an official license from the country in which he or she will be practicing (a condition acknowledged by Sharia).
Second: The physician's practice must be in alignment with the commonly agreed upon professional regulations.

[29] The English text is taken literally from the official translation. See *Islamic Code of Medical Ethics*. Kuwait: International Organization of Islamic Medicine, 1981: 93.

Third: The physician must be sincerely dedicated to his or her work, trustworthy, protective of the rights of others, and striving towards excellence and innovation.[30]

These are the three fundamental conditions in Islam. They can be summed up using two words: sincerity (*ikhlāṣ*) and professionalism (*ikhtiṣāṣ*). This was reiterated by numerous verses throughout the Qur'an. For instance, in one verse it is stated, "…'Indeed, the best one you can hire is the strong and the trustworthy'" (Qur'an 28:26). In this context, strength refers to professionalism and experience while trustworthiness refers to sincerity and honoring confidentiality.

Fourth: The physician should be knowledgeable of the legal rulings associated with medicine and treating patients.

Fifth: The physician should be characterized by Islam's noble attributes, particularly:

(i) God-consciousness, fear of God, and cognizance of God's presence throughout his or her treatment of a patient. The physician should be as the Prophet Muhammad (PBUH) described, "To worship God as if you see Him, and if you do not achieve this state of devotion, then (take it for granted that) God sees you."[31]

(ii) Humility towards God, patients, and colleagues and practicing virtue in all interpersonal relationships.

(iii) Truthfulness and absolute honesty in regards to sight, behaviors, integrity, and chastity. In addition, to refrain from cheating, betrayal, envy, malevolence, and all other diseases of the heart.

Sixth: The physician should respect his medical specialization through enhancing his interest in and study of the field and pursuing creativity and innovation. He should also respect other specializations, meaning he should not treat a disease that is beyond his area of expertise but rather

[30] For more information, see relevant papers presented by Ali Dawud Al-Jaffal, Ahmad Raja'i Al-Jindi, Abdul Sattar Abu Ghuddah, Muhammad 'Atta Al-Sayid, Muhammad Ali Al-Bar, Mustafa Abdul Ra'uf, Su'ud Al-Thubayti published in Group of Scholars (1993). *Islamic Fiqh Academy Journal*, issue 8 (3/10–407).

[31] Bukhari, *Kitāb Al-Īmān* (no. 4777) and Muslim, *Kitāb Al-Īmān* (no. 9), on the authority of Abu Hurayrah.

refer the patient to the appropriate physician or seek advice from the relevantly specialized physician. Respect for other specializations also entails that the physician refrain from practicing any profession that may conflict with his medical profession, such as simultaneously working at a pharmacy.

Seventh: The physician should honor medical confidentiality and abide by the ethical and humanitarian values ratified by Islam. In other words, the temptations of wealth, authority, and desires in this world should never affect his integrity. He should live his life committed to these superior values and not allow his conscience to be bought with anything this world can offer. This includes even the simplest of transgressions such as granting undue medical leaves or submitting false reports. This is a great responsibility that falls on the shoulders of physicians and all those working within similar professions.

Eighth: The physician should be keen on curing the patient and should not prevent treatment except in cases where there is a legal or scientific justification. In turn, a physician is in no way permitted to participate in ending a patient's life.

Ninth: The physician may not conduct any experimentation on his patients without the patient's consent or without the approval of the specialized authority.

Tenth: The physician must adhere to the laws, systems, regulations, and medical decisions issued by the specialized authorities serving to regulate matters of private and public health. This falls under the Islamic legal obligation of obeying those in authority as long as it does not conflict with any of the Sharia texts. As commanded by God, "O you who have believed, obey God and obey the Messenger and those in authority among you…" (Qur'an 4:59).

These are the 10 commandments that physicians must adhere to. They are considered a code of conduct for the medical profession and the solemn covenant (*al-mīthāq al-ghalīẓ*). They represent a binding contract and a mandatory commitment that God has commanded us to fulfill in His orders, "O you who have believed, fulfill [all] contracts…" (Qur'an 5:1) and, "…And fulfill [every] commitment. Indeed, the commitment is ever [that about which one will be] questioned" (Qur'an 17:34).

10. Confidentiality

Although confidentiality is included in the abovementioned 10 commandments, it is necessary that we discuss it further due to its particular significance. It is also often referred to as medicine-related confidential information or medical profession privacy. This ethical value implies the necessity of maintaining confidentiality regarding all matters seen or heard by the physician from the patient. The physician must not disclose any secret that may harm the patient or any related party. The scope of this concept extends to all the information related to the patient's health, personal history, sexual relations, and so forth.

Religion has categorically prohibited every type of transgression against a person's honor as it has equally prohibited transgressions against life and wealth. Basically, causing any undue harm to any human being is religiously forbidden. Therefore, disclosing confidential information is prohibited by the Sharia and is both professionally and legally liable. Further, this action is considered a betrayal of trust and hence is not a trait of true believers. Rather, God describes true believers as, "And they who are to their trusts and their promises attentive" (Qur'an 23:8). Furthermore, Prophet Muhammad (PBUH) identified betrayal of trust as one of the signs of hypocrisy.[32]

Safeguarding a patient's secrets is an integral part of all human values and is reinforced by all divine religions. Even the ancient oath of Amenhotep, one of the Ancient Egyptian pharaohs, included the statement, "Whatever I hear in my profession or outside of it which should not be disclosed, I will never reveal."[33] Following this came the Hippocratic Oath, taken by medical graduates to this day, which includes, "Whatever, in connection with my professional practice or not, I see or hear, in the life of men, which ought not to be spoken of abroad, I will not divulge, as reckoning that all such should be kept secret."[34]

---

[32] The text of the Prophetic narration states, "Signs of a hypocrite are three: If he speaks, he tells a lie; and if he promises, he breaks his promise; and if he is entrusted, he betrays [proves to be dishonest]." See Bukhari, *Kitāb Al-Īmān* (no. 33) and Muslim, *Kitāb Al-Īmān* (no. 59), on the authority of Abu Hurayrah.

[33] *Al-mawsū'ah al-ṭibbīyah al-fiqhīyah*, 556.

[34] Ali Dawud al-Jaffal (1993). Phyician ethics (Akhlāqīyāt al-ṭabīb). *Islamic Fiqh Academy Journal* 8(3): 17–18.

Early Muslim physicians similarly underscored the importance of confidentiality. In his book *The Best Accounts of the Biographies of Physicians* (*'Uyūn al-anbā' fī ṭabaqāt al-aṭibbā'*), Ibn Abi Usaybi'ah highlighted some of the oaths taken by the physicians of his era such as, "Those things that I see or hear while treating patients or at other times, which should not be disclosed, I refrain from talking about." He also mentioned some ethics associated with physicians including "perfect morality, sound mind, safeguarding patients' secrets, knowledge of Islamic law, avoiding the practice of abortion, and other similarly admirable behavior."[35]

Islam has prohibited disclosing secrets (except in cases of necessity with specific guidelines) due to the potentially harmful psychological, moral, physical, and financial consequences. In fact, breaching medical confidentiality is harmful to the medical profession itself. If a patient loses confidence in the physician, he may not reveal all the information regarding his condition, which may in turn obscure discovery of the actual disease. Islam places a strong emphasis on the issue of trustworthiness to the extent that a person is obligated to conceal what was said during a gathering if the other party indicates a desire for concealment. In this regard, it has been narrated that the Prophet (PBUH) asserted, "When a man tells someone something and then departs, it becomes a trust (*amānah*)."[36] This Prophetic narration clearly highlights that gatherings are considered trusts and that the one you consult is considered a trustee.

In its eighth session, the International Islamic Fiqh Academy issued resolution No. 79 (10/8) concerning the necessity of maintaining confidentiality in all medical professions except under exceptional cases. The exceptions under which confidentiality may be breached are:

- In cases where public interests will be preserved.
- In cases where public harm will be prevented.

The exceptional cases under which a breach of confidentiality is acceptable must be clearly stipulated in the codes of professional practice for the field of medicine as well as other professions.[37]

---

[35] *'Uyūn al-anbā' fī ṭabaqāt al-aṭibbā'*, (1/35).
[36] Narrated by Tirmidhi, no. 1882.
[37] See Group of Scholars (1993). *International Fiqh Academy Journal* 8(3).

Script of Oral Discussions (Day 3, Session 3)

After **Ali Al-Qaradaghi** presented his paper, the following discussion took place.

Abdullah Bin Bayyah

Everything we have heard so far is good, and in my opinion it is all complementary and free of contradiction. A document on ethics can be drafted out of our discussions, starting with broad principles followed by more particular issues like those outlined by Sheikh Al-Qaradaghi. This would be a very important document that could be of added value for doctors and parties responsible for drafting laws. These parties need intellectual and academic support to enable them to enforce these laws and to guide them to make the right decisions. Likewise, doctors need academic ethical documents that are in compliance with their convictions and their ethical and religious consciences.

There is nothing new that I would like to add to what my colleagues have already presented. The way I see it, the higher objectives are a field or garden for rulings and ethics are the fruits that the rulings produce. Now the soil is ready, the field is ready, and the trees are being planted; therefore, the fruits will be the noble ethics by which everyone should abide.

However, if you plan to write a report or document, you should also address other groups besides the doctors, such as pharmaceutical companies, insurance companies, and governments. You should advise these parties to limit their greediness and focus instead on the humanitarian dimension of providing assistance to people. This is especially relevant in countries that lack drugs for AIDS and other drugs due to the positions adopted by certain greedy pharmaceutical companies. How can we discuss ethics while neglecting to talk about those who deny people access to the drugs they need? Preventing drugs that are known to be effective from people who need them is like denying people food and water. It is not acceptable.

Finally, I would like to say that in many cases a doctor faces a situation where he must intervene. This puts him in a delicate situation because intervening when someone's life is in danger is obligatory according to Sharia. Thus, the role of a doctor is central in this regard. The responsibility a doctor has in front of God is immense. Indeed, the medical profession is an incredibly honorable one and the doctor is rewarded for his work. Before a doctor is dealing with patients, he is dealing with God Almighty.

Mohammed Ghaly

Do you have any comments about the inclusion of two new higher objectives of Sharia by Sheikh al-Qaradaghi, namely, the security of the society and the security of the government, especially as far as it relates to medical ethics?

Abdullah Bin Bayyah

The security of the society and the security of the government are certainly important to the matter at hand but are not at the heart or core of it. Our discussion is about biomedical ethics, and each party should do its role. Governments should pass the appropriate laws, doctors should uphold them in their profession, pharmaceutical companies and insurance companies should operate according to these ethics, and so on. Even in the face of difficulties or perceived risk, every party should hold fast to the pertinent ethical values such as justice, mercy, etc. These are major principles, but they encompass minor principles or minor objectives.

I often liken the higher objectives to a ladder, the highest rung of which is the grand higher objectives (*maqāṣid kullīyah kubrá*). Al-Shatibi says there is no higher degree above them and they govern all comprehensive principles (*kullīyāt*), including Islamic legal theory (*uṣūl al-fiqh*). The second rung includes the three categories: the necessities (*ḍarūrīyāt*), needs (*ḥājīyāt*), and luxuries (*taḥsīnīyāt*). To repeat, we have at the top of the ladder the grand higher objectives. Then in the middle of the ladder we have the higher objectives that are comprehensive (*kullī*) with respect to what is below them and particular (*juz'ī*) with respect to what is above them. And so on until you reach the lowest level of the ladder.

Mohammed Ghaly

Are the higher objectives that Sheikh Al-Qaradaghi mentioned considered among the category of grand objectives (*al-kullīyāt al-kubrá*)?

Abdullah Bin Bayyah

The higher objectives that Sheikh Al-Qaradaghi mentioned are among the necessities, which are those things whose preservation both on the individual and collective levels are necessary for a human society to exist. Scholars cite this as one of the reasons they were called "necessities." The other reason they were called "necessities" is because they were known from the religion by necessity or by default (*'ulimat min al-dīn bi-al-ḍarūrah*). And God knows best.

Hassan Chamsi-Pasha

We have nowadays the concepts of public health ethics and community medicine. Community medicine is not always conducted by physicians; it may be conducted by medical professionals and others who administer preventative medications, for example. So the field of medicine is expanding to encompass community medicine, which is included among the areas to which medical ethics apply.

Jasser Auda

Regarding the categorization of the higher objectives of Sharia, we cannot add to them except what is of their kind. The higher objectives include things like honor and wealth, etc. Adding things [explicitly] related to the society or government would be adding things of a different type altogether because the higher objectives are related to the needs of the human [as an individual]. Ibn 'Ashur had a perspective on this. He delineated within each of the five or six higher objectives two dimensions: one related to the individual and the other related to the society. So we can add a societal dimension to the preservation of life, of honor, of wealth, etc. For example, when it comes to the higher objective related to [the societal dimension of] the preservation of life, we can talk about public health. When it comes to honor, we can talk about human rights in general. By expanding the current higher objectives to the level of society we avoid introducing new higher objectives that are not of the same type and thus do not belong in the same category.

Abdullah Bin Bayyah

The higher objectives of Sharia are unrestricted and can always be added to. Any instance in which God says in the Qur'an that, "God wants…" or, "In order not to…" or anything that indicates a purpose or goal, whether in the positive or the negative sense, counts as a higher objective. In his book *The Conclusive Argument from God* (*Ḥujjat Allah al-bālighah*), Wali Allah unearthed a treasure of higher objectives. He included as higher objectives everything that could ever be imagined as such from references in the Qur'an and the Prophetic tradition. The higher objectives are in fact in every ruling of Sharia, whether it relates to a specific ruling, to a reason behind a ruling, or to a comprehensive ruling. So certainly no one can say that the higher objectives have all been found; they are unrestricted in number. However, the well-known set of five higher objectives [preserving religion, life, intellect, offspring, and wealth] will remain distinct because this set is comprehensive and complete.

"…Unquestionably, His [God's] is the creation and the command…" (Qur'an 7:54). There is wisdom behind every single cell He has created in this universe, and likewise there is wisdom behind every single ruling He has commanded Thus, I think these [five] higher objectives should be kept as they are, and we can downstream them to the rest [and in this sense consider them to be comprehensive and all-inclusive].

Abdul Sattar Abu Ghuddah

I wrote a research paper entitled, "Sharia-Based Principles for the Profession of Medicine and Medical Treatment" (*Al-mabādi' al-shar'īyah lil-taṭbīb wal-'ilāj*). The paper included a number of legal maxims relevant to the medical field, e.g. the maxim of necessities, the maxim of [avoiding] harm, the maxim of (taking) permission, the maxim of cultural norms, and others. If you find it is suitable, it can serve as the introduction to the process of practical application after we come up with what corresponds to the four principles on a theoretical level. In fact, some of the maxims may already correspond to the four principles.

Ahmed Raissouni

Our main focus is deducing some of the comprehensive principles (*kullīyāt*) or rules related to biomedical ethics and basing the process of deduction upon the higher objectives of Sharia. I agree with linking biomedical ethics to the first three necessities, which are the preservation of life, of offspring, and of intellect. It is clear that the development of the principles of biomedical ethics should be based on these three necessities in particular, and there is no exaggeration in doing so. Sheikh Al-Qaradaghi mentioned this clearly and presented practical examples of their application.

As for linking biomedical ethics with the rest of the necessities, that would entail a certain degree of exaggerative interpretation, unnecessary complications, and unreasonable generalizations. A better approach would be to choose from the higher objectives or necessities those that are relevant to medicine, and I think Sheikh Al-Qaradaghi is more inclined to this approach as well. Dr. Chamsi-Pasha touched on this: instead of talking about the security of the state and society, we will go straight to community medicine and what it requires in terms of laws and measures.

In regards to the issue of the higher objectives of Sharia in general, I agree with Sheikh Bin Bayyah and Dr. Auda that the five necessities were crafted on the basis of certain premises or were meant for certain purposes. We can add as many higher objectives as we want. This is because the needs of individuals and of societies are abundant and cannot be limited, meaning that some of them may become necessities though they were not previously considered as such. Therefore, the door is open. However, after many years of contemplating the idea, I do not think we should add anything to the set of five higher objectives of Sharia. This is because if we did, the addition would be of a type different from that of the five higher objectives.

The preservation of honor (*'irḍ*) is sometimes counted as the sixth higher objective, but I believe it is not essential. The agreed-upon higher objectives of Sharia are five [the preservation of religion (*dīn*), life (*nafs*), intellect (*'aql*), offspring (*nasl*), and wealth (*māl*)]. Muslim scholars like Ibn 'Ashur — and I agree with him — stated that the preservation of honor complements the preservation of offspring. Some Muslim scholars would replace the preservation of offspring with the preservation of lineage (*nasab*) in the set of five higher objectives of Sharia. However, others have objected by saying that lineage is not among the necessities but rather is among the needs; they raised the question, where is the necessity of people knowing that so-and-so is the son of this person or that? It is an important issue but is counted at the level of needs and not necessities; everything should be given proper prioritization.

The early scholars used to derive the necessities from the prescribed legal punishments (*ḥudūd*) and penal law (*'uqūbāt*). However, they used to cite short examples in which they hastily made these connections, without giving detailed reasoning or consideration to the matter. To be honest, that did not do justice to the necessities, and this is why Ibn 'Ashur refused the idea of making a direct link between the necessities on the one hand and the prescribed legal punishments and penal law on the other. The necessities are much broader than the penal law, and there are things more important than the penal law for preserving these necessities, especially as far as the positive obligation (*al-hifẓ al-wujūdī*) is concerned.[1]

[1] Editor's note: *Al-ḥifẓ al-wujūdī* entails taking measures to ensure that a particular higher objective is indeed preserved or upheld (e.g. facilitating learning and education for preservation of the intellect), while *al-ḥifẓ al-'adamī* entails taking measures to ensure the higher objective will not be harmed (e.g. prohibiting alcohol and other intoxicants for preservation of the intellect).

Positive obligation is the basis, and negative obligation (*al-hifẓ al-'adamī*) complements and protects the bare minimum level of preservation (*al-hifẓ al-ḍarūrī*). Positive obligation does not entail punishments in the first place, and this is why Al-Shatibi and others said, "These necessities have been arrived at by means of induction (*istiqrā'*)," and when we say induction, it means that each one of these necessities was arrived at by the examination of hundreds of texts and rulings. We need to get past the claimed link between the necessities and the penal law because we now have the ability to study the necessities and their sources in a much more comprehensive way.

As mentioned by Sheikh Al-Qaradaghi and supported by Sheikh Abu Ghuddah, the maxims related to the two concepts of harm and necessity are intimately related to the lives, bodies, and needs of human beings. These maxims themselves include what we can call "mothers" and "daughters." We start with the [broad] rules that state, "There shall be no harm nor reciprocating of harm," "harm is to be removed," etc. From those, other subrules are derived, from which we choose the most overarching and essential with respect to the medical field.

Hassan Chamsi-Pasha

The book I wrote with Dr. Al-Bar contains a chapter on the juristic rules of medicine, and we included two or three examples of practical applications under each rule so that the issues could be relevant and clear to physicians. We mentioned a total of 20 rules.

Ali Al-Qaradaghi

We all agree to compose biomedical ethics from the higher objectives of Sharia, whether from all or some of them. This requires a practical workshop that will deal specifically with this topic without touching upon topics of indirect relevance. I recommend we conclude this session and begin organizing a workshop incorporating what was said during the seminar — whether it was about three higher objectives, eight higher objectives, etc. I can present a group of recommendations to you all and then we can elaborate on them, mentioning the rules we alluded to in the seminar as well as from previously written books or studies. We can make this into a document or report, and in that way we will have presented a core text. The document should be written in a rigorous, legal style and should be constrained to a couple of pages. After that, it may be expanded upon by explanations and mention of practical applications in the scope of medical professionals, insurance companies, etc.

Mohammed Ghaly

As I was re-reading the submitted papers, I began to develop a modest conception that I would like to propose to you for feedback. The concept, as Sheikh Bin Bayyah illustrated, is in the form of a pyramid divided into top, middle, and bottom sections. Based on my readings and the ongoing discussions, the summit of the pyramid consists of the higher objectives of Sharia. These higher objectives can indeed be applied to biomedical ethics, and it appears there are no objections to doing so. The prevailing opinion seems to be that applying the higher objectives of Sharia to biomedical ethics is actually the best approach, as it would be rooted in the Islamic tradition and thus would likely not trigger a lot of debates about its Islamic character.

Following the higher objectives of Sharia, which are at the top, we arrive at what is more specific or detailed in the middle. I will now mention these specifics without ordering them in terms of priority and will leave it to you to re-arrange them as you see best. Let us talk about the ethics that will fall under a certain higher objective. For example, we can take the higher objective of preservation of life, assuming we find it relevant and applicable to the field biomedical ethics in Islam. We find under it a set of ethics related to the physician, the patient, and so on, and those ethics are directly related to the preservation of life. We put these under the higher objective.

What also come under this higher objective are the juristic rules or Islamic legal maxims — that are used to rigorously determine the method(s) of applying the higher objectives on the medical issues that we are dealing with. [This is especially important] because it is clear that one of the problematic areas of the four principles approach in the West has to do with specification and the application of these four principles to individual cases. So under this higher objective [the preservation of life], we have a certain number of rules. If we wanted to apply these rules to some particular situations, then the juristic rules will determine the method(s) of application.

To clarify: we have the ethical principles under the higher objectives; the juristic rules [that aid in the method(s) of application to specific cases] under the higher objectives; and perhaps we also have specific examples of juristic rulings. As Sheikh Al-Qaradaghi mentioned, some examples are cloning and organ donation. In this way, when the physician looks into the higher objectives and the ethics, they will not remain vague generalizations, and it will be easier to apply the higher objectives on individual cases.

I also want to touch upon the inclusion of the four principles in our endeavor. For example, we can say that under so-and-so higher objective and such-and-such principles, the principle of autonomy is included but with certain limits. It is not an open-ended inclusion; rather, we are bound by the higher objectives, the principles, and the governing ethical laws of Islam. So we will have to pay attention as to where to put and how to include the four principles.

As we lay down the higher objectives and what comes under them, we must consider who exactly will be the ones applying these ideas to specific situations. They will not always be physicians. There may be other stakeholders such as ethics committees, legislators, insurance companies, pharmaceutical companies, or individuals concerned with public health. It is critical we discuss the qualifications and credentials of different implementing parties in more detail. We have been discussing theories, and I hope we can work on papers and workshops that address the details of implementation.

Annelien Bredenoord

If you were to formulate the principles of Islamic bioethics and also formulate more specific rules, how would you position them? Would they be a particular set of ethical guidelines for the Islamic world? How would you position the Islamic medical ethics in relation to the four principles and in relation to people living in other parts of the world? I am asking this because, once again, if we discuss universality then it should be formulated in a manner that it can be shared by all of us. Is that your aim and if not, then what is the aim?

Ali Al-Qaradaghi

Al-Shatibi stated that these five necessities are part of general religion, meaning you will not find two people who differ on that matter. They are shared by all religions and are inherent to our natural disposition (*fiṭrah*). So we take these five necessities as our starting point and sometimes use the specifics of Islam to elaborate and shed further light on them. So they are a healing and mercy to all of mankind and are universal in their nature. In the case there is something specific to Islam that we think may be of benefit to others, we are happy to present it to them.

Mohammad Ali Al-Bar

How can we apply the four principles to specific cases outside the [cultural and philosophical] settings in which they originated? For example, we have different understandings of autonomy. How can we harmonize ideas from different cultural perspectives? There is difficulty in the connecting or joining of ideas that — while they do agree in many regards — are perhaps not similar enough to the point that they can be linked in the same intellectual pyramid.

Mohammed Ghaly

Of course it is a difficult task, but we need to challenge our [Islamic] scholars in this regard. I think Sheikh Al-Qaradaghi did try in his paper. For example, he placed the principle of autonomy in the scope of one of the higher objectives of Sharia, namely the intellect (*'aql*).

Jasser Auda

I suggest the pyramid be turned into a network because, in my view, the problem with the pyramid is its vertical structuring of ideas. A network, on the other hand, connects ideas across the board, which better reflects the situation here.

Hassan Chamsi-Pasha

Who is the target audience for these principles of medical ethics and bioethics? Are we addressing all doctors around the world or only Muslim doctors as a first phase? I would say we should focus on the Muslim doctors at first because, to be honest, I can tell you as an example that many doctors I have interacted with in Saudi Arabia do not immediately see the significance of the field of medical ethics or do not have a complete understanding of medical ethics.

So it is important we specify our objective. It is no doubt that Islam is a message for all mankind, but I think we have two objectives here. The immediate objective is to reach out to all Muslims doctors and encourage them to become familiar with Islamic knowledge in order to be able to practice their profession in line with the Islamic understanding of their field. Our other aim is to reach out to all of humanity and to all doctors around the world. I do not think that Beauchamp and Childress expected their book would reach a global audience — at the time they wrote it, perhaps they were addressing the American public — but eventually it did.

Tariq Ramadan

My understanding of our purpose here — and more generally at the research Center for Islámic Legislation and Ethics — is to discuss Islamic legislation and ethics from the inside, from an Islamic framework. We are not addressing the West; we are addressing ourselves first, from an Islamic point of reference. After that, we engage in dialogue with the West so that the issues may be understood from an Islamic point of reference. So the question is not who to address; rather, it is about the importance of approaching the issue through an Islamic framework. In so doing, we are not addressing Muslim doctors only; we are also addressing non-Muslim doctors so that they may understand the Islamic point of reference. I would like non-Muslim doctors to read this and realize that within the

Islamic standards and approach to biomedical ethics there exist points of agreement between us.

Hassan Chamsi-Pasha

I agree we should start with ourselves. We should deliver this message to Muslim doctors first since they are the ones most likely to use these rulings in their profession. We need them to be exemplars in the application of Islamic ethics in the medical field — indeed, what we lack is the practical application. I think this is an important part of our objective, and after that the message will spread to the rest of the world.

Ahmed Raissouni

There is not a big difference between addressing Muslims and addressing non-Muslims. Perhaps we would use clarifying terms when addressing the latter, but the core ideas are the same. Regarding structure, the two methods of using a pyramid and using a network are both possible. It is hard to tell now what the structure will end up being; upon formulation it will be clear which structure is most suitable.

Mohammed Ghaly

When Beauchamp and Childress wrote their book about the four principles, they did not read about Islam, although they have studied theology. They studied Christianity and perhaps they knew about Judaism, but I do not think they had much knowledge about Islam, Buddhism, or other religions. As Dr. Beauchamp mentioned and as we discussed in detail, the principles emerged from Western backgrounds and philosophies — Western in their founding, their form, their development, etc. However, this did not to prevent him from putting his ideas out for everybody.

My point is that "universality" does not at all mean separating ourselves from locality and from immersion in tradition. On the contrary: it is this immersion that leads to universality. If the four principles were identical [to what we have], we would have ended our discussions on the first day. In order to get to a point where we can address everyone, we must delve deep into our tradition and heritage so that we can come up with something of an Islamic nature. From this we extract what we believe is universal about it, which we introduce to the world, and then it is up to each person to decide whether or not to embrace it.

I believe the most important goal is to contribute an Islamic perspective. A big concern nowadays in both the East and the West is that we need governing principles in bioethics so that doctors practice their profession ethically because otherwise humanity will be lost. Bioethics is being discussed all around the world, and Islam should have an input. That does not mean rejecting others or simply keeping to ourselves; rather, it means we deeply examine the Islamic tradition in order to create something rooted in the Islamic tradition. Through our religion we know what is universal to humanity and what is exclusive to Islam and Muslims. For example, the ritual acts of worship like prayer and fasting are not expected of those who do not believe in Islam, and likewise certain Islamic rules cannot be generalized to all of humanity. However, other things are indeed universal, so we take from these.

We should start with doctors in the Islamic world as a matter of necessity. The West will be all right if they are not provided with our Islamic biomedical ethics because they already have biomedical ethics. Our biggest duty is towards our doctors because their general understanding of biomedical ethics is lacking in the first place.

Mohammad Ali Al-Bar

In addition, we should remember there are a large number of Muslim doctors in the West.

Mohammed Ghaly

Yes, and there are also many Western doctors in the Muslim world. There are also Muslim patients in the West who interact with doctors there.

Tariq Ramadan

I want to say that there is a big difference between initiating and responding. Are we presenting something, or are we responding to the West? We want the basis for our discussion to be that we are presenting something.

Annelien Bredenoord

Dr. Ramadan, I understand that you want an introduction rather than a response, but it is almost unavoidable that there is some kind of response because you already took notice of concepts developed in other parts of the world. So just a pure introduction without seeing what others have done is not possible. So I think it is some kind of mix.

Tariq Ramadan

It is and at the same time it is not because the whole understanding is different. What we see now with many of the things done by Muslims, especially in ethics, is that we listen to the West and we try to respond by taking and not presenting. My point is that we have a contribution to make. When we say wisdom is the believer's stray camel that he is always searching for (*al-ḥikmah ḍāllat al-mu'min*), wherever he finds it, it becomes his, we are listening and we are taking, but now we have something to give. So we build from within and not with the obsession to respond, which is completely different. This does not mean that we are not listening. We are listening, but it is dangerous for us to simply say that we have the same common principles given that the sources of the two philosophies are completely different. So it is wrong for us to keep on responding. We must listen and respond, but our response is not a response to their questions. It is a response to our questions. It is completely different.

Jasser Auda

If I may add something with regards to the philosophy of the Center, we differentiate between apologetic responses and transformational responses. We do not want to be apologetics or take what others have done and then say that we have the same thing. Rather, if we try to introduce something, then we learn from the essence of the others' philosophies and try to transform reality by introducing new ideas.

Ali Al-Qaradaghi

In regards to responding, the Noble Qur'an teaches us about two key matters. Firstly, it calls everyone to "...a word that is equitable between us and you…" (Qur'an 3:64) or in other words to the shared constants or unchanging principles. There are indeed many shared things among all of humanity, especially in medical ethics. The second thing that the Qur'an asks from us is to rise above. In the verse, "Say, 'O People of the Scripture, come [*ta'ālaw*] to a word that is equitable between us and you…'" (Qur'an 3:64), our scholars interpreted "come" [*ta'ālaw*] to mean "rise above" [the verb *ta'ālaw* can have different meanings depending on the context]. In other words, we should rise to a high level so that we accept from each other and agree with each other on the basic constants.

As Dr. Ramadan said, now we need two things. The first one is to look for the shared constants or seek the shared well-being of all people. The second thing is to rise to a high level in such a way that we do not have partisanship or discrimination.

Mohammed Ghaly

Allow me to summarize the second point so we may move to the third and last point. It is clear that the Islamic conception of formulating biomedical ethics revolves around the higher objectives of Sharia and alongside them the rules, ethics, rulings, and so on. I think this conception can assimilate the four-principle approach as well, perhaps adding to or taking away from it some things. In any case, it is clear that we will be using this conception that is based on the higher objectives.

The third and last point concerns what is next? Sheikh Al-Qaradaghi suggested having another meeting or workshop to further detail the matters we discussed and agree on how to phrase them. I would like to ask you if there are any issues or themes that should be on the agenda or if you have any other recommendations or suggestions regarding next steps.

Ali Al-Qaradaghi

I think now the vision is clear and our task has been narrowed down and specified more precisely. Biomedical ethics have been discussed and studied thoroughly, and there is plenty of great literature on the subject. Our job now is to connect the general principles of biomedical ethics that we have agreed upon to the higher objectives of Sharia. This is one, unified mission. Our goal is to produce a well-organized document that will of course require explanation, detailing, and thereafter linking the contents of the document to the fundamentals [of Islam] (*ta'ṣīl*). For this, I think we need more individuals on board. We need more physicians, Sharia scholars, and scholars of the higher objectives of Sharia.

Mohammed Ali Al-Bar

I am looking forward in the next meeting or workshop to having more of our brothers and sisters from the West or who represent Western philosophy. Dr. Bredenoord's and Dr. Beauchamp's contributions were incredibly informative and enriched the discussions. I am convinced that now we better understand one another. Dr. Beauchamp has heard criticism or reviews from the United States and from Europe; this may have been the first time Dr. Beauchamp also listened to reviews from and discussed with people from Islamic world. We also need to listen to experts of bioethics from the United States, Europe, and elsewhere who have perspectives other than the ones we have heard. Having different perspectives in this field leads to a broader outlook on biomedical ethics and a greater understanding of various topics.

Annelien Bredenoord

I certainly agree with the previous remarks. I think you can see it through in two steps. The first step would be a symposium or a conference in which the principles of Islamic biomedical ethics are formulated and discussed. I would suggest that you already have a document to discuss so that it does not remain abstract but you really have a charter or guidelines or whatever you usually produce. That would be a first kind of meeting during which you together lay things down conceptually. Then in a second meeting you could put these Islamic biomedical ethical principles into practice to see when you start to specify this whether it results in conflicts, whether it is coherent, and whether it needs adjustments. Then I think you should invite many practitioners just to discuss this with them.

You can make a document using the case-based approach. You either take one case and you give comments from different approaches, or you take different cases and you all comment from the same approach. We have a lot of case-based medical ethics textbooks, and it may be useful to see the similarities and differences.

Mohammed Ghaly

Dr. Bredenoord has previously suggested that when the document is produced, physicians should be invited to discuss the cases of ethical dilemmas they have faced. She said that when you do this, sometimes you end up prioritizing one principle and de-prioritizing another because the purpose of these principles is their application. This is similar to what we might call medical *fatwas* or medical unprecedented questions/dilemmas (*nawāzil ṭibbīyah*). She also suggested that after we agree on the principles and finalize the document, we present it at one of the bioethics conferences.

Script of Concluding Discussions: Part One (Day 2: Session 1 and Session 2)

Tariq Ramadan

Our primary purpose here at the research Center for Islamic Legislation and Ethics is to address Muslims and Muslim societies, not to address the West. The West has arrived at principles of biomedical ethics, and we as Muslims living in Muslim countries are in need of a set of universal biomedical ethics produced from an Islamic framework. This is helpful in understanding our goals during this seminar.

Jasser Auda

I agree with Dr. Ramadan and would add that we are in need of this kind of independent reasoning (*ijtihād*) in Islamic thought and in the Muslim world. Through their research, our researchers here at the Center have become deeply aware that there is a need for principles that address the issues surrounding biomedical ethics within Islamic thought because these issues are linked to policy and public interests. We do not deny that Islamic *fiqh* academies have done a great job especially in matters of medicine. Nonetheless, what we need now is not to import policies from other countries whose nature differs from that of Muslim societies in some regards. Rather, we want to add to this discipline and benefit from the wisdom and insights of others so that we may arrive at Islamic values that address policies in Muslim countries in the issues of medicine. This is our goal today.

Mohammed Ali Al-Bar

The issues we have been discussing so far present constant dilemmas for physicians nowadays. Of course the culture of physicians is Western in nature, as medical schools in the Muslim world rely upon the same curricula and philosophies as Western medical schools. However, there is a shift as many [Muslim] doctors are becoming aware of differences in ethical and Islamic legal considerations. Islamic *fiqh* academies have discussed many issues of biomedical ethics, including abortion and organ transplants, both of which are considered potentially ethically problematic. All these attempts have intended to arrive at a system that Muslim doctors could rely on and benefit from. It would be a very effective additional step for Islamic *fiqh* academies to distribute their research studies and *fatwas* on medical ethics to doctors in the Muslim world.

We tend to adopt Western culture in its entirety and simply give its ideas and notions Islamic names. People do so because they find — and accurately so — that notions of autonomy, beneficence, nonmaleficence, and justice are present in Islam as important principles as well. After all, they are notions common to all of humanity. However, many of our colleagues end up adopting these ideas emerging from the West without any modifications or amendments.

Others are critical of this trend of taking Western ideas without amendment. Dr. Abdulaziz Sachedina from the United States wrote a book that put forth a good critique of the subject in which he argued that Islam is different from Western culture in many aspects. He himself is an American Muslim living in the West. In my opinion, his book presented a balanced approach and, although I differ with him on certain details, I am in general agreement with his perspective. He basically stated that we need an Islamic legal foundation for these ethical issues.

I believe that a person's sources for morality are human natural disposition (*fiṭrah*), intellect, and religion. Human natural disposition is a topic Al-Ghazali and many other Islamic philosophers have touched upon. Ethical values are present in the human being's natural disposition, as the Qur'an indicates. God says, "...[Adhere to] the *fiṭrah* of Allah upon which He has created [all] people. No change should there be in the creation of Allah. That is the correct religion..." (Qur'an 30:30).

Ahmed Raissouni

The phrase, "that is the correct religion," indicates that this natural disposition was importantly reemphasized in religion and that there is a link between the natural disposition and religion.

Mohammed Ali Al-Bar

Yes, that is an important point.

The second source of morality is the intellect (*'aql*), to which Islam and the Qur'an pay a great deal of attention. Islam focuses on the fact that one cannot arrive at the truth without using reason and that faith or belief emerges through reason. We find many instances of verses in the Qur'an that ask, "Then will you not reason?" or "Then will you not see?" or "Then will you not give thought?", to mention few. The intellect is fundamental to arriving at the truth, whether it is ethical truth, truths about the universe, or religious truth.

Both human natural disposition and the intellect can be inhibited or distorted by a person's whims and desires. God says, "...Pharaoh said, 'I do not show you except what I see, and I do not guide you except to the way of right conduct'" (Qur'an 40:29), though Pharaoh was one of the most corrupt tyrants in history. Arrogance is the most significant example of human whims that distort sound intellect, and it is at the core of immorality. Arrogance is what caused Satan (*Iblīs*) to be expelled from Paradise: "[Satan] said, 'I am better than him [Adam]'" (Qur'an 7:12). This is why Islam focuses on purification of the soul, saving it from the shackles of arrogance, and directing it towards humility, which are essential concepts in Islamic ethics in general.

The third source of morality is religion (*dīn*), which provides needed direction and guidance since any two people's intellects will inevitably differ on some details of what is right and wrong. Of course, there are still many points of agreement: honesty is deemed good and dishonesty is deemed bad by everyone and in all religions, for example. However, there are some behaviors that all religions used to prohibit in the past but that are widely accepted by, and practiced in, societies nowadays. In other words, there is a shift in ideas, concepts, and behaviors. So my point is, because of this shift, we need an established, unchanging reference, and authority. That is religion.

In essence, there has always been one religion for us, Islam. I do not mean by that the Islam that we belong to. Rather, I mean the state of submission (*islām*) in which all human begins should submit to one God. Despite the different prophets that have been sent, they all basically preached one message, which is the oneness of God. Prophet Muhammad (PBUH) emphasized that all the prophets — including Abraham, Moses, and Jesus, peace be upon them all — are messengers of the same God.

Therefore, we need to distinguish between what is pure religion — namely, that which was revealed to mankind at different stages of their history — and the deviations that impacted these religions at the hands of human beings. For example, in the West now there exist two important philosophies, one of which is utilitarianism that can be traced back to Greek history but was more recently developed by Thomas Hobbes and other philosophers, including Jeremy Bentham. According to Bentham's description of this philosophy, if arresting and torturing a group of children belonging to our enemy will make our enemy surrender to us, then there is no ethical problem with this. Similarly, if permitting usury is in the interest of a group of people, then it is also permitted.

As an example, a study showed that if a person smokes 20 cigarettes a day for 30–40 years he would lose about 5–7 years of his life. Rothmans [Rothmans, Benson, & Hedges], the cigarette company, conducted a research study in Czechoslovakia. The study stated that people who died at the age of 70 rather than at the age of 65 would have spent those extra years retired, and the state would be required to support them financially.

They argued that if more people died at the age of 65, the state would save a lot of money since it would no longer need to support those who continued living. Hence, they claimed that smoking is important because it saves the state money and is beneficial for hospitals, insurance companies, and other similar organizations. This is a very clear example of the utilitarian philosophy, which still affects us today.

The second philosophy, that of Immanuel Kant, developed what we call "deontology" or the "philosophy of duty." He did not recognize doing actions to gain God's acceptance and pleasure. He argued that actions should emerge exclusively from a sense of duty. In other words, if a person acts in order for society or God to reward him, Kant considered his act to be unethical. Moreover, Kant believed unconditionally that truth is a virtue and lying is a vice, so much so that even if it led to the killing of an innocent person, one should not lie. For example, at the time of Nazi Germany many Jewish people escaped to Morocco from the oppression in Europe. When the Nazis arrived in Morocco they used to inspect houses, searching for Jewish people. As a result, the Muslim families there would hide their Jewish neighbors despite knowing that the penalty for this was death. When the Nazis would ask a Muslim family where their Jewish neighbor was, they used to lie since in Islam this would not be considered sinful. Although telling a lie is not virtuous, saving the life of an innocent human being is more important and in such a case one cannot claim the duty to tell the truth is an excuse for surrendering a Jewish neighbor to the Nazis.

Kant also regarded keeping promises as essential. If, for instance, I told my children that we would go on a picnic on a certain day and on that day their mother fell ill, I would have a dilemma. One duty would be to keep my promise to my children and take them on a picnic, and the other duty would be to their mother, to care for her when she falls ill. According to Kant, given that you promised your children to take them on a picnic, you should forget about anything else. Is this really logical? In my opinion, this kind of thinking lacks balance. Needless to say, being truthful and keeping promises are undoubtedly important traits. However, ultimately, it should be a question of balancing between issues depending on each one's weight. These situations are often perceived as dilemmas although they are not actually dilemmas. From my perspective, there is no dilemma in these cases and the issues are clear.

It goes without saying that there are other philosophies and many different schools of thought, but these are the ones I focused on.

Mohammed Ghaly

As Sheikh Al-Qaradaghi mentioned earlier, putting forth an Islamic alternative in the field of biomedical ethics is considered a new idea in Islamic thought. There have been many deep, thorough discussions in Islamic *fiqh* academies that were mostly focusing on details and specifics like organ donation, cloning, and abortion. However, there have not been enough analysis on and discussion about the [broader] ethical principles in biomedicine.

Sheikh Abu Ghuddah wrote a research paper a while ago entitled "Sharia-Based Principles for the Profession of Medicine and Medical Treatment" (*Al-mabādi' al-shar'īyah lil-taṭbīb wal-'ilāj*) in which he included what he also mentioned in his chapter for this seminar: it is incumbent on the physician, just like any other professional, to know the religious rulings related to his or her profession. In his earlier paper, Sheikh Abu Ghuddah clarified that since it is not reasonable to expect of every physician to know every detail surrounding religious rulings on medical practice, physicians are excused from knowing the details. His reconciliation was that physicians should know the [religious] principles related to medicine and apply them to specific cases using their own understanding and logic.

I think the first book on the principles of biomedical ethics coming from Western thought was published in the late 1970's, and it has now in 2013 reached the seventh edition. It is clear the West has more experience with biomedical ethical principles than we do in the Muslim world. Muslim physicians in the Muslim world and elsewhere already deal with these principles in one way or another, so they are in need of knowing whether these principles are compatible with Islamic teachings. Of greater importance is that Islam should have its own say in this field. Perhaps the theory of the higher objectives of Sharia can provide a solution, as Sheikh Al-Qaradaghi has suggested, because it starts from an Islamic framework and at the same time can accommodate what has come before. Sheikh Raissouni spoke about the fundamental ethics (*ummahāt al-akhlāq*) as a possible entry point for this topic. These starting points are all important, as they could help us to introduce biomedical ethical principles rooted in the Islamic tradition.

Ali Al-Qaradaghi

There are general principles — or what we can call fundamental ethics (*ummahāt al-akhlāq*) — that we can organize and structure. We want this organization and the connections therein to be well defined, not vague. In addition, standards or criteria are critically important. I understand the concept of standards through the term *al-mīzān* (scale or balance) in God Almighty's verse, "We have already sent Our messengers with clear evidences and sent down with them the Scripture and the balance [*al-mīzān*] that the people may maintain [their affairs] in justice..." (Qur'an 57:25). God did not say "the Scripture" alone; rather, He said, "the Scripture and the balance [*al-mīzān*]." In other words, it is necessary that with the Scripture comes the balance [*al-mīzān*] that informs how the Scripture should be applied.

Another important issue I mentioned in my chapter is linking the principles of biomedical ethics with the higher objectives of Sharia. If this initial idea or premise is accepted, then my chapter is open to improvements through feedback from everyone so that we may arrive at a complete and comprehensive product with legal, technical terminology that can be presented to physicians and others.

Some universities require their medical students to take a core course. At my university, this course uses the book I coauthored with Dr. Ali Al-Muhammadi, *Jurisprudence of Contemporary Medical Issues* (*Fiqh al-qaḍāyā al-ṭibbīyah al-mu'āṣirah*). It discusses various medical issues, including cardiopulmonary resuscitation (CPR) devices, DNA profiling, artificial insemination, and many other issues.

Abdul Sattar Abu Ghuddah

I would like to emphasize what was discussed previously: these principles apply to all fields, such as politics, education, economics, and so on, as much as they do to medicine. I hope each of us keeps this point in mind and extracts from the principles what he or she finds especially relevant to the medical field.

Jasser Auda

I agree with Sheikh Abu Ghuddah. Here at the Faculty of Islamic Studies, in the Department of Public Policy, we teach a course entitled "The Higher Objectives of Sharia [as a Basis] for Making Public Policy." Just like every example of public policy has a certain philosophical basis, how can the higher objectives of Sharia form that philosophical basis for making public policy? The philosophical basis here includes what gets prioritized, what themes the policy fits under, and other matters.

One element I would like to highlight is inserting and incorporating the system of Islamic legal maxims or juristic rules into the framework of the higher objectives of Sharia. In his chapter, Sheikh Al-Qaradaghi applied the rules of *tarjīḥ* (giving preference to one opinion over another) we normally apply in Islamic law — such as eliminating hardship, avoiding evil, choosing the lesser of the two evils, etc. — to the traditional set of higher objectives of Sharia. It is an added philosophical complexity but a necessary one because the philosophies that deal with such a subject consist of both principles and ways of dealing with complications and contradictions. The inclusion of the juristic rules makes the picture complete.

Mohammed Ghaly

Incidentally, the four-principle approach is very similar in that it places four relatively simple principles at high levels and then classifies issues under these principles. For example, informed consent is classified under the principle of autonomy. As for the application of these broad principles to specific cases, one can choose to go from the bottom up or from the top down. Also, as was mentioned before, it is essential for physicians to have some criteria or standards of measurement when applying ethics because otherwise decisions will be arbitrary and can be based on personal whims.

Annelien Bredenoord

One of the questions was about whether there are universal principles in bioethics or whether the four principles are universal. If there indeed are universal principles, how do they relate to religious principles (regardless of which religion they belong to)? Dr. Al-Bar said that ideas, concepts, and morals change across societies and over time so we need durable terms of reference that do not change, or at least do not change as fast as society might change. Dr. Al-Bar said that for him, that is religion — in this case, the Islamic religion — but in the end he said that he perceives all religions to be one and the same.

Mohammed Ali Al-Bar

In their origin.

Annelien Bredenoord

Yes, in their origin. If we want common principles in bioethics, then we need a common reference point — and I think this is also what Beauchamp and Childress meant — so the question is: Could this be formulated using religious language? Since two-thirds of the world is religious and one-third is not, how do we formulate the bioethical principles, given that we do not share the same moral and religious language? I would be interested in hearing your comments because I think we need to formulate them in a language that is acceptable to everybody, and it cannot be one particular religion because we do not all share it.

Another question I had about the higher objectives of Sharia is how they relate to the four principles. Can they be included or can we add them to the four principles? I am curious; maybe they are different, but maybe we are talking about the same thing.

Tariq Ramadan

I have a question [for Dr. Al-Qaradaghi]. When you mentioned that the principle of autonomy could be included under the higher objective of

Sharia related to the preservation of the intellect, were you saying that the principle of autonomy is a principle or a fundamental (*'aṣl*)? Or were you saying the principle of autonomy can itself be counted as one of the higher objectives of Sharia?

Ali Al-Qaradaghi

The preservation of the intellect consists of two aspects, positive and negative obligations. The positive or proactive aspect entails developing the mind and providing it freedom. Among the necessities of Sharia (*al-ḍarūrīyāt al-shar'īyah*) is that we protect the intellect and its freedom, creativity, and development. The negative or protective aspect entails preventing the intellect from harm of any kind.

God says, "And Allah presents an example of two men, one of them dumb and unable to do a thing, while he is a burden to his guardian. Wherever he directs him, he brings no good. Is he equal to one who commands justice, while he is on a straight path?" (Qur'an 16:76). God likens the person who chooses to be entirely dependent on his guardian to a person in whom there is no good. All scholars agree that independence and freedom of thought are fundamental to the positive side of the preservation of the intellect.

Tariq Ramadan

My question is about this: Is it a principle or a fundamental (*'aṣl*)?

Ali Al-Qaradaghi

Preservation of the intellect is a principle. If we adopt a hierarchical model, then we could consider it a general principle.

With regard to Dr. Bredenoord's question about religion, we mean by "religion" anything a person chooses to follow, whether it is truth or falsehood. Islam protects, defends, and fights for freedom of religion, even if we consider the particular religion someone chooses to be false. The first verse to be revealed concerning the protection of [the practice of] religions of all kinds is God's saying,

> Permission [to fight] has been given to those who are being fought, because they were wronged. And indeed, Allah is competent to give them victory. [They are] those who have been evicted from their homes without right — only because they say, "Our Lord is Allah." And were it not that Allah checks the people, some by means of others, there would have been demolished monasteries, churches, synagogues, and mosques in which the name of Allah is much mentioned… (Qur'an 22:39–40).

These verses are referring to all [kinds of] places of worship. This is why we mean by "the higher objective of preservation of religion" that we are not allowed to demean or belittle any religion. We must respect the creeds and beliefs of others. My personal estimation and perception of a person's religion and the ruling regarding whether it is true or false is another matter altogether. Therefore, when we use the word "religion," it should be understood to mean all religions.

In conclusion, I will say that we embrace the four principles and include them in our discussions involving the higher objectives of Sharia. If the four principles are good, useful, acceptable principles that benefit humanity, then why not make use of them? As we know from a famous Prophetic narration, wisdom is the believer's stray camel that he is always searching for (*al-ḥikmah ḍāllat al-mu'min*). Sheikh Al-Tantawi used to point out that the use of the word *ḍāllah* [literally, object or goal of persistent search or pursuit] implies that Muslims fell short in their duty to produce this knowledge or wisdom. So when someone else gets it before, it becomes the Muslims' *ḍāllah* (stray camel), and the least they can do is take it and benefit from it. So I hope we do indeed include the four principles in our discussions involving the higher objectives of Sharia.

Mohammed Ghaly

Throughout this seminar, we have been focusing on two main questions:

(1) What are the Islamic principles in the field of biomedical ethics?
(2) Are the four principles of biomedical ethics from the West universal?

Before we delve into the details of your comments on these two questions, I would like to say a few things about the issue of the search for the principles and fundamentals (*uṣūl*). Early Islamic scholars wrote about the fundamentals of ethics (*uṣūl al-akhlāq*), and Sheikh Raissouni mentioned them in his chapter when he discussed the fundamentals of noble ethics (*ummahāt makārim al-akhlāq*). The philosopher Ibn Miskawayh identified four items that he considered to be the fundamentals of ethics. They are wisdom, chastity, courage, and justice. This classification was the result of intercultural interaction with Greek philosophers, who studied the same issue.

Among the philosophers who mentioned these ethics was Socrates, who said that ethics depends on knowing the good and the evil of acts and that these four are the fundamental noble ethics. Muslim scholars, including Al-Ghazali and Ibn Miskawayh, expanded and elaborated upon these four principles by developing an Islamic foundation for them. They asked a question of utmost importance, and we asked Dr. Beauchamp the same question but he did not give a definite answer. The question was about the mechanisms through which these four principles were arrived at and on what philosophical reasoning or basis they were chosen.

When Islamic scholars took these four principles, they established mechanisms of interpretation. They said the human possesses three main powers: the first is the power of comprehension, perception, cognition, and understanding things; the second is the power to achieve what is good and beneficial to oneself; and the third is to obstruct that which is harmful and could include the power of anger, which is sometimes needed to obstruct harm. They said the first, power of comprehension, brings about knowledge or wisdom; the second brings about chastity; the third brings about courage; and balancing the three leads to justice, the fourth principle.

So they did establish philosophical reasoning for these principles. However, they also said that these four principles are not enough because they only have to do with a person's dealings with other creatures. There should be a fifth principle, servitude [to the Creator] (*'ubūdīyah*) that will govern man's relationship with his Creator, God. This is a historical example of the search for the principles and fundamentals of ethics. It involved intercultural interaction between the Islamic philosophy and

Greek philosophy. We should look at how Muslims dealt with Greek philosophy when they encountered it: they adopted some of it, changed some of it, and added to it. They also provided the basis or the mechanisms through which these four (or later, five) principles were arrived at. The parallels between then and now are clear. Our situation today is that there are four principles that are widespread and have reached Muslim doctors present in the Muslim world and elsewhere. It is incumbent that Islam interacts with them.

The first main question that we have been busy with during this seminar reads: what are the Islamic principles in the field of biomedical ethics? In addition to addressing this question, we also need to detail the mechanisms through which we will find or derive these principles. This is because, as Sheikh Raissouni mentioned in his chapter, the ethical values in Islam are numerous, and they are divided, subdivided, and branched. We could count hundreds or thousands, and it is unrealistic to expect a doctor to know them all. Thus, doctors need broad principles and fundamentals to make it easy for them. What are the mechanisms in our Islamic tradition that can help us formulate these principles?

Sheikh Raissouni suggested searching for the fundamental ethics as a mechanism for formulating these principles. He reviewed the work of Dr. Muhammad Abdullah Diraz, and he ultimately arrived at the two main ethics; mercy and God-consciousness (*taqwá*). His mechanism was as such: he researched the ethics and from the ethics arrived at the fundamental ethics and from the fundamental ethics arrived at what is relevant to the medical field. He was adamant and determined to find things of direct relevance to the medical field; he was not concerned with generalities. Sheikh Al-Qaradaghi, on the other hand, found the theory of the higher objectives of Sharia appropriate for two reasons. First, it has strong roots in the Islamic tradition and thus does not raise philosophical or religious complications. Second, it can accommodate the four principles and accept what is acceptable and reject what is not.

To summarize, the first question was: What is the ideal mechanism to use to arrive at the principles, and then what are these principles as derived through this mechanism? The second is similar to a question Al-Ghazali and Ibn Miskawayh dealt with: What is the Islamic contribution with regards to the current Western principles that have become widespread globally? It seems that Dr. Al-Bar has something to say about this particular question.

Mohammed Ali Al-Bar

The four principles were met with wide acceptance, although it was not universal acceptance. Even in the United States a group of well-known scholars had objections to these principles and preferred other ways of classifying or organizing [biomedical ethics]. Perhaps Dr. Bredenoord can provide us with more information on the Western perspective regarding these four principles.

Two of these four principles, namely beneficence and nonmaleficence, can be traced back to the days of Hippocrates. They are included in all medical codes, including those adopted by Ibn Abi Usaybi'ah, Dr. Hassan Hathout, and the Islamic Organization for Medical Sciences. There is no need for much discussion on beneficence and nonmaleficence, as they have been well established and agreed upon for over 2,000 years.

The recent additions are the principles of justice and autonomy. Nobody disagrees with justice in principle. However, unlike previous times, medicine is no longer confined to the doctor–patient relationship. Today, there are ministries of health and large companies that play important roles in our understanding of medicine. Medicine encompasses aspects such as general health services in countries where citizens have no access to medical treatment. It also includes prevention, health polices, and so on. Changes in our understanding of medicine have necessitated incorporating notions of justice and equality to ensure everyone is treated equitably.

Sheikh Abu Ghuddah clarified for us how the Islamic world upheld justice. The government would make sure that free medical services were available and accessible, even in prisons and distant villages. Sometimes the Muslim ruler would even send a team of physicians to a different nation if he heard of an epidemic happening there.

Now I will move on to the principle of autonomy. In earlier days, Hippocrates and those following his school of thought encouraged physicians to treat their patients as their own children. When a father or mother deals with their child, they do not always take the child's opinion; instead, they do what they know is in their child's best interest. Some call this paternalism. A countering philosophy, liberal capitalism, was spreading in the United States in the 1970s, when Beauchamp and Childress published their book. This philosophy questioned the notion that an authority such as a parent or doctor should impose his or her will on others and instead emphasized personal freedom and autonomy. In medicine, this meant that the patient's opinion was deemed more and more important.

The concept of autonomy existed in Islamic law very early on. Over 1,200 years ago, 'Abd Al-Malik bin Habib stated in his book on Prophetic medicine that a physician should take two permissions [to practice]: that of the government [through obtaining licensure] and that of the patient or the patient's guardian. Sheikh Al-Qaradaghi referenced the case in which the Prophet (PBUH) refused medicine forcefully administered to him. Similar occurrences that happened to others during the Prophet's (PBUH) lifetime showed clearly the importance of obtaining a patient's consent before treatment. Numerous Muslim jurists — including Ibn Al-Qayyim, Al-Ghazali, Ahmad, and others — wrote about these issues in detail, often differing on certain details. So the question of a patient's autonomy is not new to Muslims; on the contrary, there is a long history of discussion about it. However, we differ with the West about the extent of personal freedom a patient has in making medical requests in some sensitive issues like sex change and abortion.

Tunisia has now adopted the Western principles concerning abortion, without limitations or conditions that consider important factors such as the age of the fetus. A woman can go to a doctor and ask for an abortion without having any medical reason to do so. Arab countries should place conditions on aborting a child, such as the presence of medical reasons or because the pregnancy was the result of incest or rape. Although a doctor has the right to refuse to abort a woman's child, he is expected to refer her to another doctor. He does not have the right to advise a woman that abortion is right or wrong. In doing so, a doctor would have departed from [the accepted standards in] the medical field. Such a doctor would be considered paternalistic, and paternalism nowadays has become almost like a crime! It would not be unusual for such a doctor to be prevented from practicing or to be penalized in some way.

Mohammed Ghaly

Dr. Al-Bar said that beneficence and nonmaleficence are undisputed, and therefore we can consider them to be universal. He mentioned that injustices started happening because of the changes in the medical landscape, and justice was thus introduced as a principle. Sometimes a principle is formulated for the purpose of fighting an ill in society. So as we formulate biomedical ethical principles using the Islamic framework, we should take into consideration the reality of the Muslim world today. For example, the West may have the problem of equal access to medical care while the Muslim world has other problems to overcome, hypothetically speaking. Physicians are perhaps in a better position to give us examples of problems they see so that our Islamic scholars can tell us which principles to establish in order to address these problems.

The principle of justice was also introduced because of changes that made the field of medicine broader than the doctor–patient relationship. In addition, the liberal political theory inevitably had an effect on the discussions about the patient's autonomy. However, it seems there remains some confusion about the distinction between the question of patient consent and the wider issue of autonomy. Does the issue of consent fall under autonomy, or is it a synonym of autonomy? We need further explanation of the distinction between informed consent and autonomy and the relationship between them. In Islam we have no problem with the principle of consent, but we disagree on the extent to which we accept a patient's informed consent. According to the Western principle of autonomy, there are almost no limits because if the patient wants and agrees to a certain procedure the doctor should provide this service given that financial ability and other necessary resources are available. This has been a point of contention in laws in various countries.

If Dr. Bredenoord would like, perhaps she can add something in regards to the relationship between the principle of autonomy and informed consent. In addition, she may be able to comment on the question of autonomy being limited: Is autonomy limited/restricted only because of financial and logistical reasons, or is there also an ethical dimension to it?

Annelien Bredenoord

Before I discuss autonomy, what strikes me is that the two principles of beneficence and nonmaleficence are shared by everyone and are uncontested. I think this is logical given that these two principles date back to the Hippocratic tradition — the Greek source that we all share — whereas the other values, autonomy and justice, are relatively new values. Autonomy and justice were only introduced in Western medical ethics in the 1970s, so it is logical that our discussion focuses on these two values. In addition, within Western bioethics, these are the most contested values. The debates in Western bioethics are about the fitting in of justice and the fitting in of autonomy. I think everybody accepts the principles but differs on how to interpret them.

It goes without saying that everybody accepts the formal principle of justice. We agree that we should have procedures for justice such as *equals must be treated equally* and *unequals must be treated unequally for as far as they are unequal*. In other words, the formal part we all agree on. The material part of justice, the substantive accounts, is where we have huge political debates. This is because we have to decide on what justifies making a distinction between people. We have liberal theories, egalitarian theories, the Amartya Sen Capability Approach, and so on. So yes, we accept the formal principle of justice but then we do not go beyond that. Even within the egalitarian theory, for example, it may be illustrative to read the report by the World Health Organization. They issued an ethical report on what happens in the case of a pandemic, how vaccinations should be distributed, and how to allocate who gets what in situations where the vaccination [supply] is insufficient. They make a type of egalitarian account, where they provide the vaccination to adolescents, young people, and health workers while the elderly and a few other groups do not receive it. Basically, they make a decision and they have a good ethical base for it. This is a good example of how they perceive justice.

In regards to autonomy, I think it is very important to make a distinction between positive obligations and negative obligations, or positive autonomy and negative autonomy. Once again, everybody accepts negative autonomy, which refers to the right to non-interference. I will give an example from reproduction. In the European Charter of Human Rights we have negative reproductive autonomy. This means that a woman cannot be forcefully sterilized and cannot be forced to have an abortion. That is the right to be left alone and is quite uncontroversial universally.

On the other hand, there is the positive autonomy right, which refers to the right to ask for something. For example, there is the right to start a family and ask for *in vitro* fertilization (IVF) or assisted reproduction and, in fact, there is debate about this topic. It is not true that autonomy is limitless. In my opinion, negative autonomy is limitless whereas positive autonomy has many limits. These limits can be associated with issues of justice, harm to others, etc. So autonomy is a very thick concept, and we should avoid saying "autonomy" without making the distinction between positive and negative whenever it is discussed. This similarly applies to the topic of assisted death. If a patient asks a physician for euthanasia, this raises the question of positive autonomy. For example, in the Netherlands it is not obligatory for a physician to help somebody with dying. It is something you grant to a patient, but it is not something that you have to do. This highlights that there are several examples where we can distinguish between positive and negative rights.

Moving on to the question about the relationship between autonomy and informed consent, I think informed consent could be seen as an operationalization of autonomy. The principle of respect for autonomy requires you to provide information, which is the informed part, and also requires you to ask for consent — or informed refusal of treatment. In other words, autonomy is the foundation or the cornerstone, and informed consent is one of the practical operationalizations. In research ethics, informed consent was particularly emphasized in the Nuremberg Code after the Second World War. Informed consent had two main functions in this international code. The first function was respect for autonomy and the second had a protective rationale. If you as a physician want to conduct research, you have to ask if the person allows you to perform medical experiments [on him or her]. Such a person is better protected than when the physician does not have to ask. So the basis of informed consent is both protection and autonomy.

Hassan Chamsi-Pasha

I would like to add several remarks to the points raised by Dr. Al-Bar. Medicine has become a sort of trade and the doctor is viewed as a kind of service provider. Patients are perceived as clients. This can be found in many countries across the world and is also true of the companies that regulate hospitals like ISO and others. This concept is inimical to the field of medicine and to the doctor–patient relationship. Doctors as service providers compete for the clients or customers, and the result is a commercial mentality.

The second point I would like to address is the mistakes committed by doctors. We read in newspapers everyday about doctors and hospitals without any ethics, and a few weeks ago a hospital in Saudi Arabia was made to close for 2 months due to a medical mistake that had taken place. Any patient in many of the Gulf Cooperation Council (GCC) countries can place a complaint against a doctor after the doctor has treated him or her. The doctor's passport gets confiscated for 2, 3, or even 5 years until the court proceedings are completed. In the end, if the judge reaches a final decision that the doctor was not at fault, the doctor does not receive any compensation for the adversity he has gone through. This is a reality I have witnessed myself. Any person can write a letter — one letter is all that is needed — to place a complaint against the doctor. In the end it is the doctor's dignity and reputation that receive a great deal of harm. These processes must be regulated, as it is unacceptable for these types of things to take place in the medical field.

I would also like to make a comment about drug companies. These companies exert a great deal of pressure on doctors. Previously we were discussing statins, which help reduce cholesterol levels in the blood. There are several drugs of this type produced by different companies that vary in their strength and effectiveness but have comparable prices. The drug companies play an active role in directing the doctor to prescribe one drug instead of another. There needs to be a focus on the ethical aspect in this matter. How can we direct the doctor to do what is ethical in such situations?

This also applies to blood pressure medication. There are five main groups of such medication, and in each group there are several different medicines from which, according to international medical guidelines, a physician is given the liberty to choose. However, not all medicines have the same strength and effectiveness, and they have different side effects and associated complications. Hence, controls must be put in place to regulate a doctor's choice of medicine, especially as it relates to the pressure exerted on him or her by these companies. Of course, a doctor cannot be directly accused of doing anything wrong by choosing one medicine and not another. However, he or she could hypothetically choose a medicine even if it is not in the interest and benefit of the patient.

The final point I would like to refer to is the importance of focusing on preventative medicine and health education. It is one of the most important aspects of medicine, and it is not at all costly. God stated, "...and eat and drink, but be not excessive..." (Qur'an 7:31). The fields of health and nutrition are summarized in part of a Qur'anic verse. Nowadays, international guidelines encourage trying to lose weight, reducing the amount of food we consume, practicing sports, etc. Unfortunately, doctors nowadays do not spend enough time talking to their patients about taking preventative measures. We establish many health centers and cardiovascular clinics but are negligent about the preventative side of medicine.

Ahmed Raissouni

Dr. Bredenoord posed a question to Sheikh Al-Qaradaghi on how we can rely on the higher objectives of Sharia without imposing one religion, namely Islam. I would like to clarify that the higher objectives of Sharia, especially the five necessities identified by Sheikh Al-Qaradaghi and other religious scholars, are likely common to all world religions and religioethical frameworks, not just Islam. We should call them "the higher objectives of Sharias," by using "Sharia" in the plural form.

I have not consulted all other religions' views on the matter, so I cannot guarantee that the five necessities (the preservation of religion, life, offspring, the intellect, and wealth) are agreed upon by all religions. However, my point is that we can in principle identify what the higher objectives of other religions are, add them to the ones in Islam, have all higher objectives "interact" with one another, and choose from the mixture what we can call "the higher objectives of religions." As mentioned earlier, two-thirds of the world's population is religious, so it would be beneficial to identify the higher objectives that are common across all religions and adopt them or build upon them as needed.

Dr. Al-Bar's comments on autonomy as they relate to matters such as sex change, abortion, and euthanasia compelled me to consider some questions. What is medicine? What purposes does it serve? As Dr. Chamsi-Pasha asked, is medicine a business or trade? A physician has medical skills and can use those skills as he or she wishes. Will the physician use them to serve whoever can pay, regardless of what the payer asks for, as if they are engaged in business? If this indeed were medicine, then euthanasia would be accepted; any physician could easily put an end to suffering through injections or medications. A physician could change a person's gender for $10,000 or help a woman have an abortion, even when she is 8-months pregnant since these are skills the physician has similar to any other skill possessed by others. Similarly, people who know how to make a bomb could make bombs and sell them to other people simply because they possess the know-how.

What is the definition of medicine? Since many ethical issues depend on it, we need to know whether there is a universal, agreed-upon definition of medicine and whether there is universal agreement about its purposes. Is medicine a set of skills learned by the physician that he has the right to make money from as he wishes? Or is it a profession? The layman definition is that the physician treats illness. So whatever is not an illness does not require intervention by the physician. If a woman is due to give birth in a few weeks and the pregnancy is not harming her, then where is the illness that requires medical intervention? I would like to ask the physicians here especially: Is there a specific definition of medicine, its role, and its boundaries? Knowing its boundaries is especially important because many [ethical] violations — whether in business, religion, or any other field — transpire because of stepping outside the boundaries of the field.

Regarding the formulation of principles, I reiterate that we should deal with issues most relevant to medicine and medical practice and applicable to all times and places. In my opinion, we must include as the preface to the universal principles of biomedical ethics the sanctity of human life and its equal right to be protected. The principle of protecting human life may solve many challenges we come across. When a physician deals with a patient, he is dealing with a human soul, which is sanctified in all religions. God says, "Because of that, We decreed upon the Children of Israel that whoever kills a soul unless for a soul or for corruption [done] in the land — it is as if he had slain mankind entirely. And whoever saves one — it is as if he had saved mankind entirely..." (Qur'an 5:32). God expresses that this rule was initially directed at the Jews, while He is addressing Muslims. This indicates that the rule applies across time.

A physician should remember that human beings enjoy a sanctity that must be preserved, and we are all equal as far as this trait is concerned. Whether rich, poor, man, woman, young, old, princes, ministers, Muslims, non-Muslims, atheists, etc. we are to deal with all human souls equally with respect to their right to be protected. God says, "And We have certainly honored the children of Adam..." (Qur'an 17:70). In this verse God mentions the children of Adam [collectively]; being Muslim or non-Muslim is a separate matter.

The second point I would like to address is human dignity. Unfortunately in some hospitals, patients are not always treated with dignity during operations, treatments, and examinations. The physician should remember he is not dealing with merely a physical body. This body enjoys God-given sanctity and dignity. Thus, the sanctity of human life and respect for human dignity are two principles that could be considered as additions to the principles.

As for God-consciousness, which was discussed at length previously, its particularities are specific to each religion yet the concept exists in all religions. While we could try to bring out the shared notions, it may actually be that each religion has its own distinctive definition. In addition, I mentioned the concept of mercy earlier as being crucial given the nature of the medical profession and the delicacy of patients' privacy and confidentiality. If governments, ministries of health, pharmaceutical companies, and other involved entities are not merciful, they may easily find themselves operating materialistically and inhumanely and taking advantage of patients. Mercy is essential in all fields but is particularly pertinent to the medical profession.

Abdul Sattar Abu Ghuddah

I would like to reiterate that mercy killing is banned in Islam — not only for human begins but also for animals. Historically, when a horse was deemed incapable of moving, he was killed. However, in Islamic history we find an endowment that was created for disabled horses to be taken to a grazing land so they could eat and drink until they [naturally] died. In his book *Some Glorious Aspects of Our Civilization* (*Min rawā'i' ḥaḍāratina*), Dr. Mustafa Al-Siba'i described an endowment created for mutilated or disabled horses. Muslims strove to protect and preserve the sanctity of both human and animal life.

I do not know if this is the case for the four principles, but for the higher objectives of Sharia, all of them should be adopted together. We cannot activate some higher objectives and exclude others. Also, the higher objectives should serve to restrict one another. In other words, we cannot take the preservation of life and ignore the preservation of the intellect or the preservation of wealth. They have to be adopted together because they complement one another.

Also, the higher objectives of Sharia have their own hierarchy: the preservation of religion, then life, and so on, and this is significant. For example, it might be said that capital punishment as a result of equitable punishment (*qiṣāṣ*) [for homicide] or as a result of highway robbery (*ḥirābah* or *qāṭi' al-ṭarīq*) is counter to the preservation of life. However, we say that the preservation of religion takes precedence over the preservation of life.

Mohammed Ghaly

Do scholars agree upon the ordering of the higher objectives of Sharia, or are there differences of opinion about it?

Ahmed Raissouni

Differences of opinion exist only about the preservation of offspring and the preservation of the intellect. Al-Ghazali and his followers ranked the preservation of the intellect higher than the preservation of offspring.

However, Al-Amidi and his followers ranked the preservation of offspring above the preservation of the intellect because they considered the intellect to be part of both offspring and life. Scholars agreed that the preservation of religion comes first, the preservation of life second, and the preservation of wealth takes the fifth position. They only disagreed about the order of the third and fourth, which are the preservation of the intellect and offspring, but this is merely a theoretical debate and does not have practical consequences.

Jasser Auda

Al-Amidi disagreed with the very idea of ordering the higher objectives of Sharia. He cited the Prophetic narration stating that whoever is killed defending his wealth is considered a martyr and whoever is killed defending his honor (*'irḍ*) is considered a martyr.[1] The order mentioned in this narration differs from what is mentioned elsewhere. Thus, there are differing opinions as to whether the objectives can be ordered in principle and, if they can be ordered, how.

As for the chapter of Sheikh Al-Qaradaghi, I believe we have to address the kind of mechanism adopted there. The mechanism utilized in Western philosophy is very different from the mechanism we adopt in Islamic Sharia as far as higher objectives are concerned. The mechanism in Western philosophy goes back to Greek philosophy. The philosopher would look at a number of virtues and try to put them in order. He would talk about the core virtues first and then about the virtues that branched out of the core virtues. So the core virtues became what can be considered the principles or the main virtues.

In Islam, when we approach the higher objectives of Sharia, the employed mechanism is *istiqrā'*, which involves induction based on consulting the Qur'an or scriptural texts rather than depending on a self-made list of virtues as the Greeks did. This method depends on the scriptural texts, the components or details of the religious texts, and the comprehensive ideas included in these texts. When discussing the higher objectives, Al-Shatibi started his discussion with the method of *istiqrā'* and made it

[1] Al-Bukhari, *Al-Madhalim wal-ghadab* (no. 2470), on the authority of Abdullah bin 'Amr.

an integral part of his theory. From his perspective, reviewing related religious texts would enable us to extract the main objectives, which of course is different from the methods used by Greek philosophers.

Nevertheless, the search for higher objectives is something common to both Muslims and non-Muslims. Nowadays, those who examine the higher objectives and purposes in the other religions do so under the name "studies of systematic theology." They examine the Torah and the Bible in order to see what higher objectives they can infer from the legal laws they take from the Scripture. This systematic method leads to a system of higher objectives similar to what we have in Islam, with the exception of the preservation of religion. In my research on the studies conducted by systematic theologians I have not found any mention of the preservation of religion. There is, however, reference to the preservation of dignity and reason as well as progeny when talking about family. We could perhaps use this system as a means through which we can create a common background or common methodology.

Hassan Chamsi-Pasha

I have a brief comment about the preservation of honor. On a daily basis, patients in hospitals are left undressed after they have been anesthetized. Unfortunately, some physicians are lax in their concern for preserving the honor or dignity of their patients in this regard. Because this is a daily problem in many hospitals in the Arab and Muslim world, I think the higher objective regarding preservation of honor should be given particular attention.

Abdul Sattar Abu Ghuddah

The preservation of dignity differs from the issue of nakedness. The preservation of dignity entails prohibiting people from promoting ungrounded accusations against others of evil acts such as slander or fornication. As for ensuring that the body is covered, Muslim jurists have classified it among the supplementary commandments (*taḥsīnīyāt*), not from the necessities (*ḍarūrīyāt*) or needs (*ḥājīyāt*) because of the situations that necessitate undressing such as for medical purposes.

Hassan Chamsi-Pasha

However, it is no doubt that deliberately keeping a patient's body uncovered is counter to the preservation of dignity. The fact that anyone standing in an operation room can see a patient's body uncovered and later watch the patient leave the operation room does fall under the topic of the preservation of the dignity of the patient.

Annelien Bredenoord

It may be interesting to know we had an ongoing discussion about what dignity is. In the end, many scholars equated dignity with autonomy. The intrinsic worth of human beings is now quite often equated with autonomy, so now we use the word "autonomy" for dignity.

Script of Concluding Discussions: Part Two (Day 3: Session 1 and Session 2)

Mohammed Ghaly

We have been discussing the four-principle theory, which began in the West and eventually spread to the rest of the world. We will start this round of discussions with Dr. Bredenoord presenting a basic idea of the theory. If possible, she will also provide us with specific terms used in the English language and explain how we can classify them into main principles and subcategories so that we have a better understanding of some aspects about this theory that we have been struggling with so far. After Dr. Bredenoord's presentation, I will open the floor for discussion and commentary regarding the universal nature of these principles and whether they are compatible with Islam. This is the first point of discussion.

The second point is the Islamic contribution. Which general principles or fundamentals (or whatever term(s) we end up using) with relevance to biomedical ethics can we derive from the Islamic tradition? We have the three chapters presented respectively by Sheikh Raissouni, Sheikh Abu Ghuddah, and Sheikh Al-Qaradaghi that made distinctive suggestions in this regard.

Sheikh Raissouni suggested what we could call the virtue-based approach, which aims to search for the fundamental ethics (*ummahāt al-akhlāq*). We have a large collection of ethics in Islam, so how can we select from this collection the fundamental ethics? Also, what makes a particular ethical value or virtue part of the set of fundamental ethics? Sheikh Raissouni expressed his dissatisfaction with choosing a set of principles that is equally applied to politics, medicine, and all other fields. We will discuss this point: Should we take the general principles that are applicable to all fields — like the higher objectives of Sharia — and apply them to biomedical ethics? Or should we, from the beginning, choose principles that are especially relevant and applicable to biomedical ethics?

Sheikh Abu Ghuddah's suggestion was closer to the idea of the etiquettes of the physician. He mentioned God-consciousness (*taqwá*) and mercy in his chapter, and during a previous discussion, he added dignity (*karāmah*) and respect for human life. His discourse does not focus much on the patient but rather pays much consideration to issues surrounding the physician.

As for Sheikh Al-Qaradaghi, his chapter has to do with the Islamic perspective on the concept of principles and how it is related to the higher objectives of Sharia. One important question here is whether the higher objectives are ordered, especially if they are applied to matters of biomedical ethics.

We also have the idea of *ta'ṣīl* [developing a framework rooted in the Islamic tradition] and *tawṣīl* [communicating this framework to the public], in the words of Sheikh Bin Bayyah. *Ta'ṣīl* will be purely Islamic in nature, but *tawṣīl* will not necessarily be Islamic but rather universal in nature. This is why I kindly request from our Islamic scholars to discuss whether an ethical value can be inherently good (*taḥsīn*) or bad (*taqbīḥ*).

I hereby invite Dr. Bredenoord to give her presentation.

Annelien Bredenoord

I will try to briefly explain and repeat the main definitions of the four principles as well as the main problems of interpretation and what has been misunderstood or misinterpreted in the Western literature. I will then briefly speak about the process of specification or, in other words, how we apply abstract principles to concrete moral cases and finally will end with terminology.

One of the things I learned during this seminar is that the principles of beneficence and nonmaleficence are a part of the centuries-old Hippocratic tradition and that they generate the fewest debates. They are the most direct and clear. Even in Western discussions, there has not been that much discussion about beneficence and nonmaleficence. The two novel principles of autonomy and justice are the most controversial and have raised the most problems in understanding and interpretation. None of the principles alone is considered to be enough or sufficient. Rather, they form a comprehensive and complementary set of principles. I will try to demonstrate, using some examples from my own research, that if you take just one principle there will always be a conflict or a problem.

I would like to start with the principle of respect for autonomy. The concept of autonomy originally stems from the independent Greek city-states, and these Greek city-states were *autonomos*, meaning they had self-rule or self-governance. It was in Western philosophy that this concept of autonomy was applied to individuals. It was particularly the German philosopher Immanuel Kant who applied it to individuals. He literally said that persons should start to make and set their own rules and their own roles and govern themselves instead of authority or somebody else doing it for them. At a minimum level, autonomy is defined as self-rule free from both controlling interferences by others and interferences or limitations by oneself. The autonomous individual acts freely in accordance with a self-chosen plan. This is analogous to the way an independent government manages its own territory and its own policies. One has diminished autonomy when there are external or internal limitations in decision-making capacity. An example of an external limitation is when somebody is coerced to make a decision, such as when someone is put under pressure or is in prison and has to make a decision and is [thus] exploited. When one does not get full information, he or she cannot make an autonomous decision. An example of an internal limitation to autonomy is when one has mental illness or when one is seriously diseased.

I think one of the confusions in the debate on autonomy is that there is a distinction between a negative and a positive interpretation of autonomy.

In a negative or thin account, autonomy means "the right to make one's own decisions without interference or coercion from others." This is what Isaiah Berlin called "freedom from." I think this is a very important account of autonomy, but it is not enough. This is where the debate begins. Some people, perhaps particularly scholars in the United States, emphasized the negative account of autonomy, which is simply the right to make your own decisions, and that is it. I also emphasized the positive account of autonomy, which is the ability to take control of one's life and to live according to one's values, plans, and beliefs. This account is more associated with concepts such as self-governance, authenticity, self-expression, and self-rule. Taken together, you have a thick account of autonomy. However, acknowledging only the negative account is the reason why autonomy is often criticized to be superficial, individualistic, and shallow.

I will present a short example. Currently, one of the most important ethical debates in the medical literature is in genetics research. Due to novel genetic technology we can now very inexpensively map our human genome. The DNA of one person costs about $1,500 [to map], and you can do it in a couple of days. It is increasingly used in clinical medicine, in research, and in cardiology and it is also being introduced in oncology. One of the moral questions is whether we have a moral obligation to inform people about their genetic constitution. Should we provide them feedback about their DNA? Over the last 2 years only, hundreds of papers have been written about this topic.

If you apply the principles to this debate, you can use the principle of autonomy. If we consider the negative account of autonomy, you can say that it is sufficient to just inform a research participant or patient that they are part of [a] genetic sequencing [project] but that they will not receive feedback on their genetic information. Just giving them the information and letting them decide is enough. However, if you take the positive account of autonomy, you can say that simply taking somebody's informed consent is insufficient because having information about your genetic constitution may help you think about a life plan, give you existential meaning, and help you take control over your life — control over your diseases and your life plans. Hence, from a positive account you would say, yes, you have to inform people about their genetic constitution. That is basically the interpretation of these two concepts, and together we call them autonomy.

Now we will move on to the second principle, which is nonmaleficence. I think this principle is the most straightforward with the least discussion. It can be translated as, "First do not harm," and it actually requires the avoidance of causing harm to others. Harm can be defined as the setting back of interests of an individual. If we refer back to the discussion on informing patients about their genetic constitution, then you can specify this in two directions. You can say that disclosing genetics information is quite often harmful because people will get worried. It is about risk information, about probabilities rather than certainties. It has negative consequences for obtaining insurance and healthcare, and it also has psychological consequences. Given the fact that we should not do harm, we should not inform people about their DNA. This would be a line of reasoning using this principle.

I do not think there needs to be further discussion about nonmaleficence, so we can proceed to the third principle of beneficence. Actually, this is a group of principles, and it requires three things. First, it requires that we prevent harm from occurring. Second, it requires that we remove harmful conditions that could exist. Third, it requires that we promote the good of others. I believe beneficence is one of the most well-known principles in medical ethics, but there are two challenges or problems associated with this principle that need continuous consideration.

First, if you use the principle of beneficence without any limits or restrictions and without balancing it with other principles, then it may lead to paternalism. A physician could use this principle endlessly to do whatever is good for the patient and could intervene for the sake of the patient because in his or her opinion it would be good for the patient. As a result, we need autonomy to counterbalance this principle because if we only have beneficence then it is only the doctor who is doing good for the patient. So if we have beneficence we should always have some kind of autonomy to counterbalance it.

The second challenge associated with this principle is the debate regarding the scope and limits of beneficence. This is because beneficence is what we call a "maximizing principle." If you have the duty to promote the good of others, which is quite utilitarian, where does it end? Where does it stop? In principle we can endlessly promote the good of others, but then we must ask how much effort should be put forth to promote the good of your patient or your research participant. Are there any limits to it?

Here one arrives at a philosophical debate about what we can reasonably ask from other people. So here the physicians' and also the researchers' protective duties are generally quite strong and clear, but if the physicians' and researchers' duties include promoting the best interest of others, they need demarcation. For example, a demarcation could be the principle of justice or the principle of autonomy. Here again, if you ask whether we should inform people about their genetic constitution, then the principle of beneficence would say yes but only for the genetic information that is clinically relevant and useful to preventing disease or avoiding deterioration. There are also limits on the efforts the physician has to exert. I think the challenge for beneficence is in defining the scope and limits of duty.

The final principle is justice. This is one of the newest principles in medical ethics. It is also a group of principles. It requires that there be a fair distribution of benefits, risks, and costs across all parties in a given society. Justice actually defines the rules for cooperation. However, the problem with the principle of justice is that it is not an action guide. It needs filling in by a theory of justice. If we examine Western political philosophy in the 20th century we find many political philosophers who tried to find a theory of justice, John Rawls being the most well known among them. A distinction must be made between formal theories of justice and material theories of justice. A formal theory of justice just defines the procedure for treating one another fairly. It is often traced back to Aristotle, who said that a formal procedure of justice is that equals must be treated equally and unequals must be treated unequally, which is obvious for most people. So the principle is formal because it does not identify a particular respect in which equals should be treated equally, and it provides no criteria for determining whether two or more individuals are in fact equal.

The problem therefore is that the principle lacks substance. For example, if we have to treat equals equally, when is it justified to make differences between people? If there is a job vacancy, for instance, and it is accepted that we should not make distinctions based on race or gender, what are legitimate reasons for employing one person over another? In the end, formal justice will not provide an answer to this. We need substantive criteria. If you have one dialysis machine or one organ and several people who need it, in the end, the formal principle of justice will not provide an answer as to how these scarce resources should be distributed. Thus, we need a material theory of justice. We have traditional theories of justice like utilitarian, libertarian, egalitarian, and communitarian theories as well as more recent theories of justice such as the capability approach and many well-being theories. Regarding the example of genetic testing and providing DNA information to patients, whether justice requires you to provide those results completely depends on your theory of justice. In other words, the term "justice" alone is just a starting point. It is a principle literally, but then it needs interpretation. That was very briefly regarding the four principles.

The next issue I would like to address is that of specification. In the end, we have principles that are quite abstract and need to be filled in by theories. The process of translating the abstract norm into a considered judgment is what at least Beauchamp called specification. This is a time-consuming process that requires skills and needs a lot of argumentation. We cannot in just one hour specify principles or apply abstract principles to specific cases. I believe the core job of an applied ethicist is to translate principles to practical cases. It requires professionalism, some kind of craftsmanship, some sensitivity, and some experience. It involves a subjective scholarly element. One could say that a specification — a judgment — is justified if it is consistent with the norms of common morality (meaning if it does not violate common morality) and if it is internally coherent with the overall set of relevant and justified beliefs of the party carrying out this process of specification. So if I concluded in one paper that we should return genetic results to patients based on such-and-such reason, I cannot in the following paper conclude the opposite or argue for something that is internally incoherent with my own work. The same applies to everybody contributing to the process of specification.

As was said during the previous discussion with Dr. Beauchamp, there are some challenges. First, there is no accepted account on what our common morality is. What does it mean if an issue has to be consistent with common morality while we do not agree on common morality? The second problem is that we do not have a good coherence theory. We have no good account on what constitutes coherence. These are some challenges for the future.

Finally, I will discuss terminology. The resources I used in formulating term definitions are the book authored by Beauchamp and Childress, my own books, and the *Stanford Encyclopedia of Philosophy*. Clearly, these resources collide with each other, so I should include other resources to get a better overview of all the definitions. For now, I will provide the headlines of the definitions.

A *principle* can be defined as "a primary or general moral norm." *Ideals* are also principles or values, but the difference is that an ideal is "a principle or value that one actively pursues as a goal." So an ideal is something that is valuable and worth striving for. A *virtue* can be defined as "a positive trait or a quality deemed to be morally good." The opposite of a virtue is a *vice*. I think there will be agreement on the definition of this term. A *right* or *moral right* can be defined as "a justified claim." It can also be defined as "a legal, social, or ethical principle of freedom or entitlements." In other words, rights can be defined as "the fundamental normative rules about what is allowed of people or owed to people according to a certain legal system, social convention, or ethical theory." A *rule* can be defined as a standard or a norm. Here we can see the overlap between norms and standards. A *norm* can be defined in many ways. For example, in statistics a *norm* is the average. However, in ethics a *norm* is "a guide for action and behavior." Finally, *guidelines* are "statements through which to determine the course of action." So guidelines aim to streamline processes and to define norms for a certain practice.

Mohammed Ghaly

I hope the four-principle theory is getting clearer to everyone now. There are some objections about the theory from an Islamic angle; I will mention some of the ones that have been said before, especially by Dr. Al-Bar, and then will continue with what Dr. Bredenoord said.

Firstly, these theories did not materialize in vacuum. Rather, they have a philosophical background and a reality within which they were born. As Dr. Beauchamp stated in his research, reality is fundamentally changing in the medical world, and contemporary medical professionals can no longer use the medical ethics developed on the basis of Hippocratic theories to solve the ethical problems they face. This is why a new theory had to be developed.

The second point is that while principles such as autonomy, beneficence, nonmaleficence, and justice are undoubtedly in line with the spirit of Islam, they are based on Western philosophies. If problems of definition occur, then we must refer back to these philosophies to solve them. The principles are not separate or detached from the Western philosophies from which they emanated.

The third point is that these principles are general. They are intended to be general because those who set these principles wanted them to be universal and wanted their application to be left to the discretion of practitioners. This is both a positive and a negative thing. It is positive in the sense that it gives Muslims the flexibility to expand or contract certain elements without rejecting the theory. It is negative in the sense that whoever believes that the matter is in principle Islamic will be taking the theories [implicit therein]. For example, as Dr. Bredenoord mentioned, applying the principle of justice necessitates using a theory. So if Islam is absent, there will be problems during application.

I invite opinions regarding the four principles' background and application. What do we take from them, and what do we leave when applying these principles?

Abdullah Bin Bayyah

In my opinion, these principles or concepts or generalities (*kullīyāt*) — name them whatever you want — are a combination of some virtues or ethical notions that are neither Western nor Eastern; rather, they are everywhere and are shared by all humanity. Every human being loves justice and beneficence and abhors injustice and nonmaleficence. If the West has directed these virtues towards the medical field, that is good. We believe, "Indeed, Allah orders justice and good conduct and giving to relatives and forbids immorality and bad conduct and oppression…" (Qur'an 16:90). We have tens of similar texts related to ethical principles.

The arguments or details that were given are not convincing, at least for me. I find that these terms are words of connotation but not denotation, as they are not precise terms like, for example, *al-bay‘* (the process of selling), *al-nikāḥ* (marriage contract), *al-ṣalāh* (prayer), or *al-ṣiyām* (fasting) are. In other words, the terms [Dr. Bredenoord presented] are quite expansive. There is no problem with them being this way; what really matters is how medical doctors and relevant companies will apply these principles. The insurance and pharmaceutical companies are entities often forgotten, although they stand at the core of the matter. Sometimes they are the problem, while other times they end up being the solution if they behave properly. It would not be fair to push the companies aside and concentrate singularly on the doctors.

The real issue here is verifying the underlying ground or character of certain issues (*taḥqīq al-manāṭ*), meaning ensuring that a certain principle does in fact match a particular situation in reality. For example, this may involve the question, "Is this [particular reality] just or unjust?" We have numerous legal maxims or juristic rules to help us decide. Some examples are: choosing the lesser of two evils, bringing about good and avoiding evil, what to do when there is only one resource that everyone is in need of, and so on. All of this is abundantly specified in Islamic law. Muslim jurists (*fuqahā'*) can dissect these terminologies and develop their definitions [to be conveyed to a general audience]. The matter will then be in the hands of the individual or entity that will actually apply the principles to reality (*muḥaqqiq al-manāṭ*). This includes medical doctors as well as companies. They will be the ones to decide if something is just or unjust. So what we need at the end of the day is to find those with both technical expertise in their field and an alert conscience. This could be a religious conscience, which is the most awake type of conscience, or a civic conscience. What we need is the morally conscious professional to apply these principles — which do not belong to one civilization but rather are shared humanitarian principles — to reality.

Mohammed Ghaly

Sheikh Bin Bayyah has stated unambiguously that the principals are universal and belong neither to the East nor the West. Thus, he is in full agreement with Dr. Beauchamp that, in essence, the principles are universal in nature. The only variance lies in what he called verifying the underlying ground or character of certain issues (*taḥqīq al-manāṭ*) or how to apply these principles to real cases. This is where detailing would be required.

He also stated that in applying the principles to a certain context, we should be incredibly concerned as to who the person or entity applying the principle will be. The problem arises if the individual who will apply or contextualize the principle does not possess praiseworthy morals.

Annelien Bredenoord

I would like to say something about two issues that have been raised. The first is about context and specification, and the second is about terminology. I would like to start by saying something about terminology because we entered into a debate about epistemology, particularly with the discussion between Dr. Auda and Sheikh Bin Bayyah, so I would like to ask their opinion about it. You were saying something to the effect of, in the West we disagree about definitions and we have deconstructed definitions. However, ultimately, I think we should also discuss here with each other how we perceive definition. Do you see definition as something where the truth is somewhere out there and you can have objective meanings of words or definitions of things? Or is it similar to the dominant view in the West, which is that definition is a social construct and is a part of the philosophical approach of constructivism in which a definition is just a social construct, something we get consensus on? Ruth McLean, a well-known philosopher said that a definition is often more than mirror terminology. In other words, a definition is not only conceptual but is also normative. I personally think all definitions are agreements that people could reach at a certain point of time; they are professionally fixed points about which we agree, but we also acknowledge that they can be changed one day. I would be interested to hear Dr. Auda's perspective on definitions since he initiated the debate about terminology.

The second issue involves specification. Both Dr. Al-Bar and Sheikh Bin Bayyah stated that in the end we can have universal principles but the process of specification depends on context in addition to the good morals of the person responsible for specification. I think we completely agree that specification itself is something that requires skills and good thoughts.

There is a method that has been developed for this process called "wide reflective equilibrium." The method was developed by the two philosophers, John Rawls and Norman Daniels. They presented what they called a "thinker." The thinker is not a one-issue party. So it is not just an insurance company or just a medical doctor. Rather, it is somebody who takes the position of all relevant stakeholders, so it is comprehensive in nature. The thinker uses empirical research, considered judgments, principles, and values and molds them together into a coherent moral position. I do not think that the aim of principlism is to have one single issue or one party coming to a very particular point of view. The thinker needs to integrate all relevant stakeholders and all relevant interests. In his book *Justice and Justification*, Norman Daniels explained this method. I think in the end, ethics is all about justification, about whether you can justify your point of view. If it is merely one position of one single issue, then it is not justified.

Mohammed Ghaly

I invite comments on this, but I hope everyone takes into consideration Dr. Al-Bar's observation in a previous session when he said that if we do adopt an Islamic system of terminology, we should ensure it is clear and accessible to non-specialists. At the end, we are addressing physicians, not specialists in Sharia.

Jasser Auda

I want to clarify the concept of deconstruction (*tafkīk*) because it has a large impact on Western thought and, to a certain extent, also on Islamic thought through the writings of some individuals. As expressed in my books, I am totally against this concept. I have said that deconstruction results in historicism, which was called for by Mohammed Arkoun, Ebrahim Moosa, Hassan Hanafi, and Nasr Abu Zaid. This means deconstructing the authority of the text. In the philosophical sense, this is not compatible with belief in the sacredness of the words of God and His direct revelation to His Prophet (PBUH).

The outcome of such an understanding would be the loss of the religion of the Muslim nation (*ummah*) and the loss of its main source of knowledge and, consequently, its falling into the trap of blind submission to other nations. At that point, it would not distinguish between what such nations have of beneficial knowledge (and wisdom is the believer's stray camel that he is always searching for (*al-ḥikmah ḍāllat al-mu'min*) on the one hand and what such nations have of exclusively harmful knowledge on the other hand. The higher objectives of Sharia help protect the Muslim nation from that blind following, by God's will, because they assert the concepts of the intellect, justice, education, and freedom without putting them at odds with the concept of belief. Furthermore, historicism is not permissible to apply to a text that is revealed by God Almighty.

Mohammed Ghaly

I invite Sheikh Bin Bayyah to provide his remarks on the following question: If we wanted to define the term *justice*, or any of the ethical principles, should not the basis or starting point be a text from the Qur'an or the Prophetic tradition until we arrive at a definition? Or should it be based on constructivism and social constructs as Dr. Bredenoord mentioned?

Abdullah Bin Bayyah

Firstly, I agree with Dr. Bredenoord that people who have the proper knowledge and expertise should be the ones to apply these principles to the specific cases. Secondly, in regards to definitions, I do not think there is a difference between the West and Islam. A definition is a means of clarifying something, whether it is an entity, an adjective, or a state of being. A definition is also a means of illustrating an issue. This can be done in a number of different ways. For definitions in Sharia, we usually start with the linguistic definition then move onto the reality of the term within the context of the Sharia. If it is associated with norms known to people, then we also mention those. We include three elements: the term's linguistic reality, its reality in Sharia, and its customary reality. These three elements coalesce to form an illustration of the term.

For example, the word *'adālah* literally means balance. It is taken from the word *'idl*. In the language of the Arabs, *'idl* refers to one of the saddlebags Arabs would place on either side of a camel, ensuring they balanced out. This is where the word *justice* emanates from. We start from the linguistic definition of "balance" and then move to the Sharia-based definition, which is "giving all rightful owners (claimants) their rights." We then move to the normative definition or the normative reality of, "What is a right?" This is answered by Sharia on the one hand and by the customs and norms of people on the other. Therefore, the understanding we have is built of different parts: it has to do with the texts, the language, and the reality. This is how a definition is built in Islam. We have many resources to refer to about definitions in Arabic, such as *The Definitions of Al-Jurjani* (*Iṣtilāḥāt al-Jurjānī*).

Mohammed Ghaly

I invite comments from our Islamic scholars about the first question we are addressing related to the four principles, their universality, and their acceptance or rejection [from an Islamic perspective]. Sheikh Bin Bayyah said there is no disagreement regarding their universality and that their application (*tanzīl*) is where the complications lie. Dr. Bredenoord said that application or the process of specification does allow room for differences in opinion.

However, Dr. Ramadan has said there is also a problem with universality because these principles are not dry terms but rather are products of certain philosophical notions and thus we should not be deceived or deluded by the [apparent] compatibility of the terminology. I think Dr. Beauchamp also said something similar in our discussions with him. He said that we do all have to agree on the basis because the issue is an intellectual one and — as Dr. Al-Bar added — is an issue of human beings' natural disposition (*fiṭrah*).

Regarding the application of a certain principle, we have questions like: What is justice? How is justice realized in a certain context and a certain case? People differ on such questions depending on their religion and even depending on their disciplines or crafts. An economics specialist may apply the principle of justice in a way that differs from how a bioethicist would, even if the two were from the same religion, sect, nation, and society. We agree with the general understandings, but we must know that these understandings are a product of a certain philosophy, which we may agree with in some respects but not in others. If there are any additions or objections regarding the summary of what we have come to, I invite those comments now.

Ali Al-Qaradaghi

Firstly, I want to say that the generality of the principles is not problematic whatsoever, and it is impossible for anyone who adopts a general ethical rule to escape this generality. Even Sheikh Raissouni chose two general principles that are more general than the four principles. One is God-consciousness (*taqwá*), which applies to one's soul, to worship, to dealings with others, to everything. The other is mercy, which also applies to everything and everyone from human beings to animals to other things. Sheikh Abu Ghuddah also mentioned respecting rules or laws. All of these things are general. Therefore, if we accept this, then we also are saving our principles by using the same approach.

Thus, we should not object to the generality of the principles. The challenge we do have is first with the criteria or standards we use when interpreting them. The second has to do with the process of application, which includes the question of who will carry out this process. The application process should be strictly structured. As Dr. Al-Bar mentioned, we do not want to get confused and lost in discussions that most doctors may not understand. We should aim for accessibility; the Qur'an did not address people using complicated philosophical jargon but rather used a discourse close to their natural disposition (*fiṭrah*) so they may understand it. The third challenge is the ideological background, namely that the four principles are Western in their character and background.

Mohammed Ghaly

There are four points here. First, there is no disagreement about the generality and universality of the principles. Differences arise in three aspects. The first aspect is the criteria and standards. Even Dr. Bredenoord and Dr. Beauchamp acknowledged that the West itself has problems in this regard. Dr. Beauchamp said previously that there are matters that still need to be studied.

The second point of difference is the process of specification or how we should apply the principles to reality. Sheikh Bin Bayyah mentioned that this requires someone who is knowledgeable about all the relevant aspects and gathers them and studies them closely. In principle, we agree that the person who carries out the specification process should be cognizant and knowledgeable of all the principles so that one principle is not applied at the expense of others. He should also be well versed in medicine and contemporary medical issues.

The third aspect that Islam and the West differ on is the ideological background. The four principles are the fruit of a certain ideology, and similarly the Islamic principles should be born out of the Islamic tradition. How do we go about doing this? This is the subject of our second main point. I invite any comments about the first point, about the four principles, before we move on to the second.

Mohammed Ali Al-Bar

Dr. Bredenoord promised some answers to my questions related to autonomy. What do we make of the fact that some governments in the Gulf require a man and a woman to undergo blood tests for certain common diseases before they are allowed to get married?

Annelien Bredenoord

The example Dr. Al-Bar gave is a good example of why we need all four principles and why we cannot just rely on one principle. Autonomy requires that people can decide for themselves whether or not they are interested in receiving genetic information. Autonomy also requires what we call the right not to know genetic information, which is an informed refusal of information. However, if it was absolute, then patients could ask for all their DNA and genetic tests without considering the interests of their relatives or family members, even though information about their genetic constitution is relevant to what happens with the family members as well. If a state coerces you to undergo a genetic test before marriage, I think that would be a violation of autonomy, although the intention may be one of beneficence. The fact that you at least have to consider the interests of relatives is in my opinion a part of nonmaleficence and of justice as well. So I think it is a very good example of why we need the four principles.

Also, it could very well be possible that if I do the process of specification, I would use the same principle and come to a different conclusion than when you do the specification. This, however, is not a problem because we accept pluralism at the level of particular moralities. We do not accept relativism or pluralism on the common morality level, but it is acceptable if we reach different conclusions. Also, when you were talking about formulating principles from the Islamic tradition, I think that is not a problem as long as they are formulated in a way that can be accepted by all human beings. That is the idea of universality.

Mohammed Ali Al-Bar

My question was only partially answered. The governments in the Gulf area are imposing a law that anybody who wants to get married must undergo two or three blood tests in order to avoid the problems that are increasing in the community due to consanguinity. On the other hand, there are laws in the West that prevent consanguinity. This is also interference by the law with a person's autonomy. Governments constantly institute laws that may help the community as a whole but that directly interfere with [individuals'] autonomy.

I should mention that Islamic scholars have tried to stop the law that stipulates that two people cannot get married because of the results of their blood tests. They say that even if both the man and the woman are carriers of the thalassemia gene or the sickle cell anemia gene, for example, and have a substantial likelihood of bearing children with the disease, the government should not have the power to prevent their marriage. They say that the government can give them the knowledge and can provide them with counseling, but their marriage should not be prevented.

Annelien Bredenoord

This is a public health measure. As is characteristic of public health measures, there is a traditional clash between the principle of autonomy and the principle of beneficence or nonmaleficence. All public health measures like enforced vaccination of children, neonatal screening, and the obligation to wear seat belts in a car are violations of your autonomy. However, autonomy is not limitless. Our autonomy is violated every day by public policy and public health measures. I think that is unavoidable. I think society would be a disaster if we had limitless autonomy. The only question is — and this is the specification process — whether this is a justified violation of autonomy. I have to think about this more, but I imagine that you can ask people to undergo tests before they marry. However, you cannot force them to undergo tests and you cannot force them not to marry, but you can offer them certain options such as prenatal screening.

Abdul Sattar Abu Ghuddah

In the field of positive law, there is a constitution, there are codified laws, and there are explanatory notes and regulations. The four principles were presented as if they form a constitution. However, we already have the higher objectives of Sharia that serve as a more ideal constitution. Accordingly, it appears we can proceed in the following way. We can take the higher objectives of Sharia as our starting point, and it is not a problem whatsoever that they can be applied across disciplines because the scholars of the higher objectives of Sharia already intended this. After establishing the higher objectives of Sharia as our ideals or our constitution, we search for equivalences of the four principles in the Islamic tradition. The Western scholars or academics have exerted much effort in coming up with the four principles, so if we find analogues to some of them, we mention these analogues even if we end up using very different terminology.

Next, we move onto the processes of clarifying and detailing or specification. We describe the limitations of the four principles and add more principles as needed since four is a small number compared to the immense field we know biomedical ethics to be. Finally, we link the principles to our Islamic heritage and thus ensure alignment with our religious tradition.

Sheikh Bin Bayyah mentioned the work of Al-Jurjani as a good resource for terminology. I would like to mention that we also have *Kashshāf iṣṭilāḥāt al-funūn* by Al-Tahanawi, *Dustūr al-ʻulamā'*, and many others.

Mohammed Ghaly

We will now move to the second point of our discussions in this seminar so as to arrive at a number of outcomes. We distributed a document containing all relevant terminology because it appears we are not in full agreement over common descriptions or definitions. The terms include:

- Fundamental ethics (*ummahāt al-akhlāq*).
- Fundamentals (*uṣūl*).
- Comprehensive rules (*qawāʿid kullīyah*).
- Higher objectives (*maqāṣid*).
- Principles (*mabādiʾ*).

I ask our religious scholars especially to provide us with their thoughts so we may define these terms, particularly those mentioned in their research papers, and try to specify the relationship between all these terms.

Jasser Auda

So that we do not get overwhelmed by a discussion about the differences between the various terms mentioned, I suggest we focus on answering the question of what particularly we are looking for in this seminar. As we decide which term represents what we are looking for, we can arrive at a definition of that term specifically. Also, we can imagine this term being included in the title of the book we publish after the seminar.

Ahmed Raissouni

I believe we are going to have a few terms to discuss and choose from:

- The governing principles (*al-mabādiʾ al-ḥākimah*).
- The general fundamentals (*al-uṣūl al-ʿāmmah*).
- The comprehensive fundamentals (*al-uṣūl al-kullīyah*).
- The Sharia-based rules (*al-qawāʿid al-sharʿīyah*).

My own subjective choice would be to use the word *rules* (*qawāʿid*): the Sharia-based rules (*al-qawāʿid al-sharʿīyah*) or the general rules (*al-qawāʿid al-ʿāmmah*). I choose the term *rules* because it is the most authentic from the perspective of the Qur'an and its various uses. We are engaged with rules. However, the rules we have in Islamic law and the Islamic tradition differ in level; there are rules lower than other rules, and there are rules higher than others. Thus, we could make it general rules (*al-qawāʿid al-ʿāmmah*) or comprehensive rules (*al-qawāʿid al-kullīyah*).

As I was preparing my chapter, my understanding was that the medical doctor is the main component and thus I focused on ethics and on God-consciousness and mercy. It has become apparent through our discussions, including those about the four principles, that the matter extends far beyond the Arabic word *akhlāq* (ethics) since *akhlāq* pertain to the individual's conduct. Instead, the scope encompasses the society, government, and policies. The Arabic word *akhlāq* is not sufficient in this case, and I do not know whether the English word *ethics* is sufficiently inclusive. That is why in my opinion the appropriate term is rules (*qawāʿid*), meaning regulations of the society by way of governmental health policies. We could use either "Sharia-based rules" (*al-qawāʿid al-sharʿīyah*) to specify they are based on the Sharia and not something else or we could use "comprehensive rules" (*al-qawāʿid al-kullīyah*) to distinguish them from specific Islamic legal maxims or rules.

Mohammed Ghaly

So we have Sharia-based rules (*al-qawāʿid al-sharʿīyah*), general rules (*al-qawāʿid al-ʿāmmah*), or comprehensive rules (*al-qawāʿid al-kullīyah*).

Abdul Sattar Abu Ghuddah

We have a long history [in the Islamic tradition] with *qawāʿid* (rules) that we can refer to, and we can refer to relevant examples and applications from the past. Furthermore, using this term would demonstrate its rootedness in the Islamic tradition, its long history, and its importance. However, the word *mabādi'* (principles) is somewhat open-ended. Thus, *qawāʿid* (rules) is the best option in my view.

Ali Al-Qaradaghi

Although I have myself used the term *maqāṣid* (higher objectives), I do not necessarily deem it to be the best choice. It is worth noting that even if we choose the term *qawā'id* (rules), this does not negate the role of the higher objectives because these rules are nevertheless connected to the higher objectives.

There may be a juristic (*fiqhī*) problem with the term *qawā'id*: according to the manuals of [juristic] rules, *qawā'id* are defined as those which encompass or necessarily produce religious rulings (*aḥkām shar'īyah*), whether prescriptive (*taklīfī*) or contextual (*waḍ'ī*) in nature. For instance, "There should be neither harming nor reciprocating harm," is an example of what we call a rule.

Ahmed Raissouni

What you stated is the definition of a specifically juristic (*fiqhī*) rule [not a rule in general].

Ali Al-Qaradaghi

That is correct. However, I mean that any rule by definition encompasses rulings. A religious rule encompasses religious rulings; a juristic rule encompasses juristic rulings; and so on. This is why in the title of my book *Mabda' al-riḍā fī al-'uqūd* (*The Principle of Consent in Contracts*), I chose the term *principle* (*mabda'*) and not *rule*. Something like, "There should be neither harming nor reciprocating harm" is a rule, while something like "consent" or "obligation" is referred to as a principle or theory.

Moreover, the Arabic Language Academy in Cairo has endorsed the term *mabda'*, so it is accepted from a linguistic perspective. Basically, what I want to say is that a rule has to encompass a ruling whereas we are hoping to develop a theory that includes numerous rules, restrictions, and limitations. Arising from this it is perhaps best to use the term *principles*. However, if we agree that the term *qawā'id* (rules) also means *mabādi'* (principles), then I would have no objection to its use.

When it comes to specifying the rules, we should anyhow determine the source of these rules. What is their background? Their background is the higher objectives of Sharia, and this demonstrates that we indeed remain within the same circle of higher objectives.

Mohammed Ghaly

Does using the phrase "comprehensive rules" (*qawāʿid kullīyah*) absolve us of the problem with the word *qawāʿid* (rules)?

Ali Al-Qaradaghi

Using the adjective *comprehensive* serves to distinguish it from *specific* rules, but the comprehensiveness or specificity only refers to their linguistic denotation. As for what the term *qawāʿid* (rules) means to Islamic legal theorists, jurists, and religious scholars more generally, *qawāʿid* always encompass rulings — whether religious rulings, juristic rulings, rulings of Islamic legal theory, or grammar rulings. For example, in [Arabic] grammar, every subject of a verb should be in the nominative case. That is an example of a rule. Nevertheless, if the seminar participants would agree to use the term *rules* differently than what all scholars have agreed upon, I would not object.

Hassan Chamsi-Pasha

In regards to the complete title, I suggest *The Comprehensive Rules of Medical Ethics* (*Al-qawāʿid al-kullīyah fī al-akhlāqīyāt al-ṭibbīyah*). The word *comprehensive* is fitting because once we decide to use the higher objectives of Sharia, we can say that these comprehensive rules already imply them.

Mohammed Ghaly

I invite Sheikh Bin Bayyah to offer his thoughts. It seems we are trying to choose between *rules* and *principles*.

Abdullah Bin Bayyah

There is a line of Arabic poetry that reads,

> Pass from the front of the mountain or the back, for surely
> Each side has a path [you can tread securely].

I think both choices [*rules* and *principles*] are acceptable. Our early scholars used the term *rule* as something that is by definition comprehensive and can be applied to its parts. Therefore, if we choose the word *rule*, then the adjective *comprehensive* would already be included. That is why I do not see any objection in the last proposal by Dr. Chamsi-Pasha.

It is worth noting that the French word *principaux* gets translated as *qawā'id* and *mabādi'*. However, we usually translate *qā'idah* (rule) to French as *la base*. For example, we translate *al-qā'idah al-qānūnīyah* (legal rule) as *la base juridique*. Thus, *qā'idah* (rule) and *mabda'* (principle) are very similar. In *Al-baḥr al-muḥīṭ*, Al-Zarkashi defined *principles* as the boundaries and topics of a discipline that is studied, so he did define *principles* in an explicit or particular manner. However, nowadays we are in the habit of using *principles* in the sense given by the popular Western definition, which is completely fine. As Sheikh Al-Qaradaghi said, as long as the Arabic Language Academy allows the use of it in that sense, there is no problem. I do not have a decisive opinion on the matter. It would be acceptable to call them general rules (*qawā'id 'āmmah*) or comprehensive rules (*qawā'id kullīyah*) of biomedical ethics. And God knows best.

Abdul Sattar Abu Ghuddah

It is worth noting that a rule unites or links together many different branches without actually mentioning these branches. In other words, a rule is a comprehensive and uniting expression — an umbrella — that is itself derived from many rulings. Note it does not explicitly mention a ruling but rather is an umbrella for many rulings.

Hassan Chamsi-Pasha

There is one additional consideration to make about the terms we use. There is a shift in the West from using the phrase *medical ethics* to using the term *bioethics*. In Arabic, should we add what corresponds to the prefix *bio-*?

Mohammed Ghaly

In the West, they have medical ethics, bioethics, and biomedical ethics. Dr. Beauchamp stated previously that he personally did not prefer the term *bioethics*. In addition, *medical ethics* was an old term; it has been used in Hippocratic thought. Since the medical field has been through so much advancement, at one point there was a need for more modern terminology. Thus, both terms were combined to produce *biomedical ethics*. Dr. Beauchamp does not seem to object to the use of the term *bioethics*. Perhaps Dr. Bredenoord can comment on whether there are any clear-cut differences between *medical ethics*, *bioethics*, and *biomedical ethics*?

Annelien Bredenoord

Yes, there is a distinction, but this is also a contested distinction. In brief, one can say that medical ethics is a traditional domain that deals with ethical issues particularly in the physician–patient encounter or relationship. "Medical ethics" is the old term. After that we introduced the term *biomedical ethics* to emphasize biomedical technology and the rise of biomedical sciences. So if you also want to include stem cell research, genetics, and reproductive technology, then you should use the term *biomedical* because it is the focus of research. If you want to talk about research ethics and about doing experiments with human beings, you should also use the term *biomedical ethics*. So this term is broader.

Bioethics is another step broader because *bioethics* comes from *bio-* and *ethics*, meaning it is about the ethics of living things, including animal ethics. One could even say that it also includes agricultural issues about food. There is a discussion about where it ends, but bioethics is at least also about animal ethics. Most biomedical ethicists do not consider animal ethics, so it is a choice. Then there is also the problem that we have public health ethics and also healthcare ethics. I personally use "biomedical ethics" or sometimes "bioethics." I do not use the term "medical ethics."

Jasser Auda

In Arabic we could combine both and say, "medical and bioethics" (*al-ṭibbīyah wa-al-ḥayawīyah*).

Mohammed Ghaly

I believe the prefix *bio-* comes from Latin or Greek and simply means life or everything related to life. Therefore, if we say *ḥayawīyah* in Arabic, is this correct?

Mohammed Ali Al-Bar

The Arabic word *ḥayawīyah* is difficult to understand because it involves other meanings, including "active" and "lively." It would give the meaning a much wider scope. I think the expression Dr. Auda offered is easily understood by the average person because the term *ḥayawīyah* is mentioned with *ṭibbīyah* (medical) so that its intended meaning is understood.

Jasser Auda

Dr. Al-Bar, as a doctor, when you hear the title *The Principles* (*Al-mabādi'*) or *The Comprehensive Rules* (*al-qawā'id al-kullīyah*) *of Medical and Bioethics* (*lil-akhlāq al-ṭibbīyah wa-al-ḥayawīyah*), would this convey the intended meaning?

Mohammed Ali Al-Bar

This would be suitable for me because it would seem to encompass topics about animals, genetics, stem cells, and other things since it is a broad title.

Abdullah Bin Bayyah

Is *bio-* (*ḥayawīyah*) not already contained in the term *medical* (*ṭibbīyah*)?

Mohammed Ghaly

In English, *medical ethics* refers to the ethics of the doctor–patient relationship. It is about traditional medicine and does not include modern technologies that have to do with issues like stem cells, etc.

Regarding the translation of the prefix *bio-*, its Arabic translation according to the United Nations is *aḥyā'īyah* whereas *ḥayawīyah* is translated by the United Nations as "vital," meaning active and lively.

Jasser Auda

It seems *ḥayawīyah* is a commonly misplaced term, but it is important for us as a center to reach doctors and medical professionals across countries and organizations with something they understand well. A title with the term *ḥaywīyah* would be one easily understood by the target audience.

Mohammed Ghaly

We have two options, and they both have valid arguments. One is to use *aḥyā'īyah* for the sake of linguistic accuracy and with the purpose of opposing the widespread mistake that has occurred. The other is to use *ḥayawīyah* since it is widely used among people and thus would be more accessible to readers.

Ahmed Raissouni

I personally do not have a preference, but I would just like to point out that linguistically *ḥayawīyah* is not wrong since *biology* can be called the study of *al-aḥyā'* and it can be called the study of *al-ḥayāh*.

Hassan Chamsi-Pasha

I prefer using *ḥayawīyah* because it is more common among people and is easier for them to understand.

Mohammed Ali Al-Bar

I agree, especially because Sheikh Raissouni clarified that it is not incorrect.

Mohammed Ghaly

So it seems we have come to a decision. Our title is *The Principles* (*Al-mabādi'*) or *The Comprehensive Rules* (*al-qawā'id al-kullīyah*) *of Medical and Bio-ethics* (*lil-akhlāq al-ṭibbīyah wa-al-ḥayawıyah*).

Ali Al-Qaradaghi

Since *qawā'id* (rules) are by definition comprehensive, it would be redundant to add this adjective. If we chose to use *rules*, we could use the adjective *general*, and if we chose to use *principles*, we could use the adjective *comprehensive*. Thus, we have two options: *al-qawā'id al-'āmmah* (general rules) or *al-mabādi' al-kullīyah* (comprehensive principles).

Conclusion: Critical Remarks

Tariq Ramadan

Taken as a field bioethics has its own history, one inextricably linked with advances in medical science in the West. As scientific and technical mastery have grown, medical researchers and physicians have been confronted with new ethical questions. At the same time, in an increasingly secularized world, religion has proved unable to be a reference for all and to answer these questions satisfactorily. Construction of an ethical framework, of a new norm of operational responsibility for contemporary society, became an indispensable task. Thus emerged ethics, and particularly bioethics, which concern us here: constructs derived naturally from the precepts of collective rationality, as distinguished by its internal logic and its autonomous moral justification, through which, to paraphrase Rawls, overlapping consensus can be reached.

The field of bioethics is of particular interest to us, for it is in the discipline of medicine and by extension, of bioethics, that today's Muslim scholars (*Ulamā*) have made the greatest progress in the drafting of legal opinions (*fatāwā*) relevant to contemporary issues. The necessary encounter between the medical sciences in the broadest sense and Islamic thought is of course not new, as we are reminded by the wide-ranging presentations of Muslim scholars found in the preceding pages. But the nature of contemporary investigation has shifted, become more sharply focused, more specialized, and certainly more complex. One of the objectives of the Center for Islamic Legislation and Ethics (CILE) has been to facilitate encounters between *Ulamā* and scientists in a given specialty (scholars of the text and of the context) to better develop exchanges of views and to promote informed ethical reflections from within the scientific fields under study. The task has been to avoid the twin dangers of fragmentation and of the deconstruction of knowledge that would ultimately reduce ethics to a secondary or auxiliary role, where its impact would be marginal if not inexistent.

Through the papers presented and the ensuing discussions, this work has identified a certain number of major issues in this highly specialized field. It is clear that the terminology itself raises substantial problems of understanding. Bioethicists, either those trained in the West or in a disciplinary structure inspired by American or European universities, employ a vocabulary drawn from a corpus of principles and methodologies that many if not most '*Ulamā'*, who rely instead on a decontextualized definition of the discipline's concepts, notions, and specialized terminology, do not entirely grasp. Again and again in the course of debate, it became clear that respective understandings were at best partial, and even deficient, due to the existence of a "terminological hiatus" separating the two worlds of reference, the scientific and the religious.

This in turn revealed differences in understanding of the very role of ethics and the objectives of scientific knowledge: a veritable "epistemological hiatus" persists, though not always clearly visible in the apparent coherence of discussion, a recurring difficulty in agreeing upon mutually acceptable answers. '*Ulamā*', for instance, were inclined to provide extremely detailed answers to a given bioethical question while at the same time formulating a critique of "Western science" without always being able to pinpoint the exact nature of the problem (principles, methodology, or objectives). Their legal rulings (*fatāwā*), while applicable to the contingent necessities of the day, revealed a disconnection between the case-by-case approach adapted to contemporary needs, and the need for a holistic overview. It often seemed as though the urgent nature of an ethical response to the specific powers of the medical sciences over-rode or marginalized consideration of the very function of medicine (and thus of the definition of the human person and of his/her health in every sense of the word).

The third question arises from the natural evolution of the two hiatuses, terminological and epistemological, to form the "ideological hiatus" that underlies the very essence of the scientific method. Bioethics is, par excellence, the field whose methodology reveals an ideological presupposition — permanent in the West (as Muna Ali's article reminds us) — that must be understood in the light of the cultural, social, and economic factors that shape research and debate at each stage of the formation of bioethics. These three "hiatuses" functioned as a common denominator in the articles submitted by participants but even more markedly in the ensuing debates, as if to underline the complex nature of the encounter and, above all, the need for further reflection, and for developing a multidisciplinary and multidimensional approach (taking these hiatuses precisely into account).

The decision to focus discussion on Beauchamp and Childress's Four Principles (autonomy, beneficence, nonmaleficence, and justice) proved fruitful for several reasons. First, even though it constitutes a dominant trend familiar to a majority of experts, the Beauchamp–Childress doctrine has been criticized and contested by several philosophers, ethicists, and even physicians. As Muna Ali notes in her chapter, Beauchamp and Childress's theses are not unanimously accepted, and have been criticized for their presupposed rationalist/secular nature, their reductionism and their utilitarian compatibility with the quantifiable character of "ethical measurability" that tends to align them with the dominant economic order. It follows that the postulates formulated by Beauchamp and Childress, only one of many trends in the field, cannot be uncritically accepted; in like manner, debate cannot be reduced to a rejection of the West and its science, or, contrariwise, to the attempt to prove the "bio-ethical compatibility" of Islam. The overarching intention has been thus to grasp and to question the fundamental philosophical reference as well as the methodology devised by the two philosophers in order to elaborate a holistic method that respects both principles and ultimate goals.

From this perspective, Jasser Auda's exposition of the higher objectives of the *Shari'a* can be described as classical in that it refers to both the structure and the methodology of the ultimate goals-based approach. While such a framework is indeed essential, it became clear in the course of debate that greater refinement was called for; concepts must be clarified, and work must be done on both the input and output sides. In terms of input, the sources of ethics both in terms of conception and application must be determined in the clearest possible way. Definitions and methodology (with regard to applied ethics in bioethics) are directly related to this fundamental task. Both definition and methodology are functions of the output-side effort that must be focused on the ultimate objectives (*maqâsid*), general and specific, to be derived in this highly specific field. So, deductively (beginning with the sources) and inductively (proceeding from objectives), the terms of debate as well as the methodology governing the application of ethics must be postulated in the most holistic way possible, and in necessarily close relation with the other fields of knowledge.

Such is the picture that emerges from a survey of the theses put forward by the participants, and by the extremely rich nature of the ensuing debates. Islamic thought had long interpreted professional ethics by turning its attention, almost as a matter of course, to the ethical objectives of the sciences. Secularization has brought about a fracture and has, given the resulting independent status of knowledge, made it necessary to rethink the place and role of ethics (that could no longer be solely religious) *vis-à-vis* the sciences. In this sense, bioethics can be seen as an attempt to reconcile the medical sciences as they stand with the ethical imperative born of the question of the power of these very sciences and the way in which they are employed. In the course of debate it became clear that the fundamental premises and the nature of reconciliation lay at the root of the problem. The first question is key: Must we attempt to bring about reconciliation with science as it is currently constituted or must we call into question its role, its methods and its utility? Such is the necessity that emerged in the course of our exchanges, at the risk of producing an Islamic ethics that would seek no more than to create a framework adapted to contemporary issues, and whose sole real function would be to limit damage, and not to question or to reform the approach in its entirety.

There are three major challenges that must be faced, above and beyond the present work, which is best seen as a stage in an incremental process. Ultimately, there can be no question — from a bioethical point of view — of dealing with highly specialized and very specific problems without first formulating a clear conception of the human being and of health. The latter cannot, in turn, be reduced to its "chemical" negation as a determinant of the absence of illness. Over and above the quantifiable approach of the dominant trend in the West, there exists a relationship with the body, with the environment, and with the spirit (and with spirituality) that can neither be neglected nor dismissed as secondary. This holistic concept shapes and informs the higher objectives cited earlier: preservation of personal integrity (*nafs*), and thence of the person's life and health, and insistence in the most explicit manner that scientific norms and priorities be established based upon it. These three issues (define the fundamental conception, determine the higher objectives specific to the field of bioethics, develop a terminology appropriate to both conception and ultimate goals) cannot be avoided; this work reaffirms their vital importance and urgency.

Before us lies a two-pronged critical enterprise. That of which we have spoken regarding the field of bioethics itself, with the questions of terminology, its epistemological bases and its ideological substrate. Here, we must squarely confront the three hiatuses that arose in the course of our deliberations. In like manner, we must develop a critical view of the methods and categories established by the *Ulamā* over the centuries. While taking the texts seriously, so as not to betray their meaning, we must muster the courage to revisit the work of the men who have humbly attempted to answer the questions of their era, with the means at their disposal.

Our responsibility is to reconsider the sources of bioethics from an Islamic perspective, the specific objectives that must be conceived and formulated, and, of equal importance, to map out the purview of ethical authority in medical matters. What are the references and the sources; how are methodologies to be decided upon; who will make the decisions? These are the questions that were raised time and time again in the course of our deliberations. They must be dealt with one at a time, by establishing priorities and devising tools. This book is a vital first step in the pursuit of our efforts in the field of bioethics. It is to be hoped that the reader will find in these pages a source of reflection and inspiration to carry out further research and to deal in the most appropriate way with the many questions that still await answers.

Tariq Ramadan

Glossary

***Adab al-Ṭabīb*:** See Practical Ethics of the Physician.

***'Aqīdah*:** See Islamic Creed.

Bioethics: A modern term, said to be originally coined in 1971 by the American biochemist Van Rensselaer Potter. Now it refers to a well-established scholarly discipline which systematically studies human conduct in a wide range of areas, including life sciences, healthcare, and disease management, from the perspective of moral principles, values, and visions.

Casuistry: An applied ethics approach that uses case-based moral reasoning to form expert opinions for solving puzzling cases and examining how paradigm cases and moral categories can be envisaged, through which future similar cases can be easily resolved.

Common Morality: A moral theory used to clarify, describe, explain, and justify the existence of core ethical tenets that are commonly held by all persons who lead a moral life irrespective of their cultural, socio-political, or religious backgrounds. It plays a crucial role in arguing for principle-based bioethics.

***Ḍarūrīyāt*:** See Necessities.

Deontology: A moral theory which argues that there are several distinct duties and that certain kinds of acts are intrinsically right or wrong, irrespective of the nature of their consequences. Compare UTILITARIANISM.

Excellence (*Iḥsān*): An Arabic term which usually conveys the meaning of excellence and perfection. As an ethical term, it means the attainment of moral and spiritual excellence and beauty, usually combined with attaining the state of being ever conscious and mindful of God. According to some researchers, *Iḥsān* is the Arabic and Islamic equivalent of the bioethical principle "beneficence," whereas others believe that it represents a distinctively Islamic principle that can be added to the list of the well-known four principles.

***Fiqh al-Muwāzanāt*:** See Jurisprudence of Balances.

***Fiqh*:** See Islamic Law.

Four-Principle Approach: See Principlism.

***Ḥājīyāt*:** See Necessities.

Higher Objectives of Sharia (*Maqāṣid al-Sharī'ah*): An Islamic legal theory whose main premise is that God revealed the law for the sake of achieving specific higher objectives. The traditional and standard account of this theory speaks of five main objectives, namely preserving religion (*dīn*), life (*nafs*), offspring (*nasl*), intellect (*'aql*), and wealth (*māl*). Other accounts sometimes add other objectives to this list like preserving honor (*'irḍ*), preserving the integrity of the legitimate state and the integrity of society, freedom, etc. Some voices suggest employing this theory for building up the overall framework for a principle-based bioethics rooted in the Islamic tradition.

***Iḥsān*:** See Excellence.

***Ijtihād*:** See Independent Reasoning.

Independent Reasoning (*Ijtihād*): Literally, it refers to the act of exerting one's utmost effort in a particular activity. As a technical term, it means expending the maximum effort to master and apply the principles and rules of interpreting the scriptural texts and other evidences for the purpose of discovering SHARIA.

Induction (*Istiqrā'*): A common term in ISLAMIC LEGAL THEORY which signifies a form of reasoning in which general conclusions or principles can be inferred from a pool of particular instances that have been observed. Many believe that the list of the HIGHER OBJECTIVES OF SHARIA was determined by using this form of reasoning.

Islamic Creed (*'Aqīdah*): The set of beliefs, particularly what is related to the nature of God and the relationship between God and His creatures that Muslims should embrace. Various voices criticize contemporary discourse on Islam and biomedical ethics of excessively focusing on the ethico-legal aspects at the cost of the due attention to be paid to the Islamic creed.

Islamic Law (*Fiqh*): A scholarly discipline whose experts are occupied with extracting religious rulings, pertaining to conduct, from their adequate scriptural sources and evidences. Throughout Islamic history, five main schools of Islamic law proved to be dominant, namely the Hanafi, Maliki, Shafi'i, and Hanbali schools (within the Sunni tradition) and the Ja'fari school (within the Sh'ia tradition).

Islamic Legal Maxims (*Qawā'id Fiqhīyah*): A distinct genre within *FIQH* that constitute general rules that cut across all, or a great number of, areas and themes of *FIQH*. This genre is usually employed to address a wide range of modern issues including those related to bioethics. Many researchers believe that this genre can help in the construction of a principle-based bioethics rooted in the Islamic tradition.

Islamic Legal Theory (*Uṣūl al-Fiqh*): Literally means the roots or fundaments of *FIQH*. This scholarly discipline examines the body of principles and investigative methodologies through which religious rulings are developed from the foundational sources.

Jurisprudence of Balances (*Fiqh al-Muwāzanāt*): A newly introduced Islamic legal term whose advocates wanted to construct a particular branch of *FIQH* that focuses on studying the possible methods of balancing and weighting between different and competing factors. Within the context of principle-based bioethics, it is sometimes suggested that this branch can be a helpful tool for resolving the problem of conflict between some general principles.

***Maqāṣid al-Sharī'ah*:** See Higher Objectives of Sharia.

Natural Disposition (*Fiṭrah*): The innately good disposition that every human being is believed to be created with. According to some opinions, it can be a supporting source of guidance for leading a moral life.

Necessities (*Ḍarūrīyāt*): One of the traditional classifications of the HIGHER OBJECTIVES OF SHARIA is to divide them into three prioritized levels, namely necessities or essentials (*ḍarūrīyāt*), needs (*ḥājīyāt*), and luxuries or enhancements (*taḥsīnīyāt*). The first level, *ḍarūrīyāt*, includes what is essential for the achievement of human beings' spiritual and material well-being and whose absence will result in imbalance and major corruption in both this world and the Hereafter. The second level, *ḥājīyāt*, comprises the interests whose fulfillment will contribute to relieving hardship and to creating ease in the lives of people and whose absence will create difficulty in life although it will not become unbearable. The third level, *taḥsīnīyāt*, involves all what is meant to enhance and complete the fulfillment of what falls under the first two levels, i.e. necessities and needs. It includes things such as commendable habits and customs, rules of etiquette, and high moral standards.

Practical Ethics of the Physician (*Adab al-Ṭabīb*): Originally the title of one of the earliest books in Islamic history on medical ethics, attributed to the 9th century physician Al-Ruhawi. Later, it became the name of a distinct genre that focuses on the Islamic concepts of etiquette and personal ethics in a medical context.

Prima facie: A "prima facie" or "conditional" duty, especially within the context of principlism, means that an ethical principle must be fulfilled unless it conflicts with an equal or stronger principle.

Principle-Based Bioethics: See Principlism.

Principlism: An approach, sometimes known as principle-based bioethics, to biomedical ethics that uses a framework of four basic ethical principles (presented as part of people's common morality): respect for autonomy, nonmaleficence, beneficence, and justice. The history of this approach goes back to the 1970s when it was presented in Beauchamp and Childress' *Principles of Biomedical Ethics*.

Qawā'id Fiqhīyah**:** See Islamic Legal Maxims.

Sharī'ah**:** See Sharia.

Sharia (*Sharī'ah*): An Arabic word which literally means way, road, or path to a source of water. In Islamic literature, this literal meaning was metaphorically employed to mean the way assigned by God for humanity to achieve success in this life and in the Hereafter, however with wide differences in the modern discussions about the exact scope of this term.

Specification: A technical term used in the context of principlism to mcan the process of downstreaming these broad four principles and applying them to individual case studies.

Taḥqīq al-Manāṭ**:** See Verifying the True Nature.

Taḥsīnīyāt**:** See Necessities.

Uṣūl al-Fiqh**:** See Islamic Legal Theory.

Utilitarianism: A moral theory which judges the morality of actions based on an evaluation of consequences, effects, or outcomes where concepts like achieving welfare and maximizing utility usually occupy central positions. Compare DEONTOLOGY.

Verifying the Rationale (*Taḥqīq al-Manāṭ*): An Arabic term which literally means verifying the effective rationale behind certain judgments. As a technical term in ISLAMIC LEGAL THEORY, it designates a specific type of *IJTIHĀD* that focuses on the accurate perception of the empirical world and how this knowledge can help in constructing the SHARIA perspectives on modern and sophisticated questions.

Index

A

abortion, x, 19, 251, 290, 326, 328, 339, 360, 364, 373, 376, 379
abortion, *in vitro* fertilization, 41
abrogation, 69, 81–86
accountability, 130, 142, 225, 284, 310, 327
  internal accountability, 302
  religious accountability, 278
  self-accountability, 223, 225–226
Adab al-ṭabīb, 37, 241, 293–294, 419
AIDS, x, 47, 342
Al-Ghazali, Abu Hamid, 132, 183, 200, 217, 244, 253, 265, 273, 307, 323, 327, 361, 370–373, 381
Al-Ghazali, Muhammad, 75, 77
Al-Ruhawi, 43, 241–242, 244, 249, 294–295, 422
Al-Shatibi, 72, 178, 201, 212–213, 307–308, 313, 323, 343, 347, 350, 382
animals, xi, 63, 193, 201, 213–214, 228–229, 246, 250, 307, 320, 322, 329, 381, 399
  animal ethics, 408
  abortion, animal research, 111
'aql, 220, 270, 327, 346, 350, 361, 420

C

capitalism, 184, 194, 373
Center for Islamic Legislation and Ethics (CILE), xii, xv–xvii, 4, 20, 29, 33, 37–38, 41, 121, 413
children, 73, 118, 138, 180, 231, 250, 258–259, 279, 287, 290, 302, 362
Christianity, 111, 352
cloning, 65, 238, 326, 349, 364
  genetics, embryo cloning, *in vitro* fertilization, 318
cloning, abortion, 325
code of ethics, 24, 43, 93, 111, 290

Kuwait Document on the Islamic Code for the Medical Profession, 285
code of ethics
E-Health Code of Ethics, 291
International Islamic Code of Medical and Healthcare Ethics, 285
Medical Oath and the Codes of Medical Ethics, 281, 290
Moral Code in the Qur'an, 218
Nuremberg Code, 203–204, 376
Islamic Code of Medical Ethics, 291
code of "Principles of Medical Ethics", 5
comprehensive principles, 121, 217, 219, 247, 343, 345, 411
confidentiality, 20, 109, 236, 241, 243–244, 254, 268, 278–279, 285, 298–299, 336, 339, 380
medical confidentiality, 136, 337
consensus, 33, 65, 135, 185, 395, 413
culture, 4, 11, 43, 46, 58, 70, 107, 115, 117–119, 132, 150, 155, 159, 166, 169, 171, 177–179, 203, 221, 245, 250, 260
American culture, 159, 167
Arab culture, 260
culture of physicians, 360
Eastern culture, 115
non-religious culture, 59
religious culture, 222
Western culture, 114–115, 360

D

death, 8, 43, 59–60, 67, 72, 87, 124, 186, 290–291, 297, 334, 363
assisted death, 376
brain death, x, 59–61
cardiocirculatory death, 62
death of the Prophet, 10
expediting death, 186
imminent death, 269
deontology, 19, 31, 136, 319, 363, 420, 423
dignity, 8, 225, 268, 291, 294, 328, 334, 380, 383–384, 386
doctor's dignity, 377
human dignity, 54, 74–75, 380
disabled, 61, 118
disabled horses, 381
mentally disabled, 138
disagreement, 79–81, 83, 94, 107, 109–110, 312, 398–399
disclosure, 62, 95, 278–279
donation
organ transplants, 318

E

endowment, 162–163, 260, 381
environment, 48, 54–55, 67, 70, 131, 163, 185, 201, 253, 267, 270, 312, 322, 329, 417
cultural environment, 31
environmental ethics, 206
environmental security, 199, 329
psycho-socio-spiritual and physical environment, 49
social and physical environments, 50
European Council for Fatwa and Research, ix–x, 78, 326
euthanasia, 19–20, 111, 230, 239, 326, 376, 379
excellence, 26, 121, 242, 253–254, 275, 280, 288, 318, 335–336, 420

F

family, xvii, 10, 12, 22, 31, 57, 75, 95, 97, 114, 122, 131, 168–170, 227, 246, 260, 279, 294, 296, 322, 376, 383
  deceased's family, 297
  familial relationships, 320
  family affairs, 320
  family law, 73
  family matters, 157
  family members, 400
  family physician, 127
  Muslim family, 363
  patient's family, 230, 296
fasting, 73, 78, 84–85, 130, 196, 273, 353, 394
fasting, pilgrimage, 213
fatwa, ix–x, 78, 85–86, 234, 281, 298, 308–309, 311, 326, 360
  medical fatwas, 357
  Houses of Fatwa, 78
  collective fatwas, 299
Fiqh Academies
  International Islamic Fiqh Academy, ix–xiii, 23, 86, 122, 247, 279, 284, 339
  Islamic Fiqh Academy, x, 326
  Islamic Organization for Medical Sciences (IOMS), x
fundamental ethics, 260, 301–303, 335, 364–365, 371, 386, 403

G

gender, 57, 66, 142, 251, 379, 390
gene therapy, 238, 318, 329
genetic manipulation, 63, 326
genetics, xii, 56, 64, 388–389, 408
  epigenetics, 64
  Transgenetics, 63
genome, 388
genomics, xii–xiii
  human genome projects, 318
God-consciousncss, 127, 129, 211, 218–219, 223–226, 231, 244, 249, 253–256, 263, 266, 274–275, 282, 291, 301–303, 305, 309–311, 313–315, 321, 336, 371, 380, 386, 404

H

health, xii, xv, 6, 13, 15, 22, 28, 30, 43, 47–49, 51–52, 55, 64, 67, 83, 93, 95–96, 98–103, 107, 111, 123, 127, 131, 133, 135, 139, 142, 150, 158, 162–163, 166, 180, 186, 192, 196–198, 203, 231, 238, 248, 258–259, 280, 282, 285, 289–291, 293–296, 298, 372, 378, 389, 401, 404, 409, 414, 416–417, 419
  healthcare, 32, 136
  health ethics, 23
  health hazards, 65
  health insurance, 20, 160–161, 181
  health issues, xii
  health problems, 58
  health professionals, 206
  patient's health, 338
  personal health, 295
  psychological health, 231, 269
  public health, 92, 96, 98–99, 102, 122, 158, 191, 197, 280, 337, 343–344, 349, 402
health, pharmaceutical companies, 380
higher objectives, 233, 342
higher objectives of Sharia (*maqāṣid al-sharī'ah*), 29, 37, 69–71, 178, 185, 192–195, 199–201, 211, 252–253, 301, 303,

307, 314, 317, 323, 330, 345–348, 350, 355–356, 365–369, 378, 381, 386, 397, 402, 406, 420, 422
ordering the higher objectives of Sharia, 382
theory of the higher objectives of Sharia, 364, 371
Hippocrates, 170, 244, 272, 372
Hippocratic oath, 43, 122, 125, 128, 338
Hippocratic tradition, 35, 140, 190, 375, 387
Hippocratic medical ethics, 97, 117, 122
Hippocratic medicine, 250
Hippocratic theories, 392
Hippocratic thought, 408
history, 43, 52, 54, 70, 115, 119, 180, 183, 189, 206, 246, 250, 260, 278, 303, 321, 338, 361–362, 373, 404, 413
Greek history, 362
history of biomedical ethics, 92, 124
history of ethics, 116, 124
history of Islamic medicine, 250
history of medical ethics, 94
Islamic history, 31, 75, 260, 381, 421–422
hospitals, 44, 161–163, 175, 244, 258–260, 272, 274, 280, 282, 363, 377, 380, 383
public hospitals, 162
western hospitals, 150
hospitals, pharmaceutical companies, 127

I

Ibn Al-Qayyim, 132, 277, 284, 373
Ibn Miskawayh, 217, 244, 370, 371
ijtihad, 71, 77, 87, 194–195, 199, 253, 311, 359, 420, 423
collective ijtihad, 299
independent legal reasoning, 69
informed consent, 10, 62, 109, 112, 115–116, 136, 147, 158, 166, 168–170, 187, 250, 366, 374, 376, 388
waivers of informed consent, 111
International Islamic Code for Medical and Health Ethics, 23
in vitro fertilization (IVF), 376
Islamic Fiqh Academy, x
Islamic law, 5, 22, 26, 29, 31, 72–75, 83, 171, 183, 199, 230, 234, 255, 264–265, 289, 331, 333, 339, 366, 373, 394, 404, 420–421
school of Islamic law, 74, 80, 82, 84, 421
Islamic legal maxims, 5, 28–29, 32, 37, 348, 366, 404, 421, 423
Islamic legal theory, 5, 39, 193, 305, 343, 406, 421, 423
Islamic medicine, ix, 5, 8, 12, 24, 27, 241, 290–291
history of Islamic medicine, 250
Islamic Oath, 125, 128
Islamic Organization for Medical Sciences, 23, 285, 287–290, 372

J

Jews, 83, 172, 179, 249, 315, 363, 380
Judaism, 352
Jewish bioethics, 59
Judaism, Christianity, 116, 124

K

killing(s), 93, 99, 104, 125, 200, 230, 309, 311, 326, 363

mercy killing (euthanasia), 185, 230, 381
mercy killing, abortion, 197
mass killings, 180

L

luxuries, 72, 185, 195–196, 323–324, 343, 422

M

marriage, 72, 227, 400–401
marital issues, 258
marriage contract, 394
Muslim religious scholars, xv, 6, 10–11, 18, 24–25, 28, 31, 34, 37, 257

N

natural disposition, 74, 131, 193, 267, 308, 311–312, 321, 350, 361, 398–399, 422
necessities, 72–73, 75, 185, 192, 195–196, 221, 252, 323–324, 331, 343–347, 368, 383, 419–420, 422–423
basic necessities, 270
contingent necessities, 414
five necessities, 212, 220, 314, 345, 350, 378
needs, 72–73, 87, 185, 192, 195–196, 199–201, 270, 323–324, 331, 343–344, 346–347, 383, 422
contemporary needs, 414
ethical needs, 296
material needs, 289
needs of society, 296
negative obligation, 95, 324, 326–327, 347, 368, 375
noble character, 130, 216, 304, 320

O

organ donation, x, 18, 41, 49, 59–60, 65, 326, 349, 364
organ donation shortage, 63
organ transplants, 360
organ transplantation, 85

P

pain, 8, 47, 97, 105, 122, 129, 163, 170, 226, 229–231, 240, 291, 334
parents, 193, 235, 279
pharmaceutical companies, 187, 342, 349, 394
philosophy, x–xi, xiii, 41, 43, 61, 65, 67, 141, 175, 188, 263, 293, 319, 323, 354, 362, 373, 390, 392, 398
Eastern culture, 168
Greek philosophy, 124, 371, 382
Harrisian philosophy, 17, 19
Islamic philosophy, 71, 370
Ķant's philosophy, 160
liberal political philosophy, 96
moral philosophy, 57, 66, 175
political philosophy, 30, 141, 167
utilitarian philosophy, 160, 363
western philosophy, 356, 382, 387
Philosophy of Pluralism, xiv
pilgrimage, 78, 84, 273
positive obligation, 95, 99, 324, 346–347, 375
prayer, 84–85, 111, 130, 178–179, 212–213, 228, 235, 301–302, 353, 394
gregational prayer, 196
privacy, 8, 111, 136, 338, 380
psychology, 14, 138, 171, 217, 221, 223, 277, 329, 330, 335, 339, 389
psychological diseases, 326

psychological processes, 268
psychological retribution, 284
psychological state, 220

R

rationality, 192
collective rationality, 413
common rationality, 154
rituals, 84, 108, 130, 237, 320

S

soul(s), 62, 75, 200, 225, 240, 242, 273,
294–296, 311, 320–321, 326, 380, 399
purification of the soul, 76, 216, 217, 304, 361
spirituality, xi, 37, 43, 47, 48, 218, 221, 223, 236, 242, 318, 417, 422
spiritual excellence, 420
stem cell, x, xii, 318, 410
animals, genetics, stem cells, 409
stem cell research, 408

T

technology, xii, 50–51, 59, 66, 165, 190–191, 318–319
biomedical technology, 64, 67, 408
biotechnology, 60, 233
genetic technology, 388
reproductive technology, 408
terminology, 28, 75, 124, 174, 205, 218, 263, 303, 365, 387, 392, 395–396, 398, 402–403, 408, 414, 417
Islamic legal terminology, 173
theology, xii–xiv, 12, 15, 59, 155, 267, 352, 383
Islamic theology, 29, 37
theologian, 22, 38
trustworthiness, 105, 253, 255, 276–278, 306, 336, 339

U

universality, 28, 57–58, 69–70, 76, 87, 177, 245–246, 250, 350, 352, 398–399, 401
utilitarianism, 14, 19–20, 57, 100–101, 103, 126, 131, 136, 142, 154–155, 159, 164, 266, 312, 319, 362, 389, 391, 415, 420, 423
utilitarianism, deontology, virtue ethics, 134

V

vaccination, 375, 402
virtue ethics, 105

W

women, 74–75, 78, 84, 118, 194, 227, 231, 275, 290
women, animals, 80
World Health Organization, 47, 197, 259, 291, 375